Handbook of Outpatient Cardiology

Ankit A. Bhargava
Bryan J. Wells • Pablo A. Quintero
Editors

Handbook of Outpatient Cardiology

Springer

Editors
Ankit A. Bhargava
Department of Medicine
Division of Cardiology
Emory University School of Medicine
Atlanta, GA, USA

Bryan J. Wells
Department of Medicine
Division of Cardiology
Emory University School of Medicine
Atlanta, GA, USA

Pablo A. Quintero
Department of Medicine
Division of Cardiology
Beth Israel Deaconess Medical Center, Harvard Medical School
Boston, MA, USA

ISBN 978-3-030-88952-4 ISBN 978-3-030-88953-1 (eBook)
https://doi.org/10.1007/978-3-030-88953-1

This Springer imprint is published by the registered company Springer Nature Switzerland AG
The registered company address is: Gewerbestrasse 11, 6330 Cham, Switzerland

"...the practice of medicine is predominantly a humanistic act. Physicians must care about their patients, and they must constantly improve their scientific knowledge about disease. To care and not know is dangerous. To know and not care is even worse. Caring and knowing must be combined to succeed in doctoring."

–J. Willis Hurst, MD

This book is dedicated to students and trainees past, present, and future.

Ankit A. Bhargava
Bryan J. Wells • Pablo A. Quintero
Editors

Handbook of Outpatient Cardiology

Springer

Editors
Ankit A. Bhargava
Department of Medicine
Division of Cardiology
Emory University School of Medicine
Atlanta, GA, USA

Bryan J. Wells
Department of Medicine
Division of Cardiology
Emory University School of Medicine
Atlanta, GA, USA

Pablo A. Quintero
Department of Medicine
Division of Cardiology
Beth Israel Deaconess Medical Center, Harvard Medical School
Boston, MA, USA

ISBN 978-3-030-88952-4 ISBN 978-3-030-88953-1 (eBook)
https://doi.org/10.1007/978-3-030-88953-1

This Springer imprint is published by the registered company Springer Nature Switzerland AG
The registered company address is: Gewerbestrasse 11, 6330 Cham, Switzerland

"…the practice of medicine is predominantly a humanistic act. Physicians must care about their patients, and they must constantly improve their scientific knowledge about disease. To care and not know is dangerous. To know and not care is even worse. Caring and knowing must be combined to succeed in doctoring."

–J. Willis Hurst, MD

This book is dedicated to students and trainees past, present, and future.

Preface

This book serves as a companion reference to the *Handbook of Inpatient Cardiology*. A significant portion of patient care is received in the outpatient setting. Our hope is that timely interventions in the outpatient setting will help to prevent further hospital admissions. Therefore, we felt that having an easy reference handbook to help guide outpatient cardiology care was important.

The materials contained within review the fundamental, practical aspects of outpatient cardiac care using the most up-to-date guidelines. Each chapter includes a summary of the presentation, diagnosis, and management of each condition. The chapters are formatted in an easy-to-read bullet-point format that includes "clinical pearls" and "key learning points" along with figures to illustrate the salient content.

We would like to thank all the authors who contributed to the writing of this important book, which includes cardiology fellows and faculty from Emory University and Beth Israel Deaconess Medical Center/Harvard Medical School. We are forever grateful for their time and expertise.

We hope this book serves as a practical and reliable reference for anyone who cares for cardiac patients in the outpatient setting.

Atlanta, GA, USA — Ankit A. Bhargava
Bryan J. Wells
Boston, MA, USA — Pablo A. Quintero

Contents

Contributors

Akanksha Agrawal Department of Medicine, Division of Cardiology, Emory University School of Medicine, Atlanta, GA, USA

Talal Khalid Al-Otaibi Department of Medicine, Division of Cardiology, Beth Israel Deaconess Medical Center, Harvard Medical School, Boston, MA, USA

Hakeem Ayinde Departments of Heart & Vascular Institute, Novant Health Presbyterian Medical Center, Charlotte, NC, USA

Franck H. Azobou Tonleu Department of Medicine, Emory University School of Medicine, Atlanta, GA, USA

Vasilis C. Babaliaros Department of Medicine, Division of Cardiology, Emory University School of Medicine, Atlanta, GA, USA

Christine Bethencourt Emory University School of Medicine, Atlanta, GA, USA

Ankit A. Bhargava Department of Medicine, Division of Cardiology, Emory University School of Medicine, Atlanta, GA, USA

Thomas E. Bigham Department of Medicine, Emory University School of Medicine, Atlanta, GA, USA

Dimitri Cassimatis Department of Medicine, Division of Cardiology, Emory University School of Medicine, Atlanta, GA, USA

Dandan Chen Department of Medicine, Division of Cardiology, Emory University School of Medicine, Atlanta, GA, USA

Robert N. D'Angelo Department of Medicine, Division of Cardiology, Beth Israel Deaconess Medical Center, Harvard Medical School, Boston, MA, USA

Devinder S. Dhindsa Department of Medicine, Division of Cardiology, Emory University School of Medicine, Atlanta, GA, USA

Allen Dollar Department of Medicine, Division of Cardiology, Emory University School of Medicine, Atlanta, GA, USA

Logan Eberly Department of Medicine, Division of Cardiology, Emory University School of Medicine, Atlanta, GA, USA

Mikhael El Chami Department of Medicine, Division of Cardiology, Emory University School of Medicine, Atlanta, GA, USA

Mariana Garcia Department of Medicine, Division of Cardiology, Emory University School of Medicine, Atlanta, GA, USA

Michael C. Gavin Department of Medicine, Division of Cardiology, Beth Israel Deaconess Medical Center, Harvard Medical School, Boston, MA, USA

Eli V. Gelfand Department of Medicine, Division of Cardiology, Beth Israel Deaconess Medical Center, Harvard Medical School, Boston, MA, USA

Patrick Gleason Department of Medicine, Division of Cardiology, Emory University School of Medicine, Atlanta, GA, USA

Allie Goins Department of Medicine, Emory University School of Medicine, Atlanta, GA, USA

Thomas H. Hauser Department of Medicine, Division of Cardiology, Beth Israel Deaconess Medical Center, Harvard Medical School, Boston, MA, USA

Nicolas Isaza Department of Medicine, Beth Israel Deaconess Medical Center, Harvard Medical School, Boston, MA, USA

Maan Jokhadar Department of Medicine, Division of Cardiology, Emory University School of Medicine, Atlanta, GA, USA

Vladimir Kaplinskiy Department of Medicine, Division of Cardiology, Beth Israel Deaconess Medical Center, Harvard Medical School, Boston, MA, USA

Daniel Katz Department of Medicine, Division of Cardiology, Beth Israel Deaconess Medical Center, Harvard Medical School, Boston, MA, USA

Christine Kempton Department of Hematology and Medical Oncology, Emory University School of Medicine, Atlanta, GA, USA

Rachel Koch Department of Medicine, Emory University School of Medicine, Atlanta, GA, USA

Bruno B. Lima Department of Medicine, Division of Cardiology, Emory University School of Medicine, Atlanta, GA, USA

John C. Lisko Department of Medicine, Division of Cardiology, Emory University School of Medicine, Atlanta, GA, USA

Michael S. Lloyd Department of Medicine, Division of Cardiology, Emory University School of Medicine, Atlanta, GA, USA

Marvin Louis Roy Lu Department of Medicine, Division of Cardiology, Emory University School of Medicine, Atlanta, GA, USA

Gina Lundberg Department of Medicine, Division of Cardiology, Emory University School of Medicine, Atlanta, GA, USA

Anant Mandawat Department of Medicine, Division of Cardiology, Emory University School of Medicine, Atlanta, GA, USA

Winship Cancer Institute, Department of Hematology and Medical Oncology, Emory University School of Medicine, Atlanta, GA, USA

Christopher S. Massad Department of Medicine, Emory University School of Medicine, Atlanta, GA, USA

Michael McDaniel Department of Medicine, Division of Cardiology, Emory University School of Medicine, Atlanta, GA, USA

Susan McIlvaine Department of Medicine, Division of Cardiology, Beth Israel Deaconess Medical Center, Harvard Medical School, Boston, MA, USA

Faisal Merchant Department of Medicine, Division of Cardiology, Emory University School of Medicine, Atlanta, GA, USA

Roshan D. Modi Emory University School of Medicine, Atlanta, GA, USA

M. Carolina Gongora Nieto Department of Medicine, Division of Cardiology, Emory University School of Medicine, Atlanta, GA, USA

Parth Patel Department of Medicine, Division of Cardiology, Emory University School of Medicine, Atlanta, GA, USA

Duane S. Pinto Department of Medicine, Division of Cardiology, Beth Israel Deaconess Medical Center, Harvard Medical School, Boston, MA, USA

Sindhu Prabakaran Department of Medicine, Emory University School of Medicine, Atlanta, GA, USA

Pablo A. Quintero Department of Medicine, Division of Cardiology, Beth Israel Deaconess Medical Center, Harvard Medical School, Boston, MA, USA

Inbar Raber Department of Medicine, Division of Cardiology, Beth Israel Deaconess Medical Center, Harvard Medical School, Boston, MA, USA

Katharine Rainer Emory University School of Medicine, Atlanta, GA, USA

Prashant Rao Department of Medicine, Division of Cardiology, Beth Israel Deaconess Medical Center, Harvard Medical School, Boston, MA, USA

B. Robinson Williams III Department of Medicine, Division of Cardiology, Emory University School of Medicine, Atlanta, GA, USA

Marwa A. Sabe Department of Medicine, Division of Cardiology, Beth Israel Deaconess Medical Center, Harvard Medical School, Boston, MA, USA

Mariem A. Sawan Department of Medicine, Division of Cardiology, Emory University School of Medicine, Atlanta, GA, USA

Arielle M. Schwartz Department of Medicine, Emory University School of Medicine, Atlanta, GA, USA

Nikoloz Shekiladze Department of Medicine, Division of Cardiology, Emory University School of Medicine, Atlanta, GA, USA

Rachel Slappy Emory University School of Medicine, Atlanta, GA, USA

Dustin Staloch Department of Medicine, Division of Cardiology, Emory University School of Medicine, Atlanta, GA, USA

Jordan B. Strom Department of Medicine, Division of Cardiology, Beth Israel Deaconess Medical Center, Richard A. and Susan F. Smith Center for Outcomes Research in Cardiology, Harvard Medical School, Boston, MA, USA

Aneesha Thobani Department of Medicine, Division of Cardiology, Emory University School of Medicine, Atlanta, GA, USA

Mark K. Tuttle Banner Health, Cardiovascular Institute of Northern Colorado, Greeley, CO, USA

Merilyn Susan Varghese Department of Medicine, Division of Cardiology, Beth Israel Deaconess Medical Center, Harvard Medical School, Boston, MA, USA

Stephanie Wang Department of Medicine, Division of Cardiology, Emory University School of Medicine, Atlanta, GA, USA

Bryan J. Wells Department of Medicine, Division of Cardiology, Emory University School of Medicine, Atlanta, GA, USA

Nanette K. Wenger Department of Medicine, Division of Cardiology, Emory University School of Medicine, Atlanta, GA, USA

Joe X. Xie Department of Medicine, Division of Cardiology, Emory University School of Medicine, Atlanta, GA, USA

Shu Yang Department of Medicine, Division of Cardiology, Beth Israel Deaconess Medical Center, Harvard Medical School, Boston, MA, USA

An Young Department of Medicine, Division of Cardiology, Emory University School of Medicine, Atlanta, GA, USA

Peter Zimetbaum Department of Medicine, Division of Cardiology, Beth Israel Deaconess Medical Center, Harvard Medical School, Boston, MA, USA

Part I
History and Physical Exam

Chapter 1
Chest Pain

Katharine Rainer, Franck H. Azobou Tonleu, and Mark K. Tuttle

Abbreviations

ACS	Acute coronary syndrome
ASCVD	Atherosclerotic cardiovascular disease
CAD	Coronary artery disease
CP	Chest pain
DVT	Deep vein thrombosis
ECG	Electrocardiogram
GERD	Gastroesophageal reflux disease
H&P	History and physical
HCM	Hypertrophic cardiomyopathy
MI	Myocardial infarction
PCP	Primary care physician

K. Rainer
Emory University School of Medicine, Atlanta, GA, USA
e-mail: Knraine@emory.edu

F. H. Azobou Tonleu (✉)
Department of Medicine, Emory University School of Medicine, Atlanta, GA, USA
e-mail: franck.herve.azobou.tonleu@emory.edu

M. K. Tuttle
Banner Health, Cardiovascular Institute of Northern Colorado, Greeley, CO, USA
e-mail: mtuttle1@bidmc.harvard.edu

A. A. Bhargava et al. (eds.), *Handbook of Outpatient Cardiology*, https://doi.org/10.1007/978-3-030-88953-1_1

PE	Pulmonary embolism
PMH	Past medical history

Introduction

- The differential diagnosis of chest pain (CP) is broad, with etiologies ranging from life-threatening to those with low morbidity and mortality.
- CP is one of the most common complaints in the outpatient setting with a prevalence ranging from 20% to 40% depending on criteria, location, and practice [1].
- The primary care physician (PCP) is often the main point of entry to the healthcare system.
- Cardiovascular disease, the most life-threatening etiology, must be ruled out in the initial evaluation.
- Musculoskeletal or "chest wall syndrome" is the most common cause in the primary care setting [2], accounting for 20.4–50% of cases [1–3], followed by gastroesophageal reflux disease (GERD).
- The prevalence of CP due to coronary artery disease (CAD) ranges from 1.5% to 15% [3, 4].
- A detailed history and physical (H&P) of the patient's CP can limit unnecessary testing.

Initial Evaluation

- The "OPQRST" mnemonic provides a helpful framework to approach the history of present illness and narrow the differential diagnosis [5]:
  - Onset of pain
  - Provocation/palliation
  - Quality
  - Radiation
  - Site of pain
  - Timing
- The pain characteristics (3 P's) that decrease the likelihood of acute coronary syndrome (ACS) [6] are:
  - **P**leuritic pain worsened with inspiration

- **P**ositional pain worsened with lying down
- Pain reproduced by **p**alpation

- The approach to a differential diagnosis of chest pain can be divided into cardiac versus non-cardiac etiologies [7].

Clinical Pearl 1
A negative ECG and troponin do not rule out ACS.

Cardiac Etiologies of Chest Pain

- Ischemic Heart Disease
  - Ischemic heart disease is an umbrella term that includes stable angina and ACS.
  - Stable angina presents with the following characteristics:

    Substernal location
    Onset with exertion
    Improvement with rest or nitroglycerin [8]

  - If a patient presents with only two out of three characteristics, the chest pain is considered atypical. If a patient has one out of three characteristics, it is considered non-anginal chest pain. The presentation predicts the likelihood that the chest pain is due to CAD (Table 1.1).
  - ACS encompasses unstable angina (UA) and myocardial infarction (MI) [9] and presents with:

    New onset angina at rest
    Angina with minimal exertion
    Crescendo angina

  - Additional symptoms of ACS can include radiation to the arms/shoulder/jaw/neck, shortness of breath, pain similar to prior ACS (if applicable), nausea, and diaphoresis [7, 10].
  - Exam can include Levine's sign (clenching fist on chest), rales on lung exam, and hypotension [7, 11]. The

Table 1.1 Pre-test probability that CP is associated with CAD-based CP characteristic

Population	Non-anginal	Atypical	Typical
Older male (>50)	20%	65%	93%
Older female (>60)	14%	51%	86%

presence of chest wall tenderness significantly decreases the likelihood of ACS [12, 13].

- ECG and troponin (if available and risk factors present) can be used for further workup. A normal ECG does not rule out ACS.
- Risk factors include older age, hypertension, diabetes, hyperlipidemia, and tobacco use [14, 15]. However, up to 12% of patients with acute MI have no risk factors [16].
- Atherosclerotic cardiovascular disease (ASCVD) risk score can be helpful to determine one's overall risk of CAD [17, 18].

- Aortic Dissection
  - Classically presents with abrupt onset sharp/tearing/ripping chest or back pain, though presentation can be subtle [19, 20].
  - Physical exam findings include soft, high-pitched, early diastolic decrescendo murmur heard best at the third intercostal space on the left (consistent with aortic regurgitation) and pulse deficit (blood pressure difference between both arms).
  - Aortic dissection is rare [21–23], but should always be considered given its high mortality [19].

- Pericarditis
  - Classically described as acute onset of sharp, pleuritic (worse with inspiration) chest pain that is positional (worse with laying down, improved with sitting up and leaning forward).
  - May occur in the setting of flu-like symptoms or associated with a history of autoimmune disease.

- On physical exam, auscultation over the left sternal border reveals a pericardial friction rub that is best heard during expiration with the patient leaning forward [24].
- Dullness with bronchial breath sounds suggests pericardial effusion (Ewart sign).
- Assess for cardiac tamponade through inspection of jugular venous pulsations and pulsus paradoxus (decrease in systolic blood pressure greater than 10 mmHg with inspiration) [25].

• Pulmonary Embolism (PE)

  - Seventy-five percent of cases present with chest pain [26], which is generally lateral or substernal.
  - Pain is of sudden onset, sharp, and pleuritic and commonly occurs with unexplained breathlessness, cough, hemoptysis, or syncope.
  - Clinical suspicion is high according to Wells score [27], including findings suggestive of deep vein thrombosis (DVT) such as calf pain or tenderness, immobilization or surgery, hemoptysis, and previous DVT/PE.
  - PMH, family history (FH), and current medications may reveal prothrombotic risk factors.
  - Physical exam may include elevated jugular venous pulsation and loud S2 over the left upper sternal border.
  - One should always consider PE in any patient with CP, tachycardia, and tachypnea/hypoxemia, especially in patients with risk factors. These patients should be sent to the emergency department for further evaluation.

• Valvular Heart Disease

  - Aortic stenosis

    History may include exertional angina, dyspnea, decreased exercise tolerance, syncope, palpitations, or dizziness.

    Auscultation over the right second intercostal space reveals a harsh crescendo and decrescendo systolic murmur that radiates into the carotid arteries.

Palpation of the carotid upstroke during cardiac auscultation may demonstrate a weak pulse that rises slowly to a delayed peak (pulsus parvus et tardus) [28].
When grading aortic stenosis, the absence of S2 is specific for stenosis in the severe range.

- Mitral valve prolapse

  Most patients are asymptomatic, though some may experience vague chest discomfort.
  Some cases present with significant mitral regurgitation, leading to fatigue, exertional dyspnea, orthopnea, or palpitations.
  Auscultation over the apex reveals a late or mid-systolic click with a holosystolic murmur or high-pitched mid-late systolic murmur [29] that radiates to the axilla.
  The murmur is louder and occurs earlier with a Valsalva maneuver, but is softer and delayed with squatting.

- Hypertrophic Cardiomyopathy (HCM)
  - HCM with obstruction occurs due to a hypertrophied septum bulging into the left ventricular outflow tract.
  - May present with exercise intolerance, angina, or syncope.
  - HCM has an autosomal dominant pattern of inheritance with 60–70% of HCM patients having an affected family member [30].
  - Auscultation at the left sternal border reveals a systolic murmur that increases with Valsalva and with standing. The murmur decreases with passive leg raising and handgrip maneuvers.
  - To differentiate the murmur of aortic stenosis and HCM:

    Auscultate the carotid pulse and note murmur severity in response to the Valsalva and handgrip maneuvers.

Valsalva maneuver → murmur louder with HCM
Handgrip maneuver → murmur softer with HCM

- A summary of risk factors, history, and physical exam findings associated with cardiac etiologies can be found in Table 1.2.

Clinical Pearl 2
Most chest pain in primary care is non-cardiac with most common etiologies including chest wall syndrome and GERD.

Non-cardiac Etiologies of Chest Pain

- Chest Wall Syndrome
  - Chest wall pain due to costochondritis or intercostal muscle spasms are the most frequent causes of CP [31].
  - History and pain to chest wall palpation are clues to the diagnosis.
  - Pain is generally moderate, well localized, continuous or intermittent, and sometimes described as "stinging."
  - Pain is generally retrosternal and/or on the left side [31] and exacerbated by position and movement.
  - May coexist with CAD [32]. Careful assessment of risk factors and further testing may be needed to rule out cardiac etiology.
- Gastroesophageal Disorders
  - Amongst the most frequent causes of non-cardiac chest pain [33] are GERD and non-GERD esophageal disorders [34] .
  - GERD

    A common diagnosis in patients with CP [35, 36].
    Typically presents with burning retrosternal chest pain, acid regurgitation, and sour/bitter taste in the mouth [37].

TABLE 1.2 Risk factors, history, and physical exam for cardiac etiologies of CP

Diagnosis	Risk factors	Characteristics of pain	Physical exam findings
Coronary artery disease	Older age Hypertension Diabetes mellitus Hyperlipidemia Tobacco use	Substernal Improves with rest (if stable) Does not improve with rest (if unstable and MI) Radiation to right shoulder or both arms/ shoulder/ jaw/ neck Associated with nausea Diaphoresis	Levine's sign May have rales Hypotension No chest wall tenderness
Aortic dissection	Age (>65) [19, 21] Male [21] Hypertension (most important) [19, 51] Smoking [22] Aortic aneurysm [52] Bicuspid aortic valve [53, 54]	Abrupt onset Sharp/tearing/ ripping chest or back	Blood pressure difference between both arms Murmur consistent with aortic regurgitation
Pericarditis	Autoimmune disease Immunocompromised	Fairly acute onset Pleuritic Anterior Sharp Radiates to trapezius Associated with flu-like symptoms	Pericardial friction rub Dullness with bronchial breath sounds

Table 1.2 (continued)

Diagnosis	Risk factors	Characteristics of pain	Physical exam findings
Pulmonary embolism	Hypercoagulable state Immobility/recent surgery Family history	Acute onset Lateral or substernal Sharp, pleuritic Dyspnea Associated with cough, hemoptysis, syncope	Tachycardia Tachypnea Hypoxemia Neck vein distension Loud P2

Usually occurs postprandially, particularly after large fatty meals or spicy foods, and tends to worsen in supine position [38].

Risk factors include older age, obesity, and tobacco use [39].

An empiric trial of PPI can be used for diagnostic purposes [40, 41].

- Non-GERD esophageal disorders

  Present with similar symptoms as GERD, including dysphagia and globus sensation [34, 42].

  Include nutcracker esophagus (more common) and diffuse esophageal spasm [43].

  It is important to consider these disorders (and referral to GI) if patient is having symptoms despite trial of PPI.

- Pneumothorax
  - Potentially life-threatening but rare cause of CP in primary care [44].
  - Presents with sudden-onset pleuritic chest pain and dyspnea.
  - May be tachycardic, tachypneic, and hypoxic [45] on exam.

  - Lung exam may demonstrate focal decreased breath sounds with hyperresonance on percussion.
  - Chest x-ray is the initial diagnostic study and can show air in the pleural space.

- Psychosocial
  - Anxiety and depression are associated with an increased risk of reporting chest pain [46].
  - Seen as a diagnosis of exclusion and can be discerned through screening questions for anxiety and panic disorders such as the GAD-7 questionnaire [47].
  - Patients report "tightness" sensation of the chest and shortness of breath.
  - Physical exam reveals tachycardia but is otherwise normal.
  - Social history may include drugs of abuse such as cocaine and methamphetamine, which may precipitate cardiac ischemia or vasospasm.
  - Substance abuse may also present with diaphoresis and pupillary dilation.
  - If thought to be the etiology, a urine drug screen should be obtained.

- Pneumonia
  - Clinical history of fever, productive cough, pleuritic CP, shortness of breath, gastrointestinal symptoms (nausea, vomiting, diarrhea), or history of recent illness.
  - Pertinent exam findings can include decreased and/or bronchial breath sounds, coarse crackles, dullness to percussion, increased tactile fremitus, and egophony.
  - Bronchial breath sounds and dullness to percussion are highly specific findings [48].

- Herpes Zoster
  - Pain is generally described as "burning," "throbbing," or "stabbing" [49] and may develop prior to appearance of rash [50].

- Exam findings typically include erythematous vesicular rash in a unilateral dermatomal distribution.
- Thoracic and lumbar dermatomes are the most common sites leading to CP.

- A summary of risk factors, history, and physical exam findings associated with non-cardiac etiologies can be found in Table 1.3.

Clinical Pearl 3

Pleuritic CP differential includes the 5 Ps: pneumonia, pneumothorax, pericarditis, pulmonary embolism, and pleuritis.

Key Learning Points

- The best approach to chest pain is a thorough history and physical.
- The 3 P's pain characteristics that decrease the likelihood of ACS include pleuritic, positional, and reproduced by palpation.
- Patients without risk factors for CAD can still have ACS.
- ASCVD score and Wells score can be helpful to assess risk of cardiac or thrombotic etiology, respectively.

Table 1.3 Risk factors, history, and physical for non-cardiac etiologies of CP

Diagnosis	Risk factors	Characteristics of pain	Physical exam findings
Chest wall syndrome	Female gender [55] History of autoimmune or chronic pain syndrome (fibromyalgia, arthritis)	Insidious and persistent Positional and exacerbated by movement but not exertion	Reproducible pain by palpation Localized muscle tension
GERD	Older age Obesity Tobacco use	Retrosternal Acid regurgitation Sour/bitter taste in mouth Postprandial Worsens in supine position	Epigastric tenderness to palpitation
Non-GERD esophageal disorders (nutcracker esophagus and diffuse esophageal spasm)	Consider if patient is having GERD-like symptoms despite trial of PPI	Similar to GERD Also includes dysphagia and globus sensation	

Pneumothorax		Sudden onset Pleuritic Dyspnea at rest	Tachycardia Tachypnea Hypoxia Decreased breath sounds Hyperresonance on percussion
Panic attack/anxiety	Family or personal history of anxiety, depression Childhood adversity Substance use	Exacerbated by emotional stress Chest "tightness"	Tachycardia Tachypnea Otherwise normal
Pneumonia	Seasonal Prolonged hospital stay	Pleuritic with inspiration Associated with productive cough and fever	Shallow breathing Cachexia Course crackles Decreased or bronchial breath sounds Dullness to percussion
Herpes zoster	Immune status- transplant, autoimmune disease [56] Female Family history HIV [50] Age $\geq$60 [50]	Burning, stabbing, pin point pain Associated with erythematous vesicular rash	Unilateral dermatomal distribution of pain and rash

References

1. Bosner S, Becker A, Haasenritter J, et al. Chest pain in primary care: epidemiology and pre-work-up probabilities. Eur J Gen Pract. 2009;15(3):141–6.
2. Svavarsdottir AE, Jonasson MR, Gudmundsson GH, Fjeldsted K. Chest pain in family practice. Diagnosis and long-term outcome in a community setting. Can Fam Physician. 1996;42:1122–8.
3. Klinkman MS, Stevens D, Gorenflo DW. Episodes of care for chest pain: a preliminary report from MIRNET. Michigan Research Network. J Fam Pract. 1994;38(4):345–52.
4. Bosner S, Haasenritter J, Becker A, et al. Ruling out coronary artery disease in primary care: development and validation of a simple prediction rule. CMAJ. 2010;182(12):1295–300.
5. Lacasse M, Maker D. Fishing and history taking: from the net to the line. Can Fam Physician. 2008;54(6):891–2.
6. Swap CJ, Nagurney JT. Value and limitations of chest pain history in the evaluation of patients with suspected acute coronary syndromes. JAMA. 2005;294(20):2623–9.
7. Fanaroff AC, Rymer JA, Goldstein SA, Simel DL, Newby LK. Does this patient with chest pain have acute coronary syndrome?: the rational clinical examination systematic review. JAMA. 2015;314(18):1955–65.
8. Diamond GA, Staniloff HM, Forrester JS, Pollock BH, Swan HJ. Computer-assisted diagnosis in the noninvasive evaluation of patients with suspected coronary artery disease. J Am Coll Cardiol. 1983;1(2 Pt 1):444–55.
9. Hedayati T, Yadav N, Khanagavi J. Non-ST-segment acute coronary syndromes. Cardiol Clin. 2018;36(1):37–52.
10. Rouan GW, Lee TH, Cook EF, Brand DA, Weisberg MC, Goldman L. Clinical characteristics and outcome of acute myocardial infarction in patients with initially normal or nonspecific electrocardiograms (a report from the Multicenter Chest Pain Study). Am J Cardiol. 1989;64(18):1087–92.
11. Eriksson D, Khoshnood A, Larsson D, Lundager-Forberg J, Mokhtari A, Ekelund U. Diagnostic accuracy of history and physical examination for predicting major adverse cardiac events within 30 days in patients with acute chest pain. J Emerg Med. 2019;S0736-4679(19):30828–5.
12. Goodacre S, Locker T, Morris F, Campbell S. How useful are clinical features in the diagnosis of acute, undifferentiated chest pain? Acad Emerg Med. 2002;9(3):203–8.

13. Bruyninckx R, Aertgeerts B, Bruyninckx P, Buntinx F. Signs and symptoms in diagnosing acute myocardial infarction and acute coronary syndrome: a diagnostic meta-analysis. Br J Gen Pract. 2008;58(547):105–11.
14. Verdon F, Herzig L, Burnand B, et al. Chest pain in daily practice: occurrence, causes and management. Swiss Med Wkly. 2008;138(23–24):340–7.
15. Han JH, Lindsell CJ, Storrow AB, et al. The role of cardiac risk factor burden in diagnosing acute coronary syndromes in the emergency department setting. Ann Emerg Med. 2007;49(2):145–52, 152 e141.
16. Body R, Carley S, Wibberley C, McDowell G, Ferguson J, Mackway-Jones K. The value of symptoms and signs in the emergent diagnosis of acute coronary syndromes. Resuscitation. 2010;81(3):281–6.
17. Marcus GM, Cohen J, Varosy PD, et al. The utility of gestures in patients with chest discomfort. Am J Med. 2007;120(1):83–9.
18. D'Agostino RB Sr, Vasan RS, Pencina MJ, et al. General cardiovascular risk profile for use in primary care: the Framingham Heart Study. Circulation. 2008;117(6):743–53.
19. Hagan PG, Nienaber CA, Isselbacher EM, et al. The International Registry of Acute Aortic Dissection (IRAD): new insights into an old disease. JAMA. 2000;283(7):897–903.
20. Pape LA, Awais M, Woznicki EM, et al. Presentation, diagnosis, and outcomes of acute aortic dissection: 17-year trends from the international registry of acute aortic dissection. J Am Coll Cardiol. 2015;66(4):350–8.
21. Clouse WD, Hallett JW Jr, Schaff HV, et al. Acute aortic dissection: population-based incidence compared with degenerative aortic aneurysm rupture. Mayo Clin Proc. 2004;79(2):176–80.
22. Howard DP, Banerjee A, Fairhead JF, et al. Population-based study of incidence and outcome of acute aortic dissection and premorbid risk factor control: 10-year results from the Oxford Vascular Study. Circulation. 2013;127(20):2031–7.
23. Olsson C, Thelin S, Stahle E, Ekbom A, Granath F. Thoracic aortic aneurysm and dissection: increasing prevalence and improved outcomes reported in a nationwide population-based study of more than 14,000 cases from 1987 to 2002. Circulation. 2006;114(24):2611–8.
24. Spodick DH. Pericardial rub. Prospective, multiple observer investigation of pericardial friction in 100 patients. Am J Cardiol. 1975;35(3):357–62.

25. Bashore TM, Granger CB, Jackson KP, Patel MR. Pericardial effusion & tamponade. In: Papadakis MA, McPhee SJ, Rabow MW, editors. Current medical diagnosis & treatment 2021. New York: McGraw-Hill Education; 2021.
26. Nadler PL, Gonzales R. Chest pain. In: Papadakis MA, McPhee SJ, Rabow MW, editors. Current medical diagnosis & treatment 2021. New York: McGraw-Hill Education; 2021.
27. Wells PS, Anderson DR, Rodger M, et al. Derivation of a simple clinical model to categorize patients probability of pulmonary embolism: increasing the models utility with the SimpliRED D-dimer. Thromb Haemost. 2000;83(3):416–20.
28. O'Gara PT, Loscalzo J. Aortic valve disease. In: Jameson JL, Fauci AS, Kasper DL, Hauser SL, Longo DL, Loscalzo J, editors. Harrison's principles of internal medicine. 20th ed. New York: McGraw-Hill Education; 2018.
29. O'Gara PT, Loscalzo J. Mitral Valve Prolapse. In: Jameson JL, Fauci AS, Kasper DL, Hauser SL, Longo DL, Loscalzo J, editors. Harrison's principles of internal medicine. 20th ed. New York: McGraw-Hill Education; 2018.
30. Ananthasubramaniam K. Hypertrophic cardiomyopathy. In: Crawford MH, editor. Current diagnosis & treatment: cardiology. 5th ed. New York: McGraw-Hill Education; 2017.
31. Bosner S, Becker A, Hani MA, et al. Chest wall syndrome in primary care patients with chest pain: presentation, associated features and diagnosis. Fam Pract. 2010;27(4):363–9.
32. Verdon F, Burnand B, Herzig L, Junod M, Pécoud A, Favrat B. Chest wall syndrome among primary care patients: a cohort study. BMC Fam Pract. 2007;8(1):51.
33. Shrestha S, Pasricha PJ. Update on noncardiac chest pain. Dig Dis. 2000;18(3):138–46.
34. Galmiche JP, Clouse RE, Balint A, et al. Functional esophageal disorders. Gastroenterology. 2006;130(5):1459–65.
35. Eslick GD, Jones MP, Talley NJ. Non-cardiac chest pain: prevalence, risk factors, impact and consulting – a population-based study. Aliment Pharmacol Ther. 2003;17(9):1115–24.
36. Wong WM, Lai KC, Lau CP, et al. Upper gastrointestinal evaluation of Chinese patients with non-cardiac chest pain. Aliment Pharmacol Ther. 2002;16(3):465–71.
37. Zimmerman J. Validation of a brief inventory for diagnosis and monitoring of symptomatic gastro-oesophageal reflux. Scand J Gastroenterol. 2004;39(3):212–6.

38. Vakil N, van Zanten SV, Kahrilas P, Dent J, Jones R, Global Consensus G. The Montreal definition and classification of gastroesophageal reflux disease: a global evidence-based consensus. Am J Gastroenterol. 2006;101(8):1900–20; quiz 1943.
39. Eusebi LH, Ratnakumaran R, Yuan Y, Solaymani-Dodaran M, Bazzoli F, Ford AC. Global prevalence of, and risk factors for, gastro-oesophageal reflux symptoms: a meta-analysis. Gut. 2018;67(3):430–40.
40. Eslick GD, Coulshed DS, Talley NJ. Diagnosis and treatment of noncardiac chest pain. Nat Clin Pract Gastroenterol Hepatol. 2005;2(10):463–72.
41. Fang J, Bjorkman D. A critical approach to noncardiac chest pain: pathophysiology, diagnosis, and treatment. Am J Gastroenterol. 2001;96(4):958–68.
42. Kahrilas PJ, Smout AJ. Esophageal disorders. Am J Gastroenterol. 2010;105(4):747–56.
43. Katz PO, Dalton CB, Richter JE, Wu WC, Castell DO. Esophageal testing of patients with noncardiac chest pain or dysphagia. Results of three years' experience with 1161 patients. Ann Intern Med. 1987;106(4):593–7.
44. Butler KH, Swencki SA. Chest pain: a clinical assessment. Radiol Clin N Am. 2006;44(2):165–79, vii.
45. Reamy BV, Williams PM, Odom MR. Pleuritic chest pain: sorting through the differential diagnosis. Am Fam Physician. 2017;96(5):306–12.
46. Barnett LA, Prior JA, Kadam UT, Jordan KP. Chest pain and shortness of breath in cardiovascular disease: a prospective cohort study in UK primary care. BMJ Open. 2017;7(5):e015857.
47. Cao W, Fang Z, Hou G, et al. The psychological impact of the COVID-19 epidemic on college students in China. Psychiatry Res. 2020;287:112934.
48. Chapter 27 - Auscultation of the lungs. In: McGee S, editor. Evidence-based physical diagnosis. 2nd ed. Saint Louis: W.B. Saunders; 2007. p. 326–45.
49. Johnson RW, Rice AS. Clinical practice. Postherpetic neuralgia. N Engl J Med. 2014;371(16):1526–33.
50. Whitley RJ. Varicella-zoster virus infections. In: Jameson JL, Fauci AS, Kasper DL, Hauser SL, Longo DL, Loscalzo J, editors. Harrison's principles of internal medicine, 20e. New York: McGraw-Hill Education; 2018.

51. Landenhed M, Engstrom G, Gottsater A, et al. Risk profiles for aortic dissection and ruptured or surgically treated aneurysms: a prospective cohort study. J Am Heart Assoc. 2015;4(1):e001513.
52. Chau KH, Elefteriades JA. Natural history of thoracic aortic aneurysms: size matters, plus moving beyond size. Prog Cardiovasc Dis. 2013;56(1):74–80.
53. Tadros TM, Klein MD, Shapira OM. Ascending aortic dilatation associated with bicuspid aortic valve: pathophysiology, molecular biology, and clinical implications. Circulation. 2009;119(6):880–90.
54. Michelena HI, Khanna AD, Mahoney D, et al. Incidence of aortic complications in patients with bicuspid aortic valves. JAMA. 2011;306(10):1104–12.
55. Disla E, Rhim HR, Reddy A, Karten I, Taranta A. Costochondritis. A prospective analysis in an emergency department setting. Arch Intern Med. 1994;154(21):2466–9.
56. Kawai K, Yawn BP. Risk factors for herpes zoster: a systematic review and meta-analysis. Mayo Clin Proc. 2017;92(12):1806–21.

Chapter 2
Dyspnea

Rachel Koch and Dimitri Cassimatis

Abbreviations

ACS	Acute coronary syndrome
ATS	American Thoracic Society
BNP	Brain natriuretic peptide
CAD	Coronary artery disease
CBC	Complete blood count
CHF	Congestive heart failure
COPD	Chronic obstructive pulmonary disease
GERD	Gastroesophageal reflux disease
Hct	Hematocrit
Hgb	Hemoglobin
HTN	Hypertension
ILD	Interstitial lung disease
LR	Likelihood ratio
NPV	Negative predictive value
PE	Pulmonary embolism

R. Koch (✉)
Department of Medicine, Emory University School of Medicine, Atlanta, GA, USA

D. Cassimatis
Department of Medicine, Division of Cardiology, Emory University School of Medicine, Atlanta, GA, USA
e-mail: dimitri.cassimatis@emory.edu

A. A. Bhargava et al. (eds.), *Handbook of Outpatient Cardiology*, https://doi.org/10.1007/978-3-030-88953-1_2

PFT Pulmonary function test
PPV Positive predictive value

Definition and Epidemiology

- Dyspnea, or the subjective sensation of difficulty breathing, is present in up to 10% of ambulatory patients, making it one of the most common chief complaints in the outpatient setting [1].
- The American Thoracic Society (ATS) published a consensus statement in 2012 that defined dyspnea as "the subjective experience of breathing discomfort that is comprised of qualitatively distinct sensations that vary in intensity. The experience derives from interactions among multiple physiological, psychological, social, and environmental factors, and may induce secondary physiological and behavioral responses" [2].
- The five most common diagnoses causing *chronic* dyspnea in the outpatient setting are asthma, chronic obstructive pulmonary disease (COPD), interstitial lung disease (ILD), cardiac disease, and obesity or deconditioning [3].

Pathophysiology

- As defined in the ATS consensus statement, several factors contribute to the sensation of dyspnea. This sensation arises from peripheral receptors that stimulate central centers in the brainstem, which simultaneously send a signal to both the respiratory muscles to increase ventilation and to the sensory cortex that is perceived as "dyspnea" [4, 5]. Simply, the respiratory system is designed to balance oxygenation and ventilation in order to maintain PaO_2, $PaCO_2$, and pH. However, dyspnea is a *symptom*, and the *sensation* of dyspnea comes from this complex interaction between peripheral receptors and central respiratory centers.

*__Clinical Pearl:__ Clinically significant dyspnea can occur *without* derangements in oxygenation or ventilation status.

- Many different receptors are involved in the sensation of dyspnea [4]:
  - Chemoreceptors:

    Peripheral chemoreceptors, in the carotid body and aortic arch, sense changes in PaO_2, pH, and $PaCO_2$. Central chemoreceptors, in the medulla, sense changes in $PaCO_2$ and pH.
  - Mechanoreceptors:

    In the lung:

    - Pulmonary stretch receptors are stimulated by increased tension of airway walls. This allows the respiratory system the ability to detect tidal volumes.
    - Irritant receptors are stimulated by either irritants, by rapid changes in tension, or by direct mechanical stimulation.

    In the chest wall:

    - Muscle spindle receptors are stimulated by changes in length of muscle fibers, thus responding to muscle stretch.
  - Metaboreceptors:

    Present in skeletal muscle, metaboreceptors are stimulated by local ischemia or metabolic acidosis in response to decreased oxygen delivery or increased consumption [6]. This is the pathophysiology in deconditioning and anemia.
- Central respiratory centers in the brainstem compile information from all receptors and determine an expected respiratory "output" required to maintain homeostasis under identified ventilation and oxygenation conditions. Mismatch between expected and actual output leads to the subjective sensation of dyspnea, known as "neuromechanical uncoupling" [7].

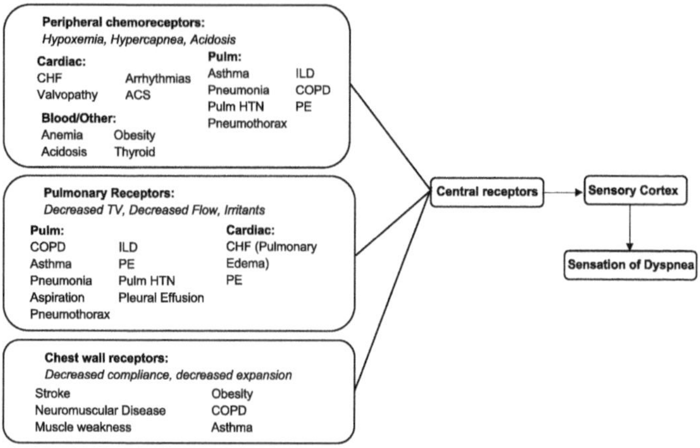

FIGURE 2.1 Differential diagnosis of dyspnea by mechanism

- For example: Decreased lung compliance leads to less-than-expected stimulation of pulmonary stretch receptors and for a given oxygenation or ventilation status.
- For example: Inability to expand the chest wall leads to less-than-expected stimulation of chest wall mechanoreceptors for a given oxygenation or ventilation status (Fig. 2.1).

History

Because dyspnea is subjective, great consideration should be given to patient's descriptions of their symptoms, as language used is often a clue to diagnosis (see Table 2.1, adapted from handbook of Inpatient Cardiology [10]):

*__Clinical Pearl:__ Racial, ethnic, and native language differences impact the terminology patients use to describe their dyspnea. In a study of patients with induced bronchoconstriction, African Americans tended to use descriptors associated with the upper airway, such as "throat/

voice tightness" and "tough breath," while Caucasian patients tended to use descriptors associated with the lungs or chest, such as "out of air," "aware of breathing," and "lightheaded" when describing their dyspnea [11].

Key historical elements to clarify:

- *Chronicity*: A critical first branch point in the history of dyspnea is the time course, as the differential diagnosis for acute-onset dyspnea (minutes to hours) is relatively limited and requires immediate action.
- *Relationship to exertion*:

*__Clinical Pearl:__ The clinician must ensure that limitations with exertion are due to dyspnea itself rather than another symptom causing the difficulty, such as musculoskeletal pain, chest pain, or weakness.

Table 2.1 Descriptors of dyspnea and clues to their potential etiology [8, 9]

Dyspnea description	Potential etiology
"My chest feels tight"	Bronchoconstriction (e.g., COPD, asthma) Cardiac ischemia
"My breathing feels shallow/rapid"	Decreased pulmonary compliance (e.g., ILD)
"I feel like I am suffocating"	Pulmonary edema (e.g., CHF)
"My breathing requires more work"	Respiratory muscle weakness (e.g., neuromuscular disease) Decreased chest wall compliance (e.g., COPD)
"I feel hunger to breathe"	Increased central respiratory drive (e.g., hypercapnia, hypoxemia, acidosis)

Adapted with permission from *Handbook of Inpatient Cardiology* [10]

  - Dyspnea not worsened by exertion is most likely due to psychogenic or musculoskeletal etiologies, as opposed to cardiopulmonary causes [3].

- *Timing/chronology of dyspnea*:

  - Intermittent: usually due to reversible causes, such as bronchoconstriction in asthma or pulmonary edema/pleural effusion in congestive heart failure (CHF).
  - Persistent/progressive: usually due to a more chronic condition, such as COPD, ILD, or pulmonary hypertension.
  - Nocturnal: causes most associated with nocturnal dyspnea are asthma, CHF, and gastrointestinal reflux disease (GERD) [3].

- *Coexisting symptoms*: careful consideration should be given to identify coexisting symptoms that could lead to a specific diagnosis:

  - Dyspnea + chest pain:

    Pleuritic chest pain: pneumonia, pulmonary embolism (PE), asthma, pneumothorax, pleural effusion.

    - ***Clinical Pearl:** Palla et al. found that pleuritic chest pain plus either tachypnea or dyspnea was present in 97% of pulmonary embolisms [12].

    Non-pleuritic chest pain: angina (from coronary artery disease [CAD], anemia, or aortic stenosis), arrhythmias, asthma, COPD.

  - Dyspnea + fever:

    Malignancy, infection (pneumonia or upper respiratory infection superimposed on chronic respiratory disease), PE.

Physical Exam

The majority of causes of dyspnea can be elucidated with careful history and physical exam.

TABLE 2.2 Physical exam findings for specific diagnoses that present with dyspnea

Physical exam finding	Possible underlying etiology
Pursed lip breathing	COPD
Cough with deep breaths	Asthma, ILD
Wheezing	Airway obstruction: asthma, COPD, airway compression, CHF, airway edema (anaphylaxis)
Crackles	"Wet" crackles: intra-alveolar fluid (pneumonia, CHF/pulmonary edema) "Dry" crackles: pulmonary fibrosis (ILD)
Localized decreased breath sounds	Pneumonia, pleural effusion, diaphragmatic paralysis, airway obstruction, pneumothorax
RV heave, loud P2	Pulmonary hypertension
S3 or S4	Systolic or diastolic dysfunction
Distant heart sounds	COPD or pericardial effusion
Elevated JVP	Right- or left-sided heart failure, pericardial tamponade
Symmetric LE edema	CHF, cirrhosis, nephrotic syndrome
Asymmetric LE edema	DVT/PE

Adapted with permission from *Inpatient Handbook of Cardiology* [10]

- Table 2.2 provides physical exam findings that give clues to the diagnosis.

*__Clinical Pearl:__ "Not all that wheezes is asthma!" The old adage attributed to Chevalier Jackson in 1865 still rings true today. The clinician must be careful not to anchor to a diagnosis of asthma or even COPD when the patient presents with wheezing on history or physical exam. One early study found that in 34 patients with a history of wheezing, only 35% were able to be diagnosed with asthma by methacholine challenge [13]. Another study found that in 441 patients with symptoms consistent with asthma, only 53% had a history of wheezing [14].

- Table 2.3 provides evidence-based metrics, such as likelihood ratios, positive predictive values, and negative predictive values, for specific common diagnoses.

Table 2.3 Likelihood ratios for specific history and physical exam findings in specific diseases [15–21]

Disease state	History and physical exam finding	Evidence Likelihood ratio (LR) Negative predictive value (NPV) Positive predictive value (PPV)
CHF	History of CHF	+LR 5.8
	Paroxysmal nocturnal dyspnea	+LR 2.6
	Orthopnea	+LR 2.2
	Presence of S3	+LR 11
	Absence of dyspnea on exertion	–LR 0.48

Table 2.3 (continued)

Disease state	History and physical exam finding	Evidence Likelihood ratio (LR) Negative predictive value (NPV) Positive predictive value (PPV)
COPD	Self-reported history of COPD	+LR 4.44
	>40 pack years of smoking	+LR 11.6
	Age >45 regardless of smoking history	+LR 2.8
	Wheezing on exam	+LR 4.0
	Max laryngeal height ≤4 cm	+LR 3.6
	Reduced breath sounds on exam	+LR 3.38
	Hoover sign (paradoxical inward movement of lower rib cage on inspiration)	+LR 4.16
Pneumonia	Respiratory rate >20	+LR 3.47
	Temperature >38 C	+LR 3.21
	Heart rate >100	+LR 2.89
	Crackles on exam	+LR 2.42
	Absence of cough	–LR 0.36
ILD	Crackles on exam	PPV 0.79 NPV 0.98
Asthma	Previous diagnosis of asthma	PPV 0.48 NPV 0.76
	History of reported wheezing	PPV 0.42 NPV 0.83
	Wheezing on exam	PPV 0.33 NPV 0.72

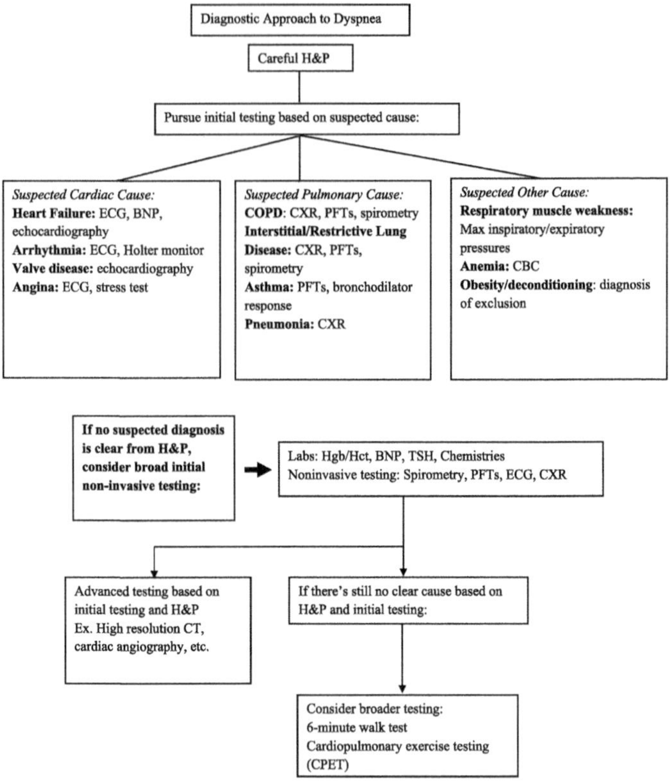

FIGURE 2.2 Diagnostic approach to dyspnea

Diagnostic Approach

- The first step in the workup of any patient with a chief concern of dyspnea should focus on vital signs, especially oxygen saturation, and the stabilization of the unstable patient.
- Careful history and physical can often elucidate the cause of dyspnea; one study indicated that physicians could identify a cause of dyspnea in 66% of cases based on clinical impression (history and physical exam) alone [20].

- The clinician should pursue initial diagnostic testing based on clinical suspicion from history and physical exam (Fig. 2.2). If no suspected diagnosis reveals itself, the clinician should pursue a set of generalized labs and noninvasive tests to further elucidate the cause. This set of tests should be performed with clinical judgment; for example, a young patient with no past medical history likely does not need a brain natriuretic peptide (BNP) in the initial round of testing.

  Specific tests:

- *BNP/NT-pro-BNP* can help identify heart failure or other cardiomyopathies as the underlying cause of a patient's dyspnea. It is also useful for ruling out heart failure as the cause of dyspnea, as a BNP <100 has a negative likelihood ratio of 0.11 [16]. BNP levels can be misleading, however, especially in female, elderly, and obese patients. One study found that 29% of patients with heart failure have a normal BNP [22].
- *Electrocardiogram (ECG)* can be helpful in identifying multiple etiologies of dyspnea, including ischemic heart disease, arrhythmias, and other cardiomyopathies. A normal ECG has 89% sensitivity for ruling out heart failure [23]. Additionally, a right heart strain pattern on ECG can point to pulmonary causes such as pulmonary hypertension, chronic thromboembolism, and severe COPD.
- *Echocardiogram* remains the preferred test for identifying cardiac pathology as the cause of dyspnea. It can identify valvular lesions, diastolic or systolic dysfunction, right ventricular overload in the setting of severe pulmonary disease, and wall motion abnormalities in the setting of ischemic heart disease. It has its limitations, however, as one study showed that up to one third of patients with heart failure with preserved ejection fraction (HFpEF) have normal diastolic function on echocardiogram [24].
- *Point-of-care ultrasound (POCUS)*, when available, can be very beneficial in identifying and/or ruling out multiple causes of dyspnea while saving the patient a trip to the radiology department. POCUS can be used to estimate

cardiac function, identify right heart strain, diagnose pneumothoraces, and identify fluid in the alveolar space. One study found that POCUS had a higher sensitivity for diagnosing pulmonary edema in patients with CHF than chest radiography (96% vs. 65%) [25].

- *Chest radiography* is one of the most useful diagnostic tests in the evaluation of chronic dyspnea. It can identify a wide variety of lung pathology, including pneumonia, pleural effusions, pneumothorax, and COPD, as well as give clues to a diagnosis of heart failure.
- *Chest computed tomography (CT)* is an important diagnostic tool in advanced evaluation of primary *pulmonary* pathology, mainly as high-resolution computed tomography (HRCT) in the diagnosis and characterization of suspected ILD. Chest CT can also be used to better evaluate equivocal findings on chest radiography.
- *Procalcitonin* has been increasingly used to aid in the diagnosis of bacterial pneumonia. In the setting of a patient with dyspnea, procalcitonin can be used to distinguish pneumonia from heart failure in patients with pulmonary edema as well as patients with acute decompensated heart failure complicated by a bacterial infection [26]. Additionally, a procalcitonin level >0.25 had a specificity of 98% in the diagnosis of bacterial pneumonia [3].
- Advanced testing can be performed if initial testing is non-diagnostic.

  – *Cardiopulmonary exercise testing (CPET)*

    Cardiopulmonary exercise testing (CPET) is gaining popularity in the continued workup of dyspnea when the diagnosis remains unclear or the patient's symptoms are out of proportion to the degree of disease. The test involves the patient undergoing physical exertion, usually using a treadmill or stationary bike, while computers monitor cardiac, ventilatory and gas exchange, and metabolic parameters. These parameters can help identify abnormalities at multiple points in the cardiopulmonary system and give insight into the patient's exercise capacity. Additionally, testing can identify if a patient's symptoms of dyspnea are out of proportion to level of measured exertion, suggesting a more functional cause of symptoms.

Key Points

- Dyspnea is a subjective sensation of difficulty breathing that can occur in patients both with and without compromise in gas exchange.
- The sensation of dyspnea arises from activation of a variety of central and peripheral locations located throughout the body that send signals to centers in the brainstem. Central respiratory centers compile this information and determine the expected respiratory "output" (i.e., diaphragmatic expansion, level of airflow, $PaO_2/PaCO_2$) for the level of input (same variables), both sensed by types of receptors. Mismatches in these factors lead to the sensation of dyspnea.
- Often the language used by patients to describe their dyspnea can give clues to the etiology. However, it is important to note that there are racial, ethnic, and cultural differences in these descriptors that can impact their interpretation by providers.
- The majority of cases of dyspnea can be diagnosed based on history and physical alone, but further testing should be chosen based on clinical suspicion of a certain etiology. Advanced testing (such as cardiopulmonary exercise testing) should be pursued if initial workup is non-diagnostic, or if the diagnosis does not fully explain the symptoms or degree of impairment.

References

1. Berliner D, et al. The differential diagnosis of dyspnea. Dtsch Arztebl Int. 2016;113(49):834–45.
2. Parshall MB, et al. An official American Thoracic Society statement: update on the mechanisms, assessment, and management of dyspnea. Am J Respir Crit Care Med. 2012;185(4):435–52.
3. Pratter MR, et al. An algorithmic approach to chronic dyspnea. Respir Med. 2011;105(7):1014–21.
4. Banzett R, Lansing R. Respiratory sensations arising from pulmonary and chemoreceptor afferents: air hunger and lung volume. Lung Biol Health Dis. 1996;90:155–80.
5. McBride B, Whitelaw WA. A physiological stimulus to upper airway receptors in humans. J Appl Physiol Respir Environ Exerc Physiol. 1981;51(5):1189–97.
6. Clark AL, Piepoli M, Coats AJ. Skeletal muscle and the control of ventilation on exercise: evidence for metabolic receptors. Eur J Clin Investig. 1995;25(5):299–305.
7. O'Donnell DE, et al. Pathophysiology of dyspnea in chronic obstructive pulmonary disease: a roundtable. Proc Am Thorac Soc. 2007;4(2):145–68.
8. Chang AS, et al. Prospective use of descriptors of dyspnea to diagnose common respiratory diseases. Chest. 2015;148(4):895–902.
9. Mahler DA, et al. Descriptors of breathlessness in cardiorespiratory diseases. Am J Respir Crit Care Med. 1996;154(5):1357–63.
10. McIlvaine S, Gelfand EV. Dyspnea. In: Handbook of inpatient cardiology. Springer Nature Switzerland; 2020. p. 441–56.
11. Hardie GE, et al. Ethnic differences: word descriptors used by African-American and white asthma patients during induced bronchoconstriction. Chest. 2000;117(4):935–43.
12. Palla A, et al. The role of suspicion in the diagnosis of pulmonary embolism. Chest. 1995;107(1 Suppl):21s–4s.
13. Pratter MR, Hingston DM, Irwin RS. Diagnosis of bronchial asthma by clinical evaluation. An unreliable method. Chest. 1983;84(1):42–7.
14. Bucca C, et al. Are asthma-like symptoms due to bronchial or extrathoracic airway dysfunction? Lancet. 1995;346(8978):791–5.
15. Htun TP, et al. Clinical features for diagnosis of pneumonia among adults in primary care setting: a systematic and meta-review. Sci Rep. 2019;9(1):7600.

16. Wang CS, et al. Does this dyspneic patient in the emergency department have congestive heart failure? JAMA. 2005;294(15):1944–56.
17. Broekhuizen BD, et al. The diagnostic value of history and physical examination for COPD in suspected or known cases: a systematic review. Fam Pract. 2009;26(4):260–8.
18. Straus SE, et al. The accuracy of patient history, wheezing, and laryngeal measurements in diagnosing obstructive airway disease. CARE-COAD1 group. Clinical assessment of the reliability of the examination-chronic obstructive airways disease. JAMA. 2000;283(14):1853–7.
19. Simon PM, et al. Distinguishable types of dyspnea in patients with shortness of breath. Am Rev Respir Dis. 1990;142(5):1009–14.
20. Pratter MR, et al. Cause and evaluation of chronic dyspnea in a pulmonary disease clinic. Arch Intern Med. 1989;149(10):2277–82.
21. Sarkar S, Amelung PJ. Evaluation of the dyspneic patient in the office. Prim Care. 2006;33(3):643–57.
22. Anjan VY, et al. Prevalence, clinical phenotype, and outcomes associated with normal B-type natriuretic peptide levels in heart failure with preserved ejection fraction. Am J Cardiol. 2012;110(6):870–6.
23. Ponikowski P, et al. 2016 ESC Guidelines for the diagnosis and treatment of acute and chronic heart failure: The Task Force for the diagnosis and treatment of acute and chronic heart failure of the European Society of Cardiology (ESC) Developed with the special contribution of the Heart Failure Association (HFA) of the ESC. Eur Heart J. 2016;37(27):2129–200.
24. Shah AM, et al. Cardiac structure and function in heart failure with preserved ejection fraction: baseline findings from the echocardiographic study of the Treatment of Preserved Cardiac Function Heart Failure with an Aldosterone Antagonist trial. Circ Heart Fail. 2014;7(1):104–15.
25. Wooten WM, Shaffer LET, Hamilton LA. Bedside ultrasound versus chest radiography for detection of pulmonary edema: a prospective cohort study. J Ultrasound Med. 2019;38(4):967–73.
26. Maisel A, et al. Use of procalcitonin for the diagnosis of pneumonia in patients presenting with a chief complaint of dyspnoea: results from the BACH (Biomarkers in Acute Heart Failure) trial. Eur J Heart Fail. 2012;14(3):278–86.

Chapter 3
Palpitations

Christine Bethencourt, Allie Goins, and Mikhael El Chami

Abbreviations

ECG	Electrocardiogram
PAC	Premature atrial contraction
PVC	Premature ventricular contraction
SVT	Supraventricular tachycardia
VT	Ventricular tachycardia

C. Bethencourt
Emory University School of Medicine, Atlanta, GA, USA
e-mail: Christine.m.bethencourt@emory.edu

A. Goins (✉)
Department of Medicine, Emory University School of Medicine, Atlanta, GA, USA
e-mail: agoins@emory.edu

M. E. Chami
Department of Medicine, Division of Cardiology, Emory University School of Medicine, Atlanta, GA, USA
e-mail: melcham@emory.edu

A. A. Bhargava et al. (eds.), *Handbook of Outpatient Cardiology*, https://doi.org/10.1007/978-3-030-88953-1_3

Background

- Palpitations are a symptom characterized by awareness of an abnormal heartbeat, often described as a sensation of unpleasant rapid pulsations in the chest area or skipped beats.
- Terms used by patients to describe palpitations often include "pounding," "flopping," "skipping," or "fluttering" in their chest or simply an awareness of their heartbeat [1]. Patients presenting with concurrent angina, syncope, lightheadedness, or dizziness should raise suspicion for an arrhythmic cause of palpitations.
- It is estimated that palpitations are the second most common reason for cardiologist visits and account for as many as 16% of visits to generalist physicians [2].
- In one study, cardiac etiologies of palpitations were identified in only 21% of outpatient visits. It is important to determine the cause of these palpitations and to distinguish between cardiac and non-cardiac causes in order to identify arrhythmias with malignant potential [3].

Etiologies

- Electrical Cardiac Abnormality
  - Palpitations are frequently caused by an underlying electrical abnormality in the heart (Table 3.1). Tachyarrhythmias are more likely to give rise to palpitations than bradyarrhythmias, and changes from normal sinus rhythm may often be triggered by non-cardiac causes (Table 3.2).
  - Atrial fibrillation and SVT are often difficult to distinguish if the arrhythmia mechanism on ECG is unclear. Determining a regular ventricular rhythm, as seen in SVT, or an irregular ventricular rhythm, as seen in atrial fibrillation, will guide diagnosis. A misdiagnosis of regular SVT is often made when atrial fibrillation with rapid ventricular response is present.

Table 3.1 Common electrical causes of palpitations

Common electrical causes of palpitations
Atrial fibrillation and flutter
Atrial premature contractions
Bradyarrhythmias
Inappropriate sinus tachycardia
Supraventricular tachycardia
Ventricular premature contractions
Ventricular tachycardia

Table 3.2 Common conditions associated with or that could trigger palpitations

Common conditions associated with or that could trigger palpitations
Structural heart disease
Psychosomatic
Medications or illicit substances
Systemic disease
Obstructive sleep apnea

  - Premature atrial or ventricular contractions are common, often benign, arrhythmia-related sources of palpitations. While both may be described by patients as "extra" or "skipped" beats, PACs are more prevalent. In PVCs, patients may describe pressure in the throat due to an ectopic systolic beat against closed heart valves.

- Structural Heart Disease
  - Mitral valve prolapse is the leading structural heart disease responsible for palpitations, affecting 1–3% of the population. Diagnosis is often made by cardiac auscultation indicating a midsystolic click followed by a late systolic murmur that can be accentuated by maneuvers such as standing or Valsalva [4].

- Common valvular causes of palpitations include mitral valve prolapse, mechanical prosthetic valves, and severe mitral or aortic regurgitation.
- Hypertrophic cardiomyopathy, arrhythmogenic right ventricular cardiomyopathy, and atrial myxomas should be considered as structural defects predisposing patients to arrhythmias and potential sudden cardiac death.
- Congenital abnormalities such as atrial septal defects, ventricular septal defects, and bicuspid aortic valves should be considered as potential etiologies for palpitations, especially in younger patients.

- Systemic Conditions
  - Palpitations caused by systemic disorders may manifest as either sinus tachycardia or increased cardiac contractility [1]. The following conditions should be considered as potential causes of palpitations given an appropriate clinical context:

    Anemia
    Arteriovenous fistula
    Electrolyte imbalance
    Fever
    Hyperthyroidism
    Hypoglycemia
    Hypovolemia
    Orthostatic hypertension
    Paget disease
    Pheochromocytoma
    Postmenopausal syndrome
    Pregnancy

- Psychosomatic Disorders
  - Psychosomatic disorders can be attributed as the cause of palpitations in up to 31% of patients, particularly in those who are younger and in women [1].
  - Psychiatric conditions, most notably anxiety, are common non-cardiac causes of palpitations. Other conditions that may present with palpitations include depression, panic attacks, and somatization.

- It is important to rule out an arrhythmia before attributing symptoms to a psychosomatic cause.

Clinical Pearl
Arrhythmic causes of palpitations can often be seen alongside psychosomatic conditions. Patients may be mistakenly diagnosed if their symptoms are attributed to established psychiatric disease; therefore, it is important to evaluate and exclude other potential causes of palpitations.

- Drug-Induced
  - Both medicinal and recreational drugs often produce changes in heart rate at varying points of their administration. It is important to construct a timeline including onset of medication use, dosage changes, and discontinuation, as well as a complete medication list.
  - Medications commonly linked to palpitations include adrenergic (sympathomimetic) drugs, hydralazine, anticholinergics, and vasodilators. Commonly used drugs such as caffeine, alcohol, nicotine, cocaine, amphetamines, and marijuana may also induce palpitations [5].
  - Beta-blocker initiation or dose increase may lead to palpitations secondary to bradycardia with increased diastolic filling time or PVCs; additionally, sudden discontinuation may lead to palpitations caused by reflex sinus tachycardia and hypertension.

Evaluation

- For the initial evaluation, all patients presenting with palpitations should undergo a focused history and physical examination to help identify the etiology of their palpitations [6–8].

- Key aspects of the history in this patient population include duration of the episodes, heart rate during the episodes, regularity of the palpitations during the episode, and association of the palpitations with stress or exercise.

  A regular rhythm is more suggestive of SVT or VT, while irregular palpitations may suggest atrial fibrillation or symptomatic PVCs.
  Palpitations that only last for an instant are more consistent with PACs or PVCs.

- It is also very important to ask patients about other associated symptoms including light-headedness, dizziness, syncope, or chest pain. If patients report associated presyncope or syncope symptoms, this could be concerning for a more serious arrhythmia, such as VT.
- Taking a detailed past medical history and family history as well as a review of the patients prescribed and over-the-counter medications can also help point towards the etiology of the palpitations and help screen patients for underlying structural heart disease and a more serious arrhythmia.

• The physical examination should focus on identifying structural heart disease (evaluating for murmurs, vascular disease, heart failure) or evidence of systemic causes of palpitations (i.e., Goiter, exophthalmos, etc.).
• The initial evaluation for patients with palpitations should also include a 12-lead ECG, as well as basic labs to rule out systemic causes of palpitations, such as hyperthyroidism and anemia [6–8].
• Patients in which your suspicion is high for structural heart disease also warrant transthoracic echocardiogram to further evaluate their palpitations. Risk factors for underlying structural heart disease in the setting of palpitations are listed below [8]:

  - Family history of hypertrophic cardiomyopathy or sudden cardiac death
  - Murmur noted on physical examination

- Abnormal ECG
- Documented frequent PVCs or atrial fibrillation

- If the patient is experiencing exertional symptoms, this patient should also be considered for exercise stress testing to rule out ischemic disease [8].

Clinical Pearl
The first step in evaluating a patient with palpitations includes a detailed history, physical examination, 12-lead ECG, and basic labs to rule out systemic etiologies (such as hyperthyroidism and anemia). If the physical exam or history is suggestive of underlying structural heart disease, a transthoracic echocardiogram is also warranted. If the patient is having symptoms triggered by exertion, an exercise stress test should also be considered.

- There are certain patients who should receive outpatient cardiac rhythm monitoring with either a 24–72 hour Holter monitor, 2–4-week event monitor, external loop recorder, or implantable cardiac monitor [8–10], (Fig. 3.1):

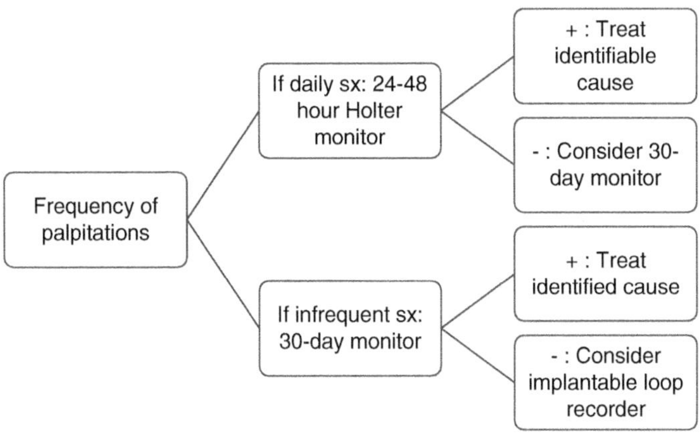

FIGURE 3.1 Algorithm for palpitation workup

- Sustained palpitations
- Palpitations due to PVCs (Determining PVC burden has implications for management.)
- Documented arrhythmia with a wearable technology (Apple watch, AliveCor, etc.) in order to confirm findings
- Palpitations associated with presyncope or syncope
- Presence of structural heart disease
- Personal or family history of arrhythmia, sudden cardiac death, or prolonged QTc

Clinical Pearl
Frequent, unexplained palpitations warrant a 24–72 hour Holter monitor as part of an in-depth workup. Infrequent palpitations are better investigated with a longer event monitor.

Management

- Management of palpitations is determined by the etiology and the severity of the symptoms.
  - If the initial evaluation suggests the palpitations are from a medication, discontinuation of the medication is key.
  - If the outpatient cardiac monitor identifies an arrhythmia, this arrhythmia should be managed as appropriate.
  - If systemic diseases are identified such as anemia or hyperthyroidism, then this underlying condition should be treated to improve the palpitations.

Key Learning Points

- Distinguishing between cardiac and non-cardiac causes of palpitations is essential to identify patients with potentially life-threatening arrhythmias.
- History, physical examination, and standard 12-lead ECG identify the etiology of palpitations in most patients.
- If patients have evidence of structural heart disease on initial evaluation or have risk factors for a more serious arrhythmia, they should also undergo trans-thoracic echocardiogram and ambulatory cardiac monitoring.
- Management of palpitations is based on the underlying etiology of palpitations, how symptomatic the patient is, and the presence or absence of structural heart disease.

References

1. Raviele A, Giada F, Bergfeldt L, et al. Management of patients with palpitations: a position paper from the European heart rhythm association. Europace. 2011;13(7):920–34.
2. Abbott AV. Diagnostic approach to palpitations. Am Fam Physician. 2005;71(4):743–50. PMID: 15742913.
3. Goyal A, Robinson KJ, Katta S, et al. Palpitations. [Updated 2020 Aug 13]. In: StatPearls [Internet]. Treasure Island (FL): StatPearls Publishing; 2020 Jan. Available from: https://www.ncbi.nlm.nih.gov/books/NBK436016/.
4. Miller, Marc A., et al. Arrhythmic Mitral Valve Prolapse: JACC Review Topic of the Week. J Am Coll Card, Elsevier, 3 Dec. 2018, www.sciencedirect.com/science/article/pii/S0735109718386923.
5. Tisdale JE, Chung MK, Campbell KB, Hammadah M, Joglar JA, Leclerc J, Rajagopalan B. Drug-induced arrhythmias: a scientific statement from the american heart association. Circulation. 2020;142(15):214–33. https://doi.org/10.1161/cir.0000000000000905.

6. Weber BE, Kapoor WN. Evaluation and outcomes of patients with palpitations. Am J Med. 1996;100(2):138–48. https://doi.org/10.1016/s0002-9343(97)89451-x. Erratum in: Am J Med 1997;103(1):86. PMID: 8629647.
7. Wexler R, Pleister A, Raman S. Outpatient approach to palpitations. Am Fam Physician. 2011;84:63–9.
8. Shen WK, Sheldon RS, Benditt DG, et al. 2017 ACC/AHA/HRS guideline for the evaluation and management of patients with syncope: executive summary. Circulation. 2017;136:e25–59. https://doi.org/10.1161/cir.0000000000000498.
9. Wolfe RR, Driscoll DJ, Gersony WM, et al. Arrhythmias in patients with valvar aortic stenosis, valvar pulmonary stenosis, and ventricular septal defect. Results of 24-hour ECG monitoring. Circulation. 1993;87:I89.
10. Giada F, Raviele A. Clinical approach to patients with palpitations. Card Electrophysiol Clin. 2018;10:387.

Chapter 4
Syncope

Shu Yang and Peter Zimetbaum

Abbreviations

ARVC	Arrhythmogenic right ventricular cardiomyopathy
AS	Aortic stenosis
BP	Blood pressure
CPVT	Catecholaminergic polymorphic ventricular tachycardia
CSP	Carotid sinus pressure
CSS	Carotid sinus syndrome
CT	Computed tomography
CVA	Cerebrovascular accident
ECG	Electrocardiogram
ED	Emergency department
ELR	External loop recorder
HCM	Hypertrophic cardiomyopathy
ILR	Implantable loop recorder
LQTS	Long QT syndrome
LVOT	Left ventricular outflow tract

S. Yang (✉) · P. Zimetbaum
Department of Medicine, Division of Cardiology, Beth Israel Deaconess Medical Center, Harvard Medical School, Boston, MA, USA
e-mail: syang2@bidmc.harvard.edu; pzimetba@bidmc.harvard.edu

A. A. Bhargava et al. (eds.), *Handbook of Outpatient Cardiology*, https://doi.org/10.1007/978-3-030-88953-1_4

MCOT	Mobile cardiac outpatient telemetry
MI	Myocardial infarction
MRI	Magnetic resonance imaging
MS	Mitral stenosis
OS	Orthostatic syncope
PCI	Percutaneous coronary intervention
PE	Pulmonary embolus
proBNP	Pro-brain natriuretic peptide
SSRI	Selective serotonin reuptake inhibitor
TdP	Torsades de pointes
TIA	Transient ischemic attack
TLOC	Transient loss of consciousness
TTE	Transthoracic echocardiogram

Introduction to Syncope

Definition

- Transient, abrupt, and self-limited loss of consciousness (LOC)
- Resolves without intervention
- Associated with loss of postural tone
- A specific form of transient loss of consciousness (TLOC) (Table 4.1)
- Should be differentiated from other causes of TLOC and pre-syncope – latter does not involve LOC, but shares similar mechanisms

Epidemiology

- Frequent reason for emergency departments (ED) referral, comprising 1–2% of hospital admissions from these settings. Annual cost of syncope-related hospitalizations nearly 2.5 billion dollars, rivaling that of asthma, HIV, and COPD, individually [2]

TABLE 4.1 Causes of syncope

Other causes of TLOC	Orthostatic syncope	Reflex syncope
Neurologic	Hypovolemia-mediated	Situational syncope
General tonic-clonic seizure	Medication-induced	Micturition syncope
Stroke/transient ischemic attack	Angiotensin-converting enzyme inhibitors (ACEis)	Swallowing-associated
Intoxications	Angiotensin receptor blockers (ARBs)	Post-exertional
Metabolic	Alpha-1 antagonists	Emotion-mediated
Hypoxia/hypercarbia	Dihydropyridine calcium channel blockers (CCBs)	Pain
Infection	Autonomic predispositions	Fear
Uremia	Diabetic neuropathy	Anxiety
Hypoglycemia	Parkinsonism	Carotid sinus syndrome
Traumatic	Multi-system atrophy	Other stimuli-driven
Concussion	Amyloidosis	
Psychiatric		
Psychogenic non-epileptic seizure		
Cataplexy		

(continued)

TABLE 4.1 (continued)

Other causes of TLOC	Orthostatic syncope	Reflex syncope
Cardiogenic syncope		
Arrhythmogenic	*Mechanical/ obstructive*	*Ischemic*
Bradyarrhythmia and heart block	Severe systolic/ diastolic cardiomyopathies	Rarely manifests as syncope
Sinus node dysfunction	Severe valvular disease	Acute ischemic systolic/diastolic dysfunction
Tachy-brady syndrome	Aortic or mitral stenosis	Malignant ventricular tachyarrhythmia
Beta blocker toxicity	Hypertrophic cardiomyopathy with LVOT obstruction	Heart block/ bradyarrhythmia
Tachyarrhythmias in the setting of:	Pericardial effusion/ tamponade	Due to transient rise in vagal tone (inferior ischemia) or necrosis of local conduction system (anterior infarction)
Channelopathies (LQTS)	Sub/massive pulmonary embolism	
CPVT	Aortic dissection	
Infiltrative disease (sarcoidosis)		

TABLE 4.1 (continued)

Other causes of TLOC	Orthostatic syncope	Reflex syncope
Cardiomyopathies (ARVC)		
Pacemaker malfunction		

Adapted from previously published table [1]
TLOC transient loss of consciousness, *LQTS* long *QT* syndrome, *CPVT* catecholaminergic polymorphic ventricular tachycardia, *ARVC* arrhythmogenic right ventricular cardiomyopathy, *LVOT* left ventricular outflow tract

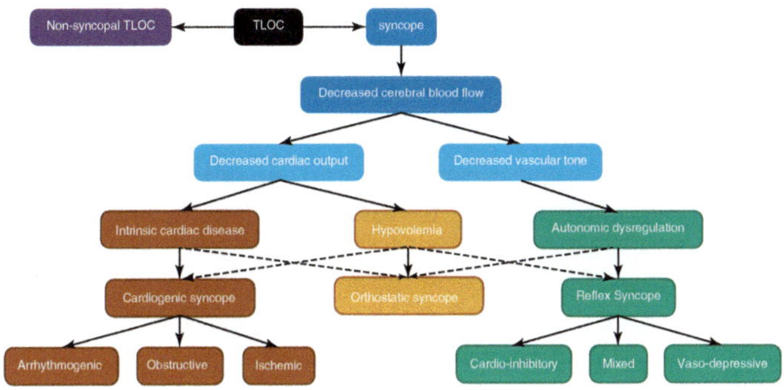

FIGURE 4.1 Mechanism of syncope. Syncope, a form of transient loss of consciousness (TLOC), results from impaired cerebral perfusion due to either decreased cardiac output or vascular resistance. Major factors (solid arrows) leading to syncope and overlapping underlying mechanisms shown (dashed arrows) [1]

Mechanisms and Causes of Syncope

- Wide array of causative conditions (Table 4.1), although 40% of cases without any identified [3, 4].
- Central mechanism is cerebral hypoperfusion.
  - Can result from inadequate cardiac output and/or inappropriately low peripheral vascular resistance
  - Can subdivide by physiologic categories, outlined below and in Fig. 4.1

- Orthostatic syncope (OS):
  - Can occur immediately following trigger (i.e., change in position from supine to standing) or in delayed fashion (i.e., after prolonged standing)
  - Hypovolemia and autonomic insufficiency predispose to OS
  - Commonly exacerbated by use of diuretic and vasoplegic agents
- Reflex (formerly vasovagal or neutrally mediated) syncope:
  - Most common form of syncope [5]
  - Occurs in response to certain stimuli
  - Characterized by exaggerated shifts in autonomic balance (increased vagal tone)
  - Three major categories:

    Cardio-inhibitory: Profound, negative chronotropic response leading to severe bradycardia and potentially asystole

    Vaso-depressive: Dysregulated vasodilatory mechanisms lead to low vascular resistance and inadequate cerebral blood flow, despite effective augmentation of cardiac output

    - Proposed mechanisms: Rapid withdrawal of sympathetic tone and abnormal baroreceptor sensitivity [6, 7]

    Mixed: Cardio-inhibition and vaso-depression both present. Upregulation of endogenous adenosine may play pathophysiologic role [8]

  - Broad range of triggers for reflex syncope (Table 4.2)
- Cardiogenic syncope:
  - Arrhythmogenic:

    Most common cause of cardiogenic syncope – 26% of all syncope [4].

TABLE 4.2 High- and low-risk features in history and exam

	Low-risk features (favoring benign etiology)	**High-risk features (favoring cardiogenic syncope)**
Clinical presentation	Prodrome typical of reflex syncope (nausea, vomiting, lightheadedness, diaphoresis, flushing)	Severe associated physical injuries, particularly with associated facial trauma
	Syncope in response to discrete trigger	Short or absent prodrome
	Abrupt change in position (orthostatic)	No clear trigger
	Prolonged standing (orthostatic or reflex)	Concurrent symptoms suggestive of:
	Strong emotion, unpleasant odor or sight, or pain (reflex)	Pulmonary embolus, gastrointestinal bleeding, myocardial infarction, aortic dissection, pulmonary embolus
	Head rotation or pressure on carotid sinuses (reflex)	Sudden/rapid recovery following event
	Micturition, defecation, vomiting (reflex)	New onset syncope
	Syncope after exercise/during recovery (reflex)	Syncope from a supine position
	Prolonged period of fatigue during recovery period (reflex)	Syncope during exercise

(continued)

Table 4.2 (continued)

	Low-risk features (favoring benign etiology)	**High-risk features (favoring cardiogenic syncope)**
Prior history	No known cardiac risk factors	History of known cardiac disease
	History recurrent syncope over long period of time (reflex)	Severe valvular disease
		Hypertrophic cardiomyopathy
		Coronary artery disease
		Cardiomyopathy
		Family history of sudden cardiac death
Exam	Orthostatic vital signs	Persistently abnormal vital signs
	Presence of carotid hypersensitivity	Systolic BP <90 mmHg
		Heart rate <40 bpm
		New systolic murmur

Adapted from previously published table [1]

Presence of structural cardiac abnormalities should raise suspicion (Table 4.1).

- Mechanical/obstructive:

  Reduced cardiac output from:

  - Primary systolic/diastolic failure
  - Physical obstruction of blood flow into systemic circulation
    - Structural cardiac pathologies: Severe aortic stenosis (AS) and mitral stenosis (MS), hyper-

trophic cardiomyopathy (HCM) with left ventricular outflow tract (LVOT) obstruction
  - Extrinsic conditions: Pericardial effusion/tamponade, sub/massive pulmonary embolism (PE)
  - Aortic dissection

    Due to complicating cardiac tamponade or massive stroke (proximal dissection extending into carotid arteries) [9]

- Ischemic:

  Acute coronary ischemia rare in patients presenting with syncope (~7%) [10]
  Potential mechanisms:

  - Acute mechanical dysfunction
  - Malignant ventricular arrhythmias
  - Heart block (more likely increased vagal tone with inferior ischemia and myocardial necrosis with anterior infarctions) [11, 12]

Clinical Pearl
Acute stroke and transient ischemic attack (TIA) infrequently cause syncope. Because cerebral blood supply is deliberately redundant with ample collateralization, syncope from cerebrovascular accidents (CVA) occurs only amidst severe, chronic multi-vessel occlusions. Vertebro-basilar insufficiency can manifest as "drop attacks," mimicking loss of postural tone and physical collapse often associated with syncope, but should not involve any LOC.

Diagnosis of Syncope

Initial Evaluation

- Include thorough *history, physical exam, and electrocardiogram (ECG)* in initial evaluation (Fig. 4.2)
- Primary goals:
  - Differentiate between cardiogenic and non-cardiogenic etiologies
  - Stratify by high- and low-risk features (Table 4.2)

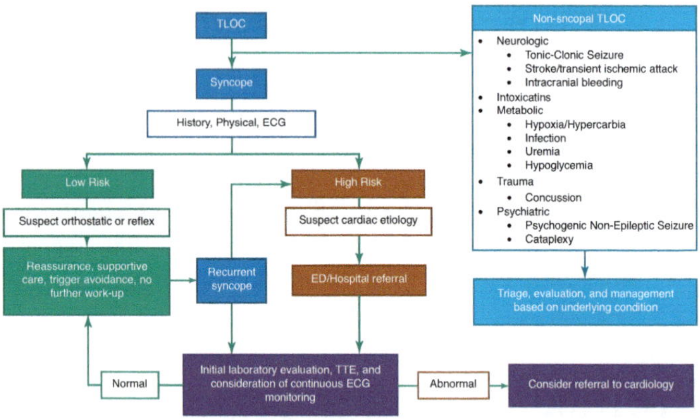

FIGURE 4.2 Diagnostic and management approach to syncope. Clinicians should begin by confirming diagnosis of syncope versus non-syncopal transient loss of consciousness (TLOC). All patients should receive thorough history, physical, and electrocardiography (ECG). If high-risk features are present or cardiogenic etiology of syncope is suspected, patients should be referred to emergency department (ED) or hospital for further evaluation. In absence of high-risk features, patients should receive reassurance and supportive care. Therapies for specific causes of syncope, such as trigger avoidance and rehydration, may also be implemented. Patients with recurrent syncope should again be screened for high-risk features at initial triage, followed by investigation with laboratory studies, imaging, and continuous ECG monitoring (discussed separately). If any abnormal results are present, clinicians should consider referral to specialist. TTE transthoracic echocardiogram

History

- Clear and accurate history critical in work-up of syncope
  - Obtain collateral information from bystanders/witnesses.
  - Confirm and distinguish syncope from other causes of TLOC.
  - Elicit potential triggers:

    Provoking events provide insight into mechanism of syncope and underlying conditions (Table 4.2).

  - Assess for pro-/post-drome:

    Absence or brief duration increases concern for significant injury and sudden death. Potential explanations:

    - Sudden onset of lethal arrhythmias
    - Inability to recognize and protect against impending LOC and physical injury

    Characteristic prodromes (nausea, vomiting, diaphoresis, flushing) carry considerable diagnostic value.

> **Clinical Pearl:** Reflex syncope is the most common form of syncope, characterized by an often prolonged period of fatigue and feeling "washed out," in direct contrast to brisk recovery seen typically in arrhythmogenic syncope [13].

  - Obtain full past medical, social, family, medication, and allergy histories:

    History of autonomic insufficiency (i.e., diabetic neuropathy or parkinsonism) increases odds of orthostatic/reflex syncope.
    Recurrent episodes over years suggest against malignant cause [14].

High-risk features supporting cardiogenic syncope:

- Significant personal history of cardiac disease [15]
- Family history of sudden/unexplained death, particularly at young age

– Elucidate other "red-flags" (Table 4.2):

Significant physical injury (i.e., facial trauma or motor vehicle accident).

- Suggests insufficient time and/or awareness to protect oneself

Syncope from supine position suggests arrhythmogenic cause.
Concomitant chest pain, dyspnea, or limb weakness points toward other medical conditions warranting urgent assessment.

Clinical Pearl: Syncope while driving is particularly concerning given risk for severe/fatal injury. This can be due to increased pressure on carotid baroreceptors by tightened seatbelts with head turning or underlying arrhythmia. However, falling asleep while driving should be considered and can be supported by descriptions of skid marks on the road (often gathered as collateral information). Drivers, who fall asleep, often have sufficient time to recover and engage the brakes, in contrast to those who suffer true syncope [16].

Physical Exam

- Beyond standard evaluation, direct attention to:

  – Abnormal vital signs:

    Persistent bradycardia (<40 beats/minute) may reflect underlying conduction disease/heart block [17].

Systolic blood pressure (BP) <90 mmHg is an independent predictor of adverse outcomes [18, 19].

- Orthostatic challenge:

  Definition: fall in systolic BP ≥20 mmHg or diastolic BP ≥10 mmHg, measured ≥2 minutes after position change [20]

  - 2018 European Society of Cardiology (ESC) guidelines added systolic BP ≤90 mmHg to criteria

  Reproducing pre-/syncope during challenge enhances post-test probability of OS [17].
  Presence of orthostatic hypotension does not preclude simultaneous cardiogenic or other causes of syncope. Red-flag features still must be assessed.

  - 10–25% of patients in ED diagnosed with cardiogenic syncope also met criteria for orthostatic hypotension [21].

- New cardiac murmur:

  Suggests structural cardiac pathology

- Carotid sinus pressure (CSP):

  Indicated if >40 years old to evaluate for carotid sinus syndrome (CSS) [17, 22]
  Diagnostic criteria (Fig. 4.3):

  - Ventricular pause >3 seconds and/or reduced systolic BP >50 mmHg following CSP
  - Reproduction of pre-/syncopal symptoms (typically requires pauses of >6 seconds) [23]

  Contraindications to CSP [17]:

  - Significant carotid bruit/stenosis
  - Recent MI
  - Prior ventricular arrhythmia

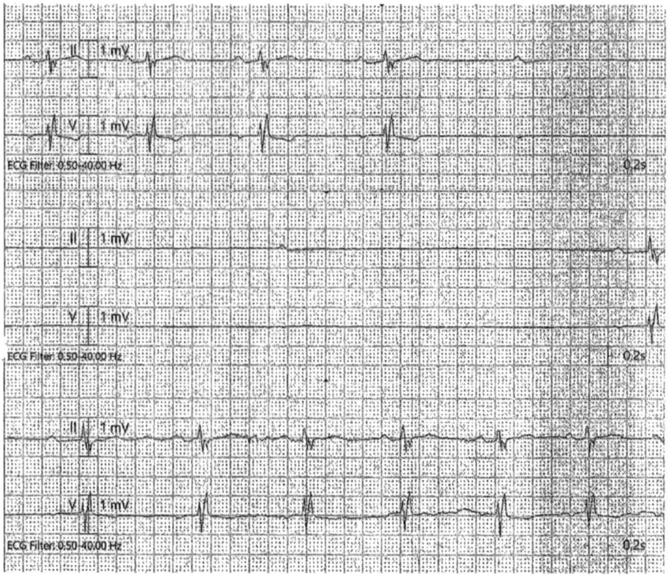

FIGURE 4.3 Carotid sinus syndrome. A 70-year-old man with a recurrent syncope of unclear etiology and unrevealing prior work-up including cardiac imaging, ischemic evaluation, and repeated ambulatory ECG monitoring. He had one prior episode of syncope while driving, prompting license suspension by state law. Upon license reinstatement, he had another episode of syncope while driving. This telemetry strip was obtained during application of carotid sinus pressure, which produced an 8.8 second pause and syncope, making the diagnosis of carotid sinus syndrome, treated with implantation of a dual-chamber pacemaker [1]

Electrocardiogram

- Obtain resting 12-lead ECG for all patients.
- Evaluate for presence/absence of:
  - Acute cardiac ischemia, arrhythmia, or conduction disease
  - Evidence of underlying structural heart disease, cardiomyopathies, or channelopathies [17, 22]

– High-risk electrocardiographic features (detailed in Table 4.3)

Table 4.3 High-risk features on ECG [1]

Concerning electrocardiographic (ECG) findings
Heart rates <40 bpm
Sinus rhythm or otherwise
Changes consistent with acute ischemia
Evidence of prior infarction-associated ECG changes
Evidence of infranodal conduction disease
Bundle branch blocks, intraventricular conduction delays
ECG evidence of structural heart disease
Left/right ventricular hypertrophy, hypertrophic cardiomyopathy, infiltrative disease
Atrioventricular block
Mobitz type II, high grade, and complete heart block
Ventricular arrhythmias
Sustained and non-sustained ventricular tachycardia (VT)
Risk factors for ventricular arrhythmias
Brugada pattern
Pre-excitation pattern
Long QTc
Short QTc
Arrhythmogenic right ventricular cardiomyopathy (ARVC)
Presence of dysfunctional cardiac implantable electronic device (CIED)
Involving permanent pacemakers (PPMs) or implantable cardioverter-defibrillators (ICD)

Clinical Pearl
QT prolongation (>450 ms in men, >460 ms in women) is associated with increased risk for arrhythmogenic syncope, specifically from torsades de pointes (TdP). Long QT can be hereditary or acquired – latter largely due medication effect (namely, anti-arrhythmic, anti-microbial, anti-psychotic, and anti-depressive classes). Incidence of TdP with medication-induced long QT is not well-defined, but likely low. Extrapolating from studies performed with dofetilide, a reasonable threshold for discontinuing QT-prolonging medications is 500ms [24].

Further Evaluation

- Consider additional testing if:
  - Diagnosis is inconclusive following routine evaluation (and cardiogenic syncope suspected).
  - Syncope recurs after initial diagnosis/treatment.
  - High-risk features are identified.

Laboratory Studies

- Start with basic chemistry panel, complete blood cell count to assess for metabolic abnormalities, anemia, or infection.
- If clinically indicated, perform cardiac biomarkers, pro-brain natriuretic peptide (proBNP), d-dimer, coagulation studies, liver function tests, and targeted culture studies.
- In women of childbearing age, pregnancy testing can inform risk stratification, diagnosis, and management [25].

Continuous Electrocardiographic Monitoring (Fig. 4.4)

- Ambulatory ECG monitoring indicated for recurrent or unexplained syncope, especially if palpitations present [26]
- External ambulatory monitors:
  - Holter monitors:

    Continuous ECG monitors, typically 24–72 hours

    - Arrhythmias, syncopal episodes unlikely to recur during monitoring period
    - Only identified arrhythmias in 2% of patients with unexplained syncope [27]
    - Reported diagnostic yield 15%, but only 2% of patients had concurrent symptoms [28]

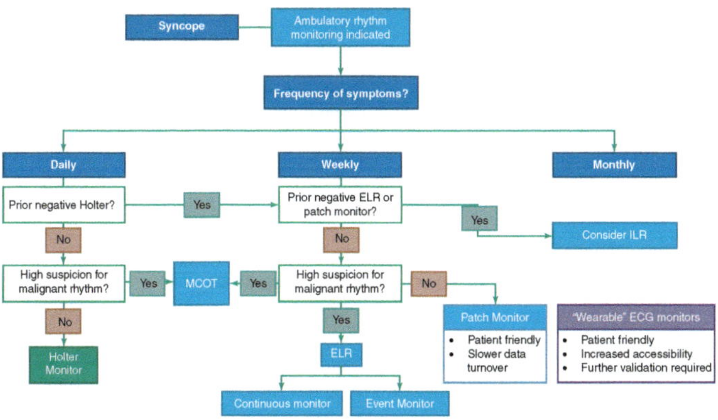

Figure 4.4 Choosing rhythm monitoring modality. Frequency of symptoms largely dictates optimal modality of ambulatory monitoring. Prior negative results and suspicion for malignant arrhythmia also influence monitor choice. While "wearable" devices offer accessible and potentially useful alternatives to traditional monitors, further research needed to delineate precise clinical roles. ECG, electrocardiogram; ELR, external loop recorder; ILR, implantable loop recorder. (Adapted from previously published figure [1])

Most useful with near-daily symptoms to assess arrhythmic culpability

- External loop recorders (ELR):

  Longer monitoring duration (up to a month)
  Improved diagnostic yield 25–88% compared with Holter monitors, but includes symptomatic/asymptomatic arrhythmias and symptoms with normal ECG [29, 30]
  Reasonable if symptoms occurring weekly

- Mobile cardiac outpatient telemetry (MCOT):

  Similar size to ELRs
  Constant link via cellular (versus analog) technology to monitoring units, staffed 24 hours/day by trained technician
  Patient activation not required for real-time event transmission (in contrast to Holter and ELR)
  Particularly useful if high-risk arrhythmias suspected
  Similar/superior diagnostic yield as ELRs [31, 32]

- External patch monitors (i.e., Zio XT patch):

  Increasing frequency of use for ambulatory ECG monitoring
  Small size, convenient for patients
  Continuously records over 2-week period; reported diagnostic yield ~74% [33].
  Major limitation: no real-time data transmission

- Commercial "wearable" ECG monitors (e.g., Apple Watch):

  Various "wearable" single-lead ECG monitors with built-in arrhythmia-detection algorithms available
  Convenient, accessible for patients
  LIVMOR only FDA-approved device for atrial fibrillation detection; data support role in QT-interval monitoring [34]
  Promising potential, but utility still undefined [26]

Clinical Pearl
Holter monitors and ELRs are capable of transmitting recorded ECG data remotely, but necessitate manual transmission via analog phone. In contrast, MCOTs automatically relay real-time information via cellular technology, facilitating detection of malignant arrhythmias and more timely response/intervention. Patch monitors (e.g., Zio XT patch) do not possess this functionality, and results can take weeks to return. The utility of "wearable" ECG monitors requires further validation prior to routine medical use.

- Implantable loop recorders (ILR):
  - Subcutaneously implanted, leadless devices, allowing long-term (up to 2–3 years) monitoring
  - More invasive and expensive than external monitors; useful if recurrent, but infrequent syncopal episodes
  - Diagnostic yield 83–88% in patients with syncope of unclear etiology [35, 36]

Imaging Studies

- Echocardiography:
  - Low overall diagnostic utility
  - Avoid use in routine syncope evaluation, but helpful when structural heart disease suspected [22]

Clinical Pearl: The diagnostic yield of echocardiogram in syncope is estimated to be ~3%, while cost per diagnosis made with echocardiography is >$34,000 [36, 37].

- Cardiac computed tomography (CT) and magnetic resonance imaging (MRI):
  - Useful in specific conditions, but should not be routinely pursued

Tilt Table Testing

- Consider in suspected, but unproven reflex syncope
  - Sensitivity 26–80%, specificity 90% [38]
- Can be positive in reflex, unexplained, and cardiac syncope [39]
  - Limited ability to distinguish between etiologies
  - Can identify high susceptibility to orthostatic stress [17]

Ischemic Evaluation

- Exercise stress testing:
  - Risky in exertional syncope as contraindicated in certain high-risk causes (severe AS, severe MS, or HCM with LVOT obstruction, sympathetically stimulated ventricular arrhythmias, and rarely heart block) [22]
  - Must be done with extreme caution in appropriately equipped environment
- Coronary angiography:
  - Reasonable to pursue +/– percutaneous coronary intervention (PCI) if acute coronary syndrome or ischemia-induced arrhythmia present; otherwise adds little value [40]

Management of Syncope

Orthostatic and Reflex Syncope

- Primary aim to improve symptoms and avoid complicating falls/injuries
  - Non-pharmacologic interventions first-line [22, 41]

    Increase fluid and salt intake (absent medical contraindications)
    Lower extremity compression garments and abdominal binders to prevent venous pooling
    Avoid vasoplegic medications
    Employ counter-pressure maneuvers and adaptive behaviors (e.g., changing positions more slowly)
    Increase exercise and physical therapy

  - Pharmacologic therapies:

    Fludrocortisone and midodrine used for orthostatic and reflex syncope. Both increase BP and reduce symptoms, but cause fluid retention and postural hypertension, respectively [42–44]

  - OS-specific:

    Droxidopa (norepinephrine pro-drug) can improve autonomic insufficiency and functional status; causes supine hypertension [45].
    Consider pyridostigmine as third-line therapy [46].

  - Reflex syncope-specific:

    Beta-blockers and selective serotonin reuptake inhibitors (SSRIs) may benefit certain populations [22].
    Pacemaker placement indicated in cardio-inhibitory syncope and CSS, especially with prolonged spontaneous sinus pauses and recurrent symptoms refractory to noninvasive therapies [47].

Cardiogenic Syncope

- Treatments tailored to specific underlying diagnoses

Driving After Syncope

- Without significant prodromes, avoidable triggers, and treatable causes, driving poses significant risk of harm to self and others.
- State laws frequently impose post-syncopal driving restrictions.
  - Can interfere with personal, family, occupational obligations
- Clinicians should be aware of local policies and engage in conversation with patients incorporating state-, occupational-, and person-specific factors [22].

Key Learning Points

- Syncope is a common and costly problem. It is often conflated with non-syncopal causes of transient loss of consciousness, for which diagnostic and management strategies are vastly different.
- Transient cerebral hypoperfusion leads to syncope and is mechanistically caused by a combination of decreased cardiac output and vascular tone.
- Routine work-up of syncope should include a complete and thorough history (utilizing patient and collateral report), physical exam, and electrocardiogram. Evaluation should focus on identifying high-risk features and patients, who require more aggressive and timely management.
- Ambulatory ECG monitoring can be useful in evaluating recurrent and unexplained syncope. Optimal modality choice depends on frequency of symptoms,

suspicion for malignant etiology of syncope, and urgency, with which study results are needed.

- Treatment of syncope relies heavily on the underlying cause. When possible, non-pharmacologic interventions should be employed first, followed by pharmacologic therapies and more invasive measures (such as pacemaker implantation). Clinicians should recognize and pre-emptively address driving restrictions following syncope given the potentially enormous personal, societal, legal, and occupational ramifications.

References

1. Yang S, Zimetbaum P. Syncope. In: Wells BJ, Pinzon PQ, Southmayd G, editors. Handbook of inpatient cardiology. First ed. Springer International Publishing: Switzerland, AG. 2020.
2. Sun BC, Emond JA, Camargo CA. Direct medical costs of syncope-related hospitalizations in the United States. Am J Cardiol. 2005;95(5):668–71.
3. Schnipper JL, Kapoor WN. Diagnostic evaluation and management of patients with syncope. Med Clin N Am. 2001;85(2):423–56.
4. Soteriades ES, Chen L. Incidence and prognosis of syncope. N Engl J Med. 2002;8.
5. Kapoor WN. Syncope. N Engl J Med. 2000;343(25):1856–62.
6. Morillo CA, Eckberg DL, Ellenbogen KA, Beightol LA, Hoag JB, Tahvanainen Kari UO, et al. Vagal and sympathetic mechanisms in patients with orthostatic vasovagal syncope. Circulation. 1997;96(8):2509–13.
7. Thomson HL, Karen W, Michael F. Baroreflex sensitivity in patients with vasovagal syncope. Circulation. 1997;95(2):395–400.
8. Saadjian AY, Lévy S, Franceschi F, Zouher I, Paganelli F, Guieu RP. Role of endogenous adenosine as a modulator of syncope induced during tilt testing. Circulation. 2002;106(5):569–74.
9. Nallamothu BK, Mehta RH, Saint S. Syncope in acute aortic dissection: diagnostic, prognostic, and clinical implications. ACC Curr J Rev. 2003;12(2):17.

10. Georgeson S, Linzer M, Griffith JL, Weld L, Selker HP. Acute cardiac ischemia in patients with syncope. J Gen Intern Med. 1992;7(4):379–86.
11. Mitrani RD, Hendel RC. The appropriateness of an ischemia evaluation for syncope. Circ Cardiovasc Imaging. 2013;6(3):358–9.
12. Zimetbaum PJ. Use of the electrocardiogram in acute myocardial infarction. N Engl J Med. 2003;8
13. Shukla GJ, Zimetbaum PJ. Syncope. Circulation [Internet]. 2006 Apr 25 [cited 2019 Oct 23];113(16). Available from: https://www.ahajournals.org/doi/10.1161/CIRCULATIONAHA.105.602250.
14. Arthur W, Kaye GC. The pathophysiology of common causes of syncope. Postgrad Med J. 2000;76(902):750–3.
15. Albassam OT, Redelmeier RJ, Shadowitz S, Husain AM, Simel D, Etchells EE. Did this patient have cardiac syncope?: the rational clinical examination systematic review. JAMA. 2019;321(24):2448.
16. Zimetbaum PJ, Josephson ME. Practical clinical electrophysiology. Lippincott Williams & Wilkins; Philadephia, PA. 2009. 330 p.
17. Brignole M, Moya A, de Lange FJ, Deharo J-C, Elliott PM, Fanciulli A, et al. 2018 ESC Guidelines for the diagnosis and management of syncope. Eur Heart J. 2018;39(21):1883–948.
18. Saccilotto RT, Nickel CH, Bucher HC, Steyerberg EW, Bingisser R, Koller MT. San Francisco Syncope Rule to predict short-term serious outcomes: a systematic review. CMAJ. 2011;183(15):E1116–26.
19. Thiruganasambandamoorthy V, Kwong K, Wells GA, Sivilotti MLA, Mukarram M, Rowe BH, et al. Development of the Canadian Syncope Risk Score to predict serious adverse events after emergency department assessment of syncope. CMAJ. 2016;188(12):E289–98.
20. Freeman R, Wieling W, Axelrod FB, Benditt DG, Benarroch E, Biaggioni I, et al. Consensus statement on the definition of orthostatic hypotension, neurally mediated syncope and the postural tachycardia syndrome. Clin Auton Res. 2011;21(2):69–72.
21. Schaffer JT, Keim SM, Hunter BR, Kirschner JM, De Lorenzo RA. Do orthostatic vital signs have utility in the evaluation of syncope? J Emerg Med. 2018;55(6):780–7.
22. Shen W-K, Sheldon RS, Benditt DG, Cohen MI, Forman DE, Goldberger ZD, et al. 2017 ACC/AHA/HRS guideline for the evaluation and management of patients with syncope: a report of the American College of Cardiology/American Heart Association Task Force on Clinical Practice Guidelines and the

Heart Rhythm Society. Circulation [Internet]. 2017 Aug [cited 2019 Jul 19];136(5). Available from: https://www.ahajournals.org/doi/10.1161/CIR.0000000000000499.

23. Wieling W, Krediet CTP, Solari D, de Lange FJ, van Dijk N, Thijs RD, et al. At the heart of the arterial baroreflex: a physiological basis for a new classification of carotid sinus hypersensitivity. J Intern Med. 2013;273(4):345–58.
24. Al-Khatib SM, LaPointe NMA, Kramer JM, Califf RM. What clinicians should know about the QT interval. JAMA. 2003;289(16):2120–7.
25. Incidence of Syncope During Pregnancy: Temporal Trends and Outcomes [Internet]. [cited 2020 Dec 11]. Available from: https://www.ahajournals.org/doi/epub/10.1161/JAHA.118.011608.
26. Steinberg JS, Varma N, Cygankiewicz I, Aziz P, Balsam P, Baranchuk A, et al. 2017 ISHNE-HRS expert consensus statement on ambulatory ECG and external cardiac monitoring/telemetry. Heart Rhythm. 2017;14(7):e55–96.
27. Gibson TC, Heitzman MR. Diagnostic efficacy of 24-hour electrocardiographic monitoring for syncope. Am J Cardiol. 1984;53(8):1013–7.
28. Bass EB, Curtiss EI, Arena VC, Hanusa BH, Cecchetti A, Karpf M, et al. The duration of holter monitoring in patients with syncope: is 24 hours enough? Arch Intern Med. 1990;150(5):1073–8.
29. Gula LJ, Krahn AD, Massel D, Skanes A, Yee R, Klein GJ. External loop recorders: determinants of diagnostic yield in patients with syncope. Am Heart J. 2004;147(4):644–8.
30. Linzer M, Pritchett ELC, Pontinen M, McCarthy E, Divine GW. Incremental diagnostic yield of loop electrocardiographic recorders in unexplained syncope. Am J Cardiol. 1990;66(2):214–9.
31. Joshi AK, Kowey PR, Prystowsky EN, Benditt DG, Cannom DS, Pratt CM, et al. First experience with a Mobile Cardiac Outpatient Telemetry (MCOT) system for the diagnosis and management of cardiac arrhythmia. Am J Cardiol. 2005;95(7):878–81.
32. Zimetbaum P, Goldman A. Ambulatory arrhythmia monitoring: choosing the right device. Circulation. 2010;122(16):1629–36.
33. Reed MJ, Grubb NR, Lang CC, Gray AJ, Simpson K, MacRaild A, et al. Diagnostic yield of an ambulatory patch monitor in patients with unexplained syncope after initial evaluation in the emergency department: the PATCH-ED study. Emerg Med J. 2018;35(8):477–85.

34. Validating QT-interval measurement using the Apple watch ECG to enable remote monitoring during the COVID-19 pandemic [Internet]. [cited 2020 Dec 11]. Available from: https://www.ahajournals.org/doi/epub/10.1161/CIRCULATIONAHA.120.048253.
35. Krahn AD, Klein GJ, Skanes AC, Yee R. Use of the implantable loop recorder in evaluation of patients with unexplained syncope. J Cardiovasc Electrophysiol. 2003;14(s9):S70–3.
36. Krahn AD, Klein GJ, Yee R, Mandab V. The high cost of syncope: cost implications of a new insertable loop recorder in the investigation of recurrent syncope. Am Heart J. 1999;137(5):870–7.
37. Recchia D, Barzilai B. Echocardiography in the evaluation of patients with syncope. J Gen Intern Med. 1995;10(12):649–55.
38. Flevari P, Leftheriotis D, Komborozos C, Fountoulaki K, Dagres N, Theodorakis G, et al. Recurrent vasovagal syncope: comparison between clomipramine and nitroglycerin as drug challenges during head-up tilt testing. Eur Heart J. 2009;30(18):2249–53.
39. Brignole M, Gianfranchi L, Menozzi C, Raviele A, Oddone D, Lolli G, et al. Role of autonomic reflexes in syncope associated with paroxysmal atrial fibrillation. J Am Coll Cardiol. 1993;22(4):1123–9.
40. Anderson LL, Dai D, Miller AL, Roe MT, Messenger JC, Wang TY. Percutaneous coronary intervention for older adults who present with syncope and coronary artery disease? Insights from the National Cardiovascular Data Registry. Am Heart J. 2016;176:1–9.
41. Lanier JB, Mote MB, Clay EC. Evaluation and management of orthostatic hypotension. AFP. 2011;84(5):527–36.
42. Low PA, Gilden JL, Freeman R, Sheng K-N, McElligott MA. Efficacy of midodrine vs placebo in neurogenic orthostatic hypotension: a randomized, double-blind multicenter study. JAMA. 1997;277(13):1046–51.
43. Sheldon R, Raj SR, Rose MS, Morillo CA, Krahn AD, Medina E, et al. Fludrocortisone for the prevention of vasovagal syncope: a randomized, placebo-controlled trial. J Am Coll Cardiol. 2016;68(1):1–9.
44. Wright RA, Kaufmann HC, Perera R, Opfer-Gehrking TL, McElligott MA, Sheng KN, et al. A double-blind, dose-response study of midodrine in neurogenic orthostatic hypotension. Neurology. 1998;51(1):120–4.
45. Biaggioni I, Arthur Hewitt L, Rowse GJ, Kaufmann H. Integrated analysis of droxidopa trials for neurogenic orthostatic hypoten-

sion. BMC Neurol [Internet]. 2017 May 12 [cited 2019 Oct 30];17. Available from: https://www.ncbi.nlm.nih.gov/pmc/articles/PMC5427571/.

46. Singer W, Sandroni P, Opfer-Gehrking TL, Suarez GA, Klein CM, Hines S, et al. Pyridostigmine treatment trial in neurogenic orthostatic hypotension. Arch Neurol. 2006;63(4):513–8.
47. Varosy PD, Chen LY, Miller AL, Noseworthy PA, Slotwiner DJ, Thiruganasambandamoorthy V. Pacing as a treatment for reflex-mediated (vasovagal, situational, or carotid sinus hypersensitivity) syncope: a systematic review for the 2017 ACC/AHA/HRS guideline for the evaluation and management of patients with syncope: a report of the American college of cardiology/American heart association task force on clinical practice guidelines and the heart rhythm society. J Am Coll Cardiol. 2017;70(5):664–79.

Chapter 5
The Cardiovascular Physical Exam

Roshan D. Modi, Christopher S. Massad, and B. Robinson Williams III

Abbreviations

bpm	Beats per minute
CE	Cardiac examination
CVP	Central venous pressure
DBP	Diastolic blood pressure
JVP	Jugular venous pressure
LVH	Left ventricular hypertrophy
PMI	Point of maximal impulse
SBP	Systolic blood pressure

R. D. Modi
Emory University School of Medicine, Atlanta, GA, USA
e-mail: roshan.modi@emory.edu

C. S. Massad (✉)
Department of Medicine, Emory University School of Medicine, Atlanta, GA, USA

B. Robinson Williams III
Department of Medicine, Division of Cardiology, Emory University School of Medicine, Atlanta, GA, USA
e-mail: brwilli@emory.edu

A. A. Bhargava et al. (eds.), *Handbook of Outpatient Cardiology*, https://doi.org/10.1007/978-3-030-88953-1_5

Vital Signs

Heart Rate

- The accurate measurement of resting heart rate is central to cardiac output and an important indicator of overall cardiac function.
- Resting heart rate for most individuals will be between 60 and 100 beats per minute (bpm), and an elevated resting heart rate is associated with increased risk of cardiovascular disease and mortality [1]. Commonly, athletes may have resting heart rates below 60 bpm.
- It is important to note that resting heart rates vary among patients based on their age, sex, physical conditioning, comorbid conditions, etc. For example, a well-trained athlete can have a normal resting heart of 45 bpm and be considered tachycardic at 90 bpm.

Blood Pressure

- The accurate measurement of systolic blood pressure (SBP) and diastolic blood pressure (DBP) is essential for diagnosis and management of hypertension. The 2017 ACC/AHA guidelines establish normal SBP and DBP as <120 mmHg and <80 mmHg, respectively, and hypertensive SBP and DBP as ≥140 mmHg and ≥90 mmHg, respectively [2].
- Measure blood pressure with the patient's unclothed arm at heart level. The patient's arm should either be resting on a table or supported at the fourth intercoastal space at the sternum with the bladder of the cuff centered over the brachial artery [1].
- Taking multiple averaged measurements will improve precision, particularly if using automated blood pressure devices [3]. Higher arm levels while recording will underestimate the blood pressure, while recording at lower lev-

els will overestimate. Blood pressure should be checked in both arms, and the higher reading should be recorded.

Jugular Venous Pressure

- Assessment of the jugular venous pressure (JVP) is a central component of the cardiovascular physical exam and provides an accurate estimation of central venous pressure (CVP) [4, 5]. Observation of changes in the JVP provides useful information about disorders that involve changes in volume status and/or cardiac function [1, 6].
- Clinically, a decreased JVP may indicate hypovolemia or decreased venous vascular tone, while an increased JVP may indicate heart failure [1, 7], pulmonary hypertension, tricuspid stenosis, AV dissociation, increased venous vascular tone, or pericardial compression or tamponade [1].
- To measure the JVP, elevate the exam table to 30–45° and turn the patient's head slightly to the left. The JVP is estimated to be the vertical distance between the highest point of the jugular vein pulsation and the center of the right atrium [1]. Working downwards from the earlobe, look for the highest point of pulsation of the jugular vein and measure the vertical distance from this point to the sternal angle as depicted in Fig. 5.1. The right atrium is an estimated 5 cm from the sternal angle which is added to this measured vertical distance to estimate the CVP in cm H_2O. A JVP measured at greater than 3 cm above the sternal angle, or more than 8 cm in total distance above the right atrium, is considered elevated [1].
- The elevation of the head of the bed or examining table may need to be adjusted depending on the patient's blood volume status. In hypovolemic individuals, the JVP will be lower than usual and the bed may need to be lowered to accurately observe the highest point of pulsation [1]. Conversely, in individuals with a high central venous pressure, the patient may need to be sitting upright to find the venous pulsation.

Clinical Pearl
Jugular vein pressure is directly related to the hemodynamics of the right atrium and a reflection of the pressures of the right side of the heart.

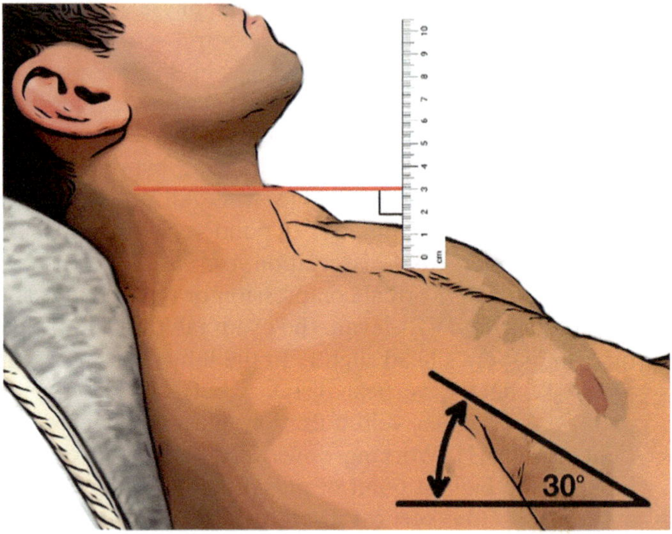

FIGURE 5.1 Illustration of JVP assessment by vertical measurement from sternal angle to highest jugular vein pulsation. Illustration depicts an elevation of 3 cm from sternal angle for a total of CVP estimation of 8 cm H_2O

Palpation

Pulses

- Palpation and assessment of the various pulses provide valuable information about cardiac activity including aortic valve disease, left ventricular function, pulmonary disease, and pericardial disease [1].

Point of Maximal Impulse

- The point of maximal impulse (PMI) represents pulsation of the left ventricle during contraction [1].
- To palpate the PMI, lay the patient supine and turn the patient on his or her left side [1]. It is particularly important to evaluate the location of the PMI, duration of the PMI in relation to the cardiac cycle, and the area in which the PMI can be felt [1, 8]. The PMI should be felt at the fifth intercostal space along the left mid-clavicular line. Any downward and lateral displacement is suggestive of left ventricular hypertrophy (LVH) or dilation.
- A PMI with a diameter greater than 4 cm significantly increases the likelihood of ventricular overload [8].
- To assess duration, simultaneously auscultate heart sounds while palpating the PMI.

Clinical Pearl
In conjunction with a displaced PMI, a sustained, high-amplitude impulse that lasts into the second heart sound also increases the likelihood of LVH [1, 8].

Carotid Pulse

- Palpation of the carotid pulse can provide valuable qualitative information regarding cardiac dynamic and arterial compliance [1, 9]. Complete assessment of the carotid pulse includes palpation and auscultation of the carotid arteries.
- Palpation of the carotid pulse is best measured with the patient sitting slightly reclined and palpating over the bifurcation or just proximal to the mandibular angle [1, 9].
- As a note of caution, especially in elderly patients, palpation or kneading of the carotids can produce a vagal response or release a plaque embolus.
- In general, a hyperkinetic or bounding carotid pulse indicates an increase in stroke volume as in fevers, exercise, anxiety, thyrotoxicosis, aortic regurgitation, or a large ventricular septal defect.
- A hypokinetic or weak carotid pulse is suggestive of a reduced stroke volume such as in hypovolemia, left ventricular failure, or mitral stenosis. In its extreme form, a weak and delayed arterial pulse in relation to the PMI, known as *pulsus parvus et tardus*, is characteristic of severe valvular aortic stenosis.

Pulsus Alternans

- Alternations in the force of an arterial pulse with regular rhythm indicate *pulsus alternans* – a sign of left ventricular dysfunction [1]. These alternations are typically best felt by applying light pressure on the radial or femoral arteries.
- A blood pressure cuff should be used to confirm the finding by lowering the pressure of the cuff slowly and listening for alternately loud and soft Korotkoff sounds, or a sudden doubling of the apparent heart rate [1].

Thrill

- With the palm placed flat over the precordium, palpate for thrills that last longer and feel different than the PMI, which signifies turbulence over a major cardiac defect.
- Though the presence of a thrill is not specific for a particular lesion, it does usually indicate a pathologic finding such as a ventricular septal defect or severe valvular regurgitation or stenosis.

Auscultation

- Proficiency in auscultation of both the heart and carotid arteries continues to be a critical component of cardiovascular disease diagnosis. It is important to identify the anatomical location of impulses, heart sounds, and murmurs and where they may fall in the cardiac cycle.

Carotid Arteries

- Auscultate each carotid artery to listen for bruits, murmur-like sounds that indicate turbulent blood flow [1, 10]. In order to accurately auscultate the carotid arteries, ask the patient to hold his or her breath while listening with the diaphragm of the stethoscope [1].
- The diaphragm should be placed near the upper end of the thyroid cartilage below the angle of the jaw, which overlies the carotid artery bifurcation into the internal and external carotid arteries [1]. More severe stenosis may have lower frequency sounds and thus require the bell to be used for auscultation [1, 11].
- Although auscultation is not sufficient to exclude stenosis [12], the detection of a bruit through physical exam can be used as a marker for total body atherosclerotic disease [13].

Heart Sounds

Where to Listen

- Auscultate the heart starting at the apex and moving to the base following the pattern illustrated in Fig. 5.2 [1]. Note the relative intensity of each valve at different anatomic locations.

How to Listen

- It is important to distinguish between the diaphragm and the bell of the stethoscope. The diaphragm is better for auscultating the high-pitched sounds of S1 and S2, murmurs of aortic and mitral regurgitation, and pericardial friction rubs [1]. The bell is more suited to the low-pitched S3 and S4 sounds as well as mitral stenosis murmurs [1]. Some modern stethoscopes do not have a bell but rather a

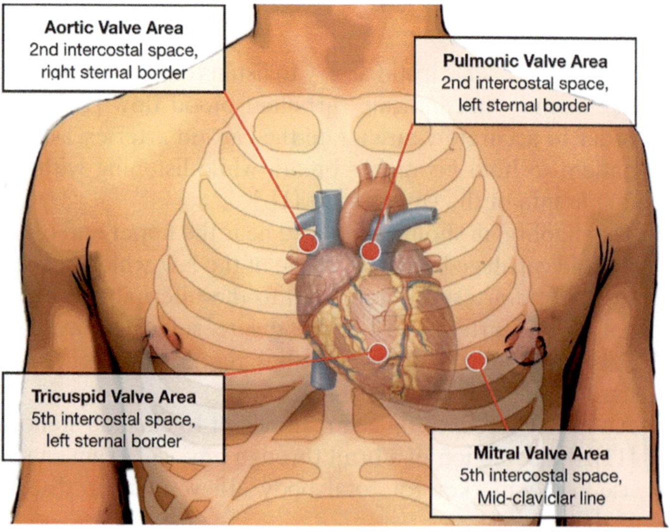

FIGURE 5.2 Optimal listening areas for auscultation of heart valves

pressure-sensitive diaphragm that functions as both a diaphragm and bell depending on the pressure applied [14].

Interpretation of Heart Sounds

- As the heart valves close, heart sounds can be heard across various areas of the chest wall. In patients with normal heart function, identification of the S1 and S2 sounds that mark the beginning and end of systole, respectively, is relatively easy.
- At normal heart rates, the diastolic interval between S2 and S1 should be longer than the systolic interval between S1 and S2 [1]. The S1 sound is typically louder than S2 at the apex of the heart, while the reverse is true at the base [1].
- Two extra sounds, S3 and S4, may occur during diastole and are usually pathologic in adults over the age of 40 [1]. The S3 sound, sometimes called an "S3 gallop," corresponds to an abrupt deceleration of ventricular filling through the mitral valve. The S4 sound corresponds to augmented ventricular filling as a result of atrial contraction into a noncompliant left ventricle [1, 9].
- Table 5.1 details possible causes for variations in the different heart sounds.

Interpretation of Murmurs

- Correctly interpreting heart murmurs requires a systematic approach in identifying timing, shape, radiation, intensity, pitch, and quality of the murmur.
- The shape of systolic, diastolic, and continuous murmurs and their likely causes is depicted in Table 5.2.
- Systolic murmurs are more common but not always pathologic. Differentiating between benign and pathologic murmurs can be challenging.

Table 5.1 Various heart sounds and their possible causes

Findings	Possible causes
Prominent S1	Mitral stenosis, increased cardiac output or contractility
Diminished S1	Mitral regurgitation, reduced left ventricular contractility, first-degree AV block
Prominent S2 (right second intercostal space)	Increased systemic vascular resistance, aortic root dilatation
Diminished S2 (right second intercostal space)	Static or calcified aortic valve
Prominent P2	Pulmonary hypertension, atrial septal defect, pulmonary artery dilatation
Diminished P2	Pulmonic stenosis
S3	Ventricular overload, as in congestive heart failure or mitral regurgitation Normal variant in children, young adults, and athletes
S4	Stiff ventricular wall from hypertensive heart disease, aortic stenosis, or hypertrophic cardiomyopathy
Systolic click	Mitral valve prolapse
Opening snap	Mitral stenosis
Physiologic split S2 – Widens with inspiration	Physiologic
Paradoxical Split S2 – Narrows with inspiration	Delayed closure of aortic valve from reduced contractility as in reduced ejection fraction, left bundle branch block, or severe aortic stenosis
Fixed split S2 – Does not vary with inspiration	Atrial septal defect (most likely), right bundle branch block, pulmonary valve stenosis
Wide split S2 – Varies with inspiration	Right bundle branch block, pulmonary valve stenosis

TABLE 5.2 List of possible causes for various murmur timing, shape, and pitch

	Likely causes
Mid-systolic 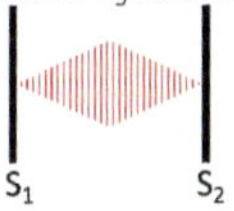	Benign flow murmurs from increased flow across a normal valve as in pregnancy, anemia, sepsis, etc. Aortic stenosis Aortic valve abnormalities (sclerosis, bicuspid, dilated aortic root) Hypertrophic cardiomyopathy Pulmonic stenosis
Pansystolic 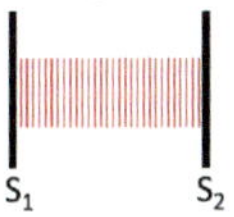	Mitral regurgitation Tricuspid regurgitation Ventricular septal defect
Late systolic 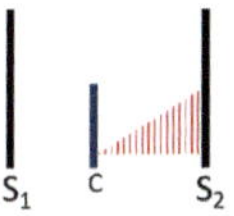	Mitral valve prolapse with a mid-systolic click (C)
Early diastolic 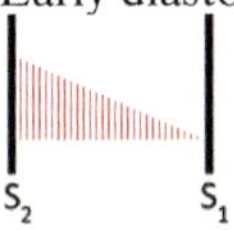	Aortic insufficiency
Mid-diastolic 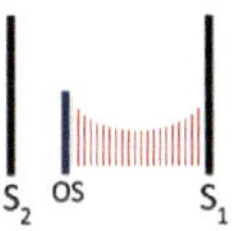	Mitral stenosis, possibly with an opening snap (OS)
Continuous 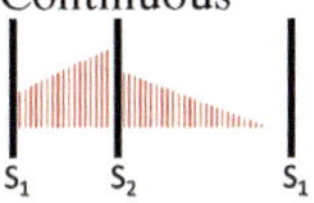	Patent ductus arteriosus (typically machine-like)
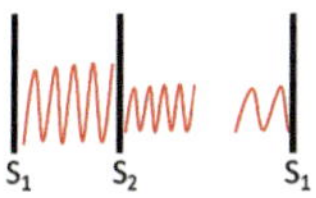	Pericardial friction rub, often with 1 to 3 distinct components

Clinical Pearl
Diastolic murmurs are less common and always pathologic.

Clinical Pearl
In general, a systolic murmur is more likely to be pathologic when [15] it is loud [16], it continues through most of systole [17], a thrill is present, or [18] it peaks in late systole (severe aortic stenosis or hypertrophic cardiomyopathy with obstruction). Table 5.2 depicts the shape and likely causes of various murmurs.

Clinical Pearls
- Jugular vein pressure is directly related to the hemodynamics of the right atrium and a reflection of the pressures of the right side of the heart.
- In conjunction with a displaced PMI, a sustained, high-amplitude impulse that lasts into the second heart sound also increases the likelihood of LVH [1, 8].
- Diastolic murmurs are less common and always pathologic.
- In general, a systolic murmur is more likely to be pathologic when [15] it is loud, [16] it continues through most of systole, [17] a thrill is present, or [18] it peaks in late systole (severe aortic stenosis or hypertrophic cardiomyopathy with obstruction). Table 5.2 depicts the shape and likely causes of various murmurs.

Key Learning Points

- It is important to consider a patient's age, comorbidities, and functional capacity during an exam. For example, a heart rate of 90 bpm in a young marathon runner may be abnormally high but normal in a middle-aged female. Similarly, a patient with tricuspid regurgitation may have a chronically elevated JVP without elevated right-sided pressures.
- Auscultating heart sounds is but one component of the cardiovascular exam. Vitals signs; JVP assessment; and palpation of central pulses, peripheral pulses, and PMI can provide in-depth information on the cardiovascular system.
- Correctly diagnosing murmurs via auscultation and palpation can be difficult. It is more important to know when a murmur may be pathologic and requires further evaluation rather than correctly diagnosing a murmur.

References

1. Bickley LS, Szilagyi PG, Hoffman RM. Bates' guide to physical examination and history taking. 2017.
2. Muntner P, Shimbo D, Carey RM, et al. Measurement of blood pressure in humans: a scientific statement from the american heart association. Hypertension. 2019;73(5):e35–66.
3. Powers BJ, Olsen MK, Smith VA, Woolson RF, Bosworth HB, Oddone EZ. Measuring blood pressure for decision making and quality reporting: where and how many measures? Ann Intern Med. 2011;154(12):781–8, w-289-790.
4. Rizkallah J, Jack M, Mahwash S, Shafer LA, Vo M, Tam J. Non-invasive bedside assessment of central venous pressure: scanning into the future. PLoS One. 2014;9(10):e109215.
5. Devine PJ, Sullenberger LE, Bellin DA, Atwood JE. Jugular venous pulse: window into the right heart. South Med J. 2007;100(10):1022–7. quiz 1004

6. Conn RD, O'Keefe JH. Simplified evaluation of the jugular venous pressure: significance of inspiratory collapse of jugular veins. Mo Med. 2012;109(2):150–2.
7. Drazner MHMD, Rame JEMDM, Stevenson LWMD, Dries DLMDMPH. Prognostic importance of elevated jugular venous pressure and a third heart sound in patients with heart failure. N Engl J Med. 2001;345(8):574–81.
8. Logar HBZ, Medvescek NR, Rakovec P. Standardization of the apex beat in the full left lateral position and its diagnostic value in detecting left ventricular dilatation. Acta Cardiol. 2011;66(4):459–64.
9. Michaels AD, Khan FU, Moyers B. Experienced clinicians improve detection of third and fourth heart sounds by viewing acoustic cardiography. Clin Cardiol. 2010;33(3):E36–42.
10. Grossberg JAMD, Potter NSMDP, Jayaraman MVMD. Asymptomatic carotid stenosis: screening and management. Med Health Rhode Island. 2011;94(4):89–91.
11. Sandercock PAG, Kavvadia E. The carotid bruit. Pract Neurol. 2002;2(4):221.
12. Ratchford EV, Jin Z, Di Tullio MR, et al. Carotid bruit for detection of hemodynamically significant carotid stenosis: the northern Manhattan study. Neurol Res. 2009;31(7):748–52.
13. Pickett CA, Jackson JL, Hemann BA, Atwood JE. Carotid bruits as a prognostic indicator of cardiovascular death and myocardial infarction: a meta-analysis. Lancet. 2008;371(9624):1587–94.
14. Irwin. Cardiopulmonary physical therapy. 4th ed. Mosby; 2004.
15. Elder A, Japp A, Verghese A. How valuable is physical examination of the cardiovascular system? BMJ. 2016;354:i3309.
16. Vukanovic-Criley JM, Criley S, Warde CM, et al. Competency in cardiac examination skills in medical students, trainees, physicians, and faculty: a multicenter study. Arch Intern Med. 2006;166(6):610–6.
17. Mangione S, Nieman LZ. Cardiac auscultatory skills of internal medicine and family practice trainees: a comparison of diagnostic proficiency. JAMA. 1997;278(9):717–22.
18. Vukanovic-Criley JM, Hovanesyan A, Criley SR, et al. Confidential testing of cardiac examination competency in cardiology and noncardiology faculty and trainees: a multicenter study. Clin Cardiol. 2010;33(12):738–45.

Part II
Imaging and Noninvasive Testing

Chapter 6
ECG Interpretation

Arielle M. Schwartz and Nanette K. Wenger

Abbreviations

AV	Atrioventricular
BBB	Bundle branch block
CAD	Coronary artery disease
LAD	Left axis deviation
LVH	Left ventricular hypertrophy
RAD	Right axis deviation
RCA	Right coronary artery
RVH	Right ventricular hypertrophy
SA	Sinoatrial

A. M. Schwartz (✉)
Department of Medicine, Emory University School of Medicine, Atlanta, GA, USA
e-mail: amschw2@emory.edu

N. K. Wenger
Department of Medicine, Division of Cardiology, Emory University School of Medicine, Atlanta, GA, USA
e-mail: nwenger@emory.edu

A. A. Bhargava et al. (eds.), *Handbook of Outpatient Cardiology*, https://doi.org/10.1007/978-3-030-88953-1_6

Standard Approach to ECG Assessment

Rate

- Heart rate (HR) = (Total # QRS complexes on 10-second ECG) × 6.
- For regular rhythms, follow the 300–150–100-75-60-50 rule (see Fig. 6.1).

Rhythm

- Consider if the rhythm is regular or irregular.
- If the rhythm is a narrow complex (<100 ms), the conduction originates from above or within the AV node.
- A broad complex (>100 ms) may either indicate the conduction is originating within the ventricle, or there may be a supraventricular conduction with aberrancy (Fig. 6.2).

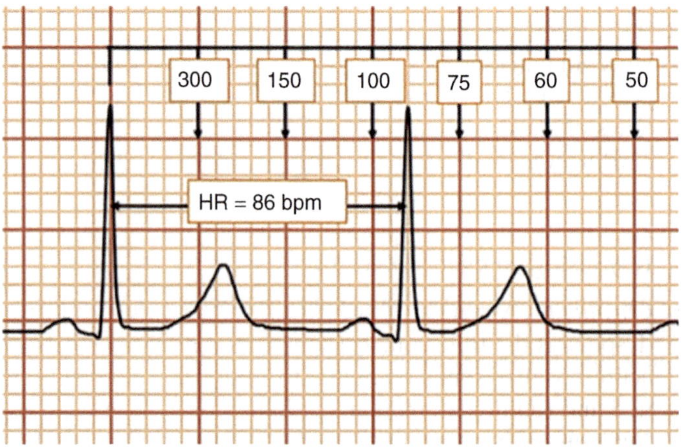

Figure 6.1 Large box method to assess heart rate. (Adapted with permission from the Emory University School of Medicine Cardiology elective lecture series)

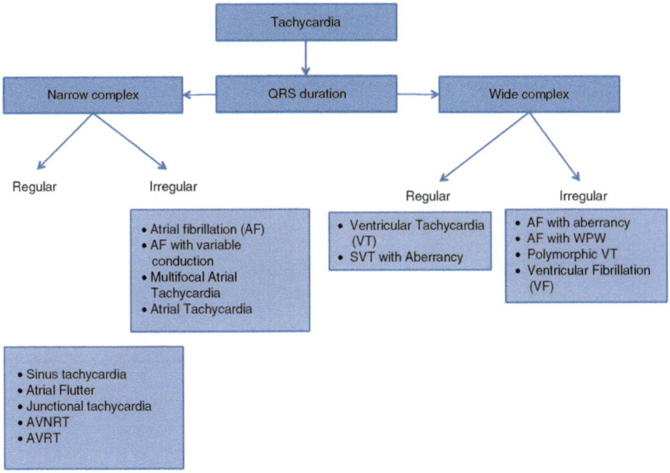

FIGURE 6.2 Differential diagnosis algorithm of tachycardia. (Adapted with permission from the Emory University School of Medicine Cardiology elective lecture series)

Axis

- Represents the cumulative electrical vector within the cardiovascular conduction system.
- A normal QRS axis is between –30° and + 90°.
- Left axis deviation (LAD) indicates the QRS axis falls between –30° and –90°.
- Right axis deviation (RAD) indicates the QRS axis falls between +90° and 180° (Fig. 6.3).

Clinical Pearl

A QRS that is positive in lead I and positive in lead aVF indicates a normal axis (0–90°). A QRS positive in lead I and negative in lead aVF has an axis between 0 and 90° and may indicate LAD (–30° to –90°). A QRS negative in lead I and positive in aVF indicates RAD (+90° to 180°).

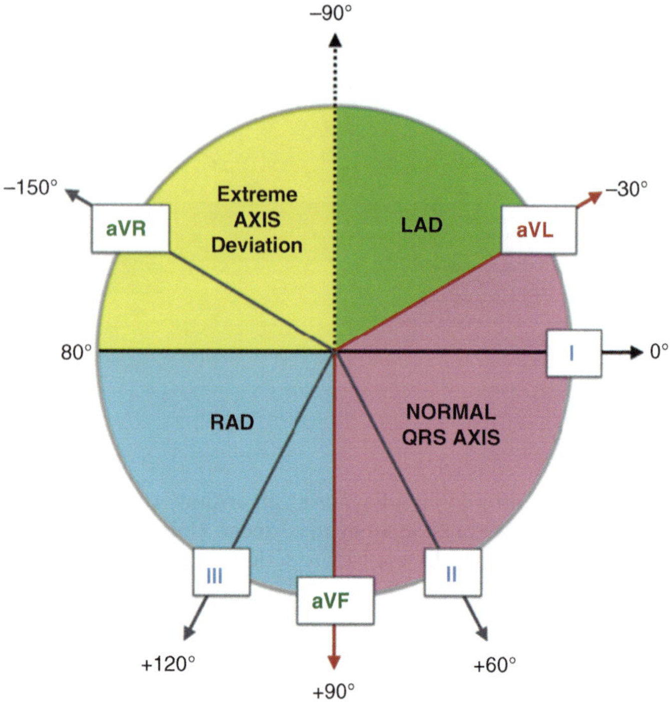

Figure 6.3 ECG axis interpretation. (Adapted with permission from the Emory University School of Medicine Cardiology elective lecture series)

P-Waves and Atrial Abnormalities

	Vector	V1	II	Criteria/findings
Normal	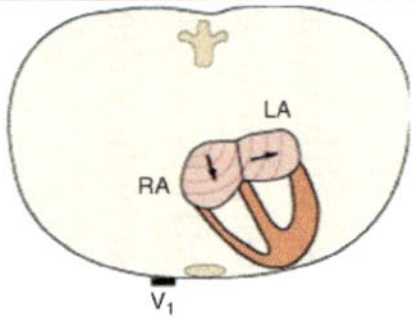	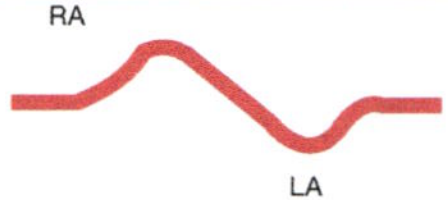	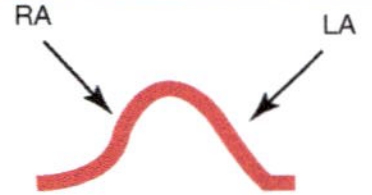	*Amplitude:* <2.5 mm in limb leads <1.5 mm in precordial leads *Duration:* <120 ms *Axis:* 45–60°
Right atrial abnormality	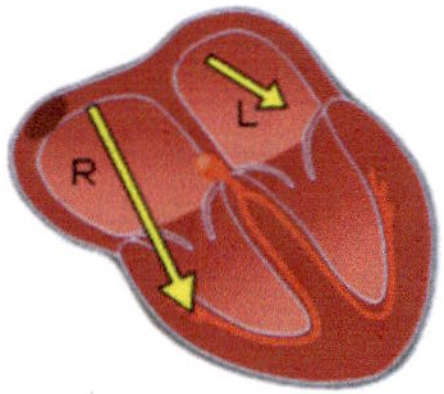	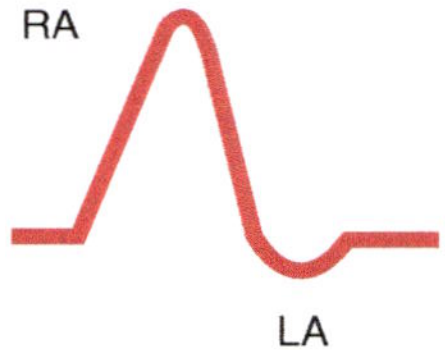	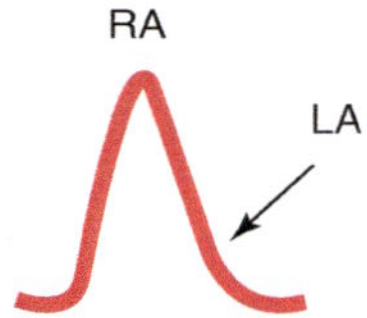	Amplitude of >2.5 mm in II Or Initial positive deflection in V1 > 1.5 mm in amplitude
Left atrial abnormality	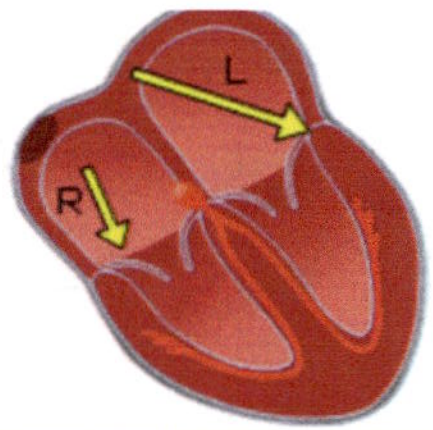	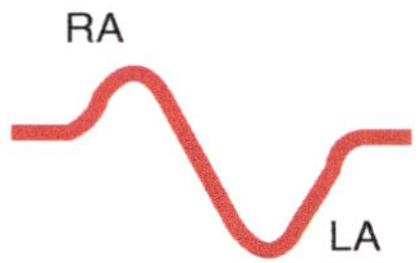	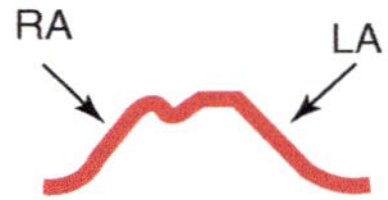	Duration ≥120 ms Negative wave in V1 with duration >40 ms and amplitude >1 mm deep

- The P-wave describes atrial depolarization, which is initiated in the sinoatrial (SA) node, located in upper the right atrium near the superior vena cava.
- Depolarization occurs initially in the right atrium, followed by the left atrium.
- Normal P-waves have characteristic axis, contour, amplitude, and duration. Variance of these characteristics may indicate specific atrial abnormalities, which may be caused by enlargement, hypertrophy, blocks, or repolarization abnormalities.

Clinical Pearl
A long P-wave indicates LAE, whereas a tall P-wave indicates RAE.

Atrioventricular Block

- Atrioventricular (AV) block refers to the disruption of the impulse from the SA node to the ventricles, which can occur due to conduction cells that are refractory or from tissue that is unable to conduct because of fibrosis or scarring.
- AV block is characterized by first degree, second degree (Mobitz I or Mobitz II), or third degree based on the anatomical site and functional characteristics and can be distinguished by ECG findings.
- There are a variety of etiologies of AV block, with ischemic disease underlying about 40% of all cases. Most commonly, an inferior myocardial infarction (MI) is responsible since the right coronary artery (RCA) supplies the AV node in 90% of the population.
- Second-degree Mobitz I is usually asymptomatic. Mobitz II involves failure of the AV node to conduct the impulse from the atria to the ventricles and is a sign of severe conduction system disease involving the His-Purkinje system. This often progresses to complete heart block.

AV block	Diagnostic criteria	EKG
1st degree	PR interval >0.20 seconds All impulses are conducted (QRS after every P)	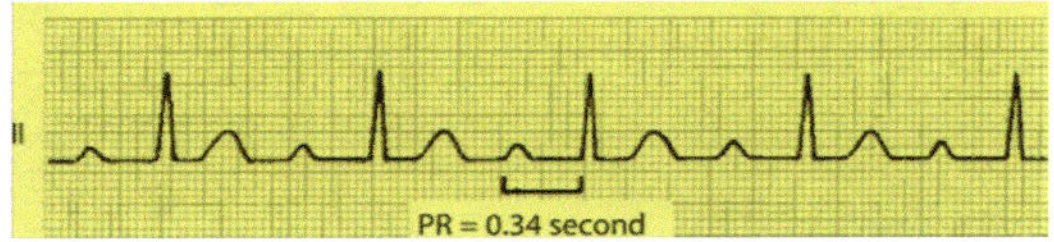
2nd degree Mobitz I/ Wenckebach	Progressive PR prolongation followed by non-conducted P-wave PR is longest in beat before dropped beat and shortest in the first beat of cycle	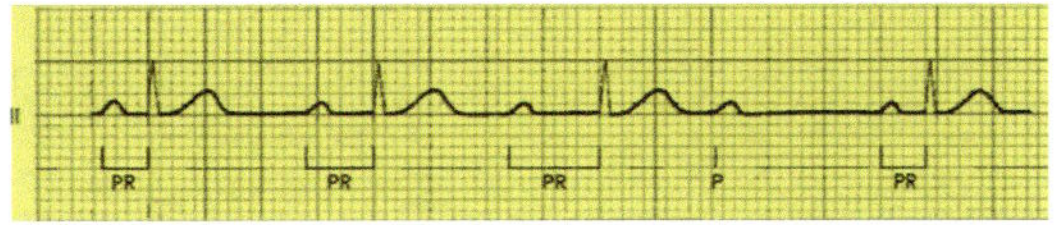
2nd degree Mobitz II	Sudden appearance of a single, non-conducted sinus P-wave without prolongation of PR interval or shortening of PR interval in the beat after non-conducted P	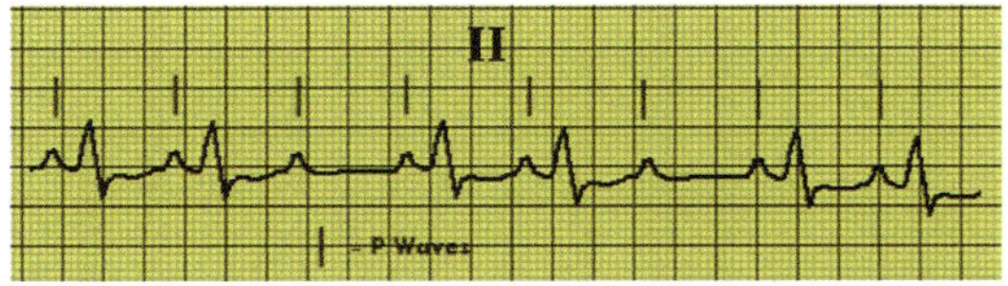
3rd degree	P-waves present with regular atrial rate faster than ventricular rate. If a junctional focus is present, QRS complexes are narrow. With a ventricular focus, QRS is wide and the ventricular rate is slower No correlation between P and QRS	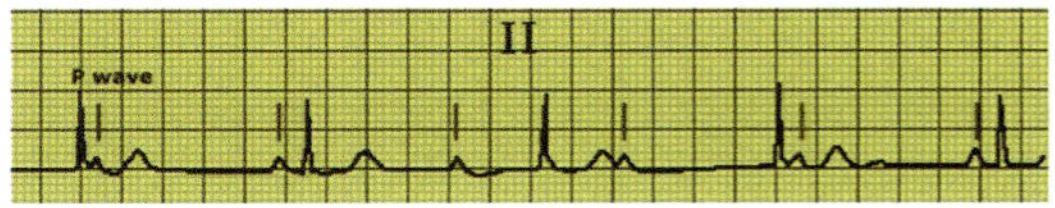

Clinical Pearl
First-degree AV block and second-degree AV block Mobitz I, also known as Wenckebach phenomenon, do not typically require therapeutic pacing, whereas second-degree AV block Mobitz II and third-degree AV block usually require therapeutic pacing.

Bundle Branch Block (BBB)

- BBBs occur when there is an injury to a branch of the His-Purkinje system, resulting in impaired electrical conduction with slowed propagation of impulses and resulting ventricular dyssynchrony.
- BBBs can be clinically significant if they lead to a substantial decrease in cardiac output, which may warrant cardiac resynchronization therapy (CRT).

	Vector	ECG features	ECG
RBBB	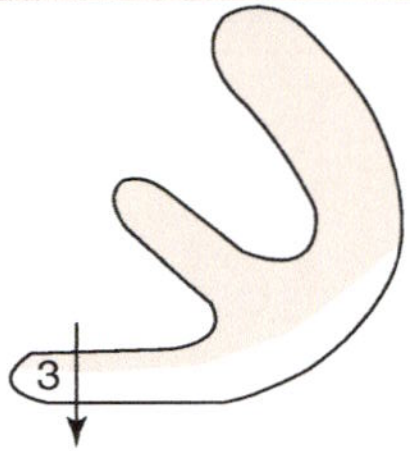	Broad QRS ≥120 ms RSR' pattern in V1–V3 (M-shaped QRS complex) Wide, slurred S wave in the lateral leads (I, aVL, V5–6)	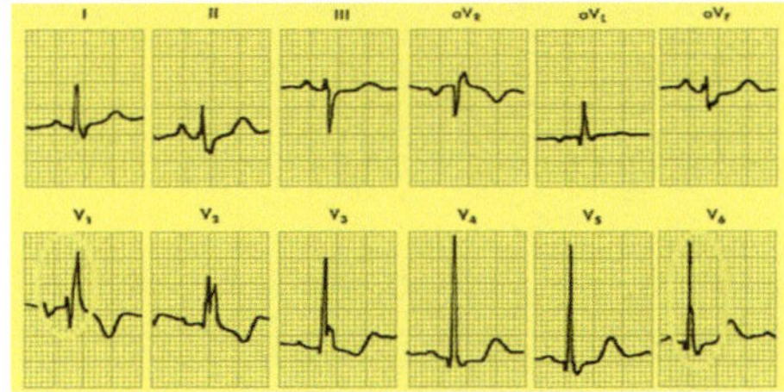
LBBB	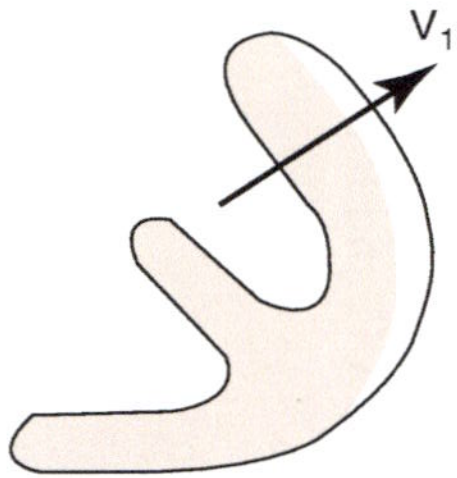	Broad QRS ≥120 ms Dominant S wave in V1 Broad monophasic R wave in lateral leads (I, aVL, V5–V6) Absence of Q waves in lateral leads (small Qs allowed in aVL) Prolonged R wave peak time >60 ms in left precordial leads	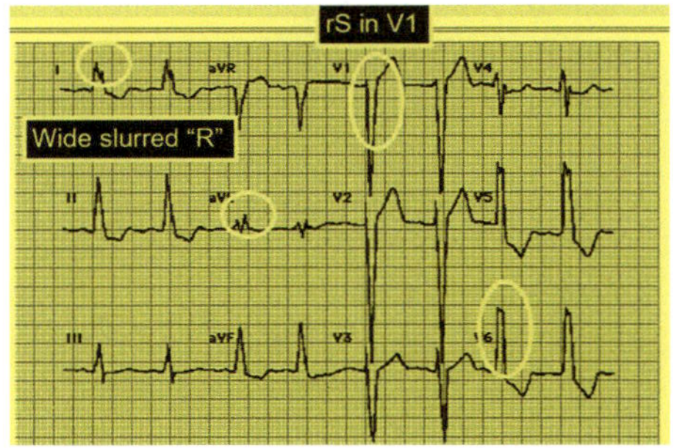

Clinical Pearl
Right bundle branch block (RBBB) can occur as a normal variant with incidence increasing with age, but the most common cause is coronary artery disease (CAD). It can also occur in any condition causing RV dilation or hypertrophy. Left bundle branch block (LBBB) is almost always associated with underlying cardiac disease such as CAD, hypertension, conduction disease, and/or cardiomyopathy.

Ventricular Hypertrophy

- ECG criteria for ventricular hypertrophy are not sensitive, however fairly specific.
- Left ventricular hypertrophy (LVH) is an independent risk factor for sudden cardiac death (SCD), acute myocardial infarction, and overall CV morbidity and mortality.
- Ventricular hypertrophy results in two main changes on ECG: increase in amplitude due to the ventricles generating more current and voltage and a shift in axis due to the total electrical current moving through a thickened wall.
- LVH can be diagnosed using a number of different ECG diagnostic criteria with varying sensitivities and specificities. These details will not be described here for the sake of simplicity.
- Here we review ECG findings typically observed in patients with LVH and RVH.

	Image	Suggestive ECG findings	ECG
Normal	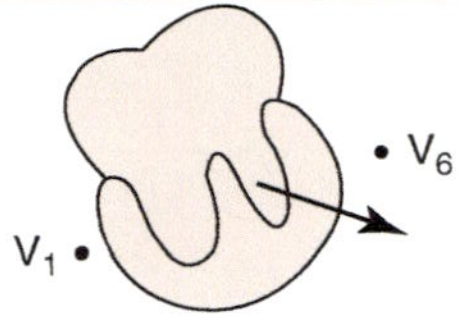	R waves become taller, while S waves become smaller from V1 to V6 ST segments are isoelectric and may slant upward to the T and are not depressed T waves in same direction as QRS and upright in V2–V6	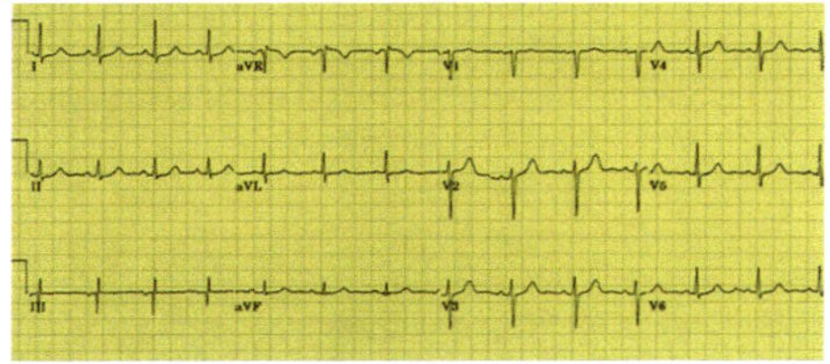
LVH	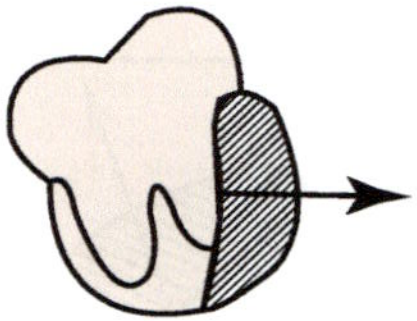	Large R waves in left and posterior leads (I, aVL, V5, V6) Large S waves in right and anterior leads (V1, V2) ST and T wave abnormalities, esp. in I, aVL, V5, V6 LA abnormality	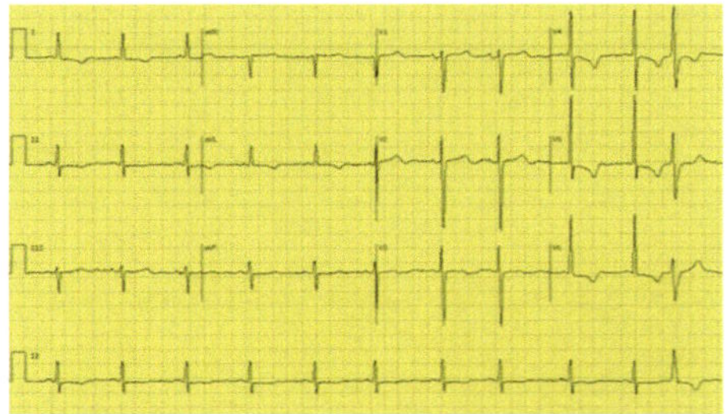

	Image	Suggestive ECG findings	ECG
RVH	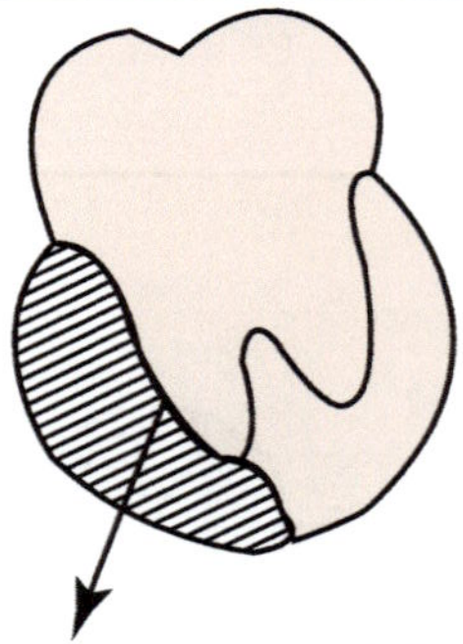	Large R waves in right and anterior leads (V1, V2, aVR) Deep S waves, small R waves in left leads (V5, V6, I, aVL) Right axis deviation T wave inversion in right to mid-precordial leads Right atrial abnormality RBBB	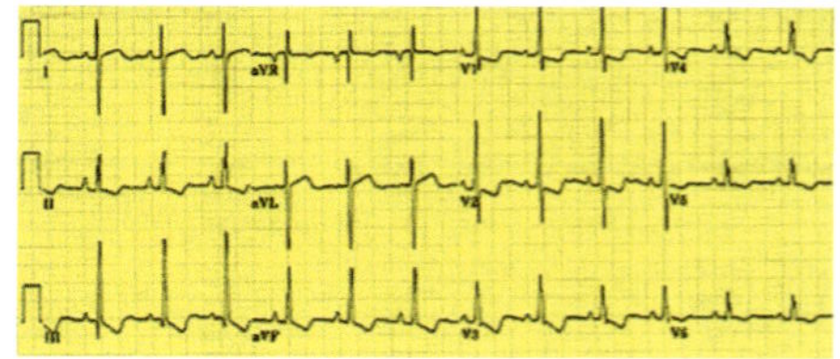

Key Learning Points

- The approach to the ECG assessment should include evaluation of rate, rhythm, and axis, intervals, chamber enlargement, and relationship between atrial rates and ventricular rates.
- Atrial enlargement, atrioventricular blocks, bundle branch blocks, and ventricular hypertrophy have characteristic ECG findings as outlined above.

Chapter 7
Stress Testing (Treadmill, Echocardiography, SPECT, PET, and Cardiac MR)

Talal Khalid Al-Otaibi and Thomas H. Hauser

Abbreviations

ABI	Ankle–brachial pressure index
ARVC	Arrhythmogenic right ventricular cardiomyopathy
AVB	Atrioventricular block
CAD	Coronary artery disease
DTS	Duke Treadmill Prognostic Score
ECG	Electrocardiogram
EGE	Early gadolinium enhancement
EIBBB	Exercise induced bundle branch block
EMB	Endomyocardial biopsy
HR	Heart rate
HRR	Heart rate recovery
LBBB	Left bundle branch block
LGE	Late gadolinium enhancement

T. K. Al-Otaibi (✉) · T. H. Hauser
Department of Medicine, Division of Cardiology, Beth Israel Deaconess Medical Center, Harvard Medical School, Boston, MA, USA
e-mail: talotaib@bidmc.harvard.edu; thauser@bidmc.harvard.edu

A. A. Bhargava et al. (eds.), *Handbook of Outpatient Cardiology*, https://doi.org/10.1007/978-3-030-88953-1_7

LVEF	Left ventricular ejection fraction
LVH	Left ventricular hypertrophy
MET	Metabolic equivalent of task
MI	Myocardial infarction
PAD	Peripheral arterial disease
Qp/Qs	Pulmonary-to-systemic shunt ratio
RV	Right ventricular
SBP	Systolic blood pressure
SE	Stress echocardiography
SSFP	Steady-state free precession
V-paced	Ventricular paced rhythm
WMA	Wall motion abnormality
WPW	Wolf Parkinson White syndrome

Stress Test

A stress test is performed using either standardized exercise protocols or a pharmacological agent.

1. Exercise Stress Test.

   Preferred if patient can reach an acceptable workload (85% of predicted maximum HR) achieved by treadmill, stationary cycle, or arm ergometry if patient unable to walk.

2. Pharmacologic Stress Test (see Table 7.1).

   - Use if unable to exercise or unable to reach goal HR.

Table 7.1 Type of pharmacological stress

Pharmacological stress	
Coronary vasodilator	Induces coronary vasodilation. Diseased vessels do not dilate causing coronary flow heterogeneity (rarely causes ischemia due to coronary steal). Agents available: adenosine, dipyridamole (increases circulating adenosine), or regadenoson (selective adenosine A2A receptor agonist)
Chronotropes/ inotropes	Dobutamine increases heart rate and myocardial demand which is more physiologic but arrhythmogenic

- Similar sensitivity and specificity to exercise stress testing but without the hemodynamic or symptomatic information.
- Preferred in LBBB or V-paced due to false-positive exercise imaging (artifactual septal perfusion defect).

Indications/Contraindications

Stress testing is indicated to either establish a diagnosis (e.g., intermediate pretest probability of CAD) or identify prognosis (e.g., known CAD) (see Table 7.2).

Table 7.2 Summary of indications/contraindications of exercise stress test

Indications	**Contraindications**
Coronary artery disease	*Absolute*
Symptomatic with chest pain (or anginal equivalent) and intermediate likelihood of obstructive CAD, management of stable CAD, following myocardial infarction, limited usefulness in patients who are post-PCI	Acute myocardial infarction (within 48 hours) High-risk unstable angina Uncontrolled arrhythmia with hemodynamic compromise
Peripheral arterial disease	
Assessment of questionable PAD, functional assessment in known PAD, evaluation post-surgical or endovascular revascularization procedures	Active endocarditis Symptomatic severe aortic stenosis Decompensated heart failure
Valvular heart disease	
Assessing functional capacity in patients with valvular heart disease	Acute pulmonary embolism Acute myocarditis or pericarditis Acute aortic dissection

(continued)

TABLE 7.2 (continued)

Indications	Contraindications
Hypertrophic cardiomyopathy	*Relative*
Risk stratification and functional assessment	Known left main coronary artery stenosis
Heart rhythm disorders	Hypertrophic cardiomyopathy with a severe resting gradient
Evaluation of exercise-induced arrhythmias, evaluation of medical or ablative therapy, chronotropic response	Severe hypertension >200/100 mmHg
Adult congenital heart disease	High-grade AV block
Functional assessment of congenital heart disease associated with pulmonary hypertension	

Assessment of Coronary Artery Disease

- Sensitivity of 68% and specificity of 77% in the general population. Exercise test has a higher sensitivity with LMCA or triple-vessel disease than in those with single-vessel disease.
- Exercise capacity is the most important prognostic variable; patients able to perform >10 METs are at low risk for cardiovascular events.

Hemodynamic Response

- *Maximum Heart Rate*: an adequate study is defined by achieving 85% of the age-predicted maximum heart rate [predicted maximum HR = 220 – age; for patients with coronary artery disease (CAD) on BB predicted maximum HR = 164 – (0.7× age)]. It is important to identifying the level of workload at which symptoms appear [7].
- *Systolic Blood Pressure:*
  - *Exaggerated SBP Response:* SBP >210 mmHg in men and >190 mmHg in women during exercise. It is indicative of the future development of hypertension in normotensive patients [2].

- *Exercise-Induced Hypotension:* SBP falls below resting systolic pressure during exercise. This is a poor prognostic indicator and suggests severe multivessel CAD with left ventricular dysfunction. This is also seen in patients with cardiomyopathy, left ventricular outflow tract obstruction, enhanced vagal tone, hypovolemia, antihypertensive medications, and arrhythmias.

- *Heart Rate Recovery HRR*: Normal recovery is defined as decrease of >12 beats/min after 1 minute with post-exercise cool down or >18 beats/min after 1 minute with immediate cessation of movement. HRR of 12 beats or less predicts an increased relative risk of sudden cardiac death and all-cause mortality independent of CAD severity [1].

Electrocardiographic Responses

- ST-segment evaluated 80 ms after the J point.
- ST depression does not localize ischemia, whereas ST-segment elevation localizes to the vascular region (STE elevation in AVR associated with LMC/ostial LAD stenosis, lead V5 is the most sensitive) [5].
- *Downsloping* or *horizontal* ST depression (≥1 mm) predictive of CAD, whereas upsloping ST depression is less specific.
- Presence of ventricular ectopy during exercise recovery is an indicator of worse prognosis [4].
- Exercise-induced BBB (EIBBB) may suggest CAD (especially at HR <125 bpm) or conduction disease. ST-segment changes before onset of the EIBBB are still interpretable [3].

Multivariable Score

- Duke Treadmill Prognostic Score DTS (see Table 7.3):
  - DTS = Exercise time − (5 × ST deviation [mm]) − (4 × Angina index [0 for no chest pain, 1 for chest pain, 2 for chest pain that stops the test]).
  - Does not include clinical variables (age, HR, etc.)

- Cleveland Clinic Prognostic Score:
  - Includes most clinical and exercise prognostic variables.

Table 7.3 DUKE treadmill score

DTS	One-year mortality
≤−11	5.0%
Between +4 and − 10	1.25%
≥ + 5	0.25%

Assessment of Peripheral Arterial Disease (PAD)

Evaluate functional limitations caused by PAD and the response to therapy.

Post-exercise ankle brachial index (ABI): will show a decrease in ABI (greater than a 5% drop in post-exercise ABI from resting levels) and also a prolonged recovery time in patients with PAD [9].

Exercise Stress Testing in Women

Exercise stress testing without imaging is less sensitive and specific in women while still providing valuable information in evaluating symptomatic patients [6].

Clinical Pearl

Beta-blockers may be held for modalities that rely on chronotropic response for diagnosis, such as in exercise or dobutamine stress. Beta-blockers should not be held in patients with known CAD when attempting to assess the quality of medical management.

Stress Echocardiography (SE)

- Negative SE test has a low annual risk of subsequent events <1% (exercise) or <2% (dobutamine), whereas a positive study has a 10–30% 1-year event rate of MI, PCI, CABG, or death [10].
- For patients undergoing major noncardiac surgery, a negative dobutamine SE is associated with a high negative predictive value of death and MI (Table 7.4).

Table 7.4 Different myocardial response to stress

	Response to stress
Normal	Hyperdynamic/normal wall motion
Ischemia	Deterioration of segmental wall motion or thickening
Viable (hibernation)	Wall motion abnormality with rest, improvement of segmental wall motion
Scar	Wall motion abnormality at rest, no change or worsening in segmental wall motion

Evaluation of CAD

- Typically performed with exercise or dobutamine stress.
- For SE, a new or worsening wall motion abnormality (WMA) during peak stress is indicative of ischemia.
- SE has sensitivity of 75–87% and specificity of 74–80% in detecting CAD.

Viability Assessment

- Viable myocardium is defined as an increase in wall thickening (≥2 segments) with low-dose dobutamine (5 μg/kg/min).
- Viable segments may show a biphasic response (improvement at low dose and then worsening at high dose) due to ischemia with higher dose of dobutamine [11].

Nuclear Cardiology

Indications/Contraindications (See Table 7.5)

Causes of a False-Positive Study

- Attenuation (breast, diaphragmatic)
- Coronary vasospasm

TABLE 7.5 Summary of indications/contraindications of nuclear stress test

Indications	Contraindications
Diagnosis of CAD Sensitivity 73–92%, specificity 63–88%, PET has increased accuracy [13]. In general, best used to evaluate patients at intermediate risk for CAD **Risk assessment** [15] Stratify risk in patient with chest pain – reversible defect indicates ischemia; fixed defect suggests scar Predictor of subsequent infarction or death. Normal findings suggest a yearly mortality <1% (in normal left ventricular ejection fraction (LVEF)), extended "warranty period" indicating low risk for several years Undergoing noncardiac operation [18] **Identification of prior myocardial infarction (MI)** [16] **Assessment of LV function** First pass radionuclide angiocardiography, useful in evaluating right ventricular function MUGA, used less b/c of echocardiography and CMR **Assessment for ischemia/viability?** [17] Eligible for revascularization	**Contraindication to stress** See Table 7.2 **Contraindication to nuclear study** I131 therapy within 12 weeks Tc99m study within 48 hours (bone, lung, MUGA, renal, tagged RBC, liver) **Contraindication to dipyridamole, adenosine, or regadenoson** Allergy Theophylline therapy within 36 hours Uncontrolled asthma Significant AV block, bradycardia, or hypotension Caffeine within 12–24 hours Acute myocardial infarction (within 48 hours)

- Anomalous coronary circulation
- Cardiomyopathy
- Conduction defect (e.g., LBBB)

Causes of a False-Negative Study

- Submaximal exercise stress
- Anti-ischemia medications
- Collateral circulation
- Balanced ischemia

Clinical Pearl
Perfusion defects for patients with left main or multivessel disease may be absent in the setting of balanced ischemia. Important signs for the presence of left main or multivessel CAD include transit ischemic dilation (TID) of the left ventricle, reversible right ventricular uptake, and/or a decline in the LVEF after stress.

Cardiac MRI

MRI provides:

- High spatial resolution images
- Quantitative assessment of ventricular function
- Myocardial viability assessment
- Quantification of intra- and extracardiac shunts
- Measurements of valvular velocities and gradients
- Contrast-enhanced angiography without the use of ionizing radiation

Clinical applications of cardiac MRI are summarized in Table 7.6.

Clinical Pearl
Avoid gadolinium when there is impaired renal function (eGFR <30) to avoid nephrogenic systemic fibrosis.

TABLE 7.6 Common clinical applications of cardiac MRI

Coronary artery disease
Myocardial infarction: Assess ventricular function, late gadolinium enhancement (LGE) for myocardial infarction-induced fibrosis, infarct size, and complications from MI
Assessment of myocardial viability: Dobutamine-induced systolic wall thickening; the presence and extent of LGE involvement (<50% transmurality cutoff for viability) can be used to predict contractile recovery
Myocardial ischemia [20]: Stress CMR imaging is performed using pharmacologic agents; a negative CMR MPI predicts an annualized cardiac event rate of less than 1% [19]. Compared to SPECT it is not limited by attenuation artifacts, has no radiation, takes a shorter time, and has higher spatial resolution

Table 7.6 (continued)

Cardiomyopathy [16]
Hypertrophic cardiomyopathy [21]: Detection of LVH where a max wall thickness (>30 mm) is specific for SCD. Presence and quantification of LGE, systolic anterior motion (SAM) of the mitral valve, and apical aneurysms *Arrhythmogenic right ventricular cardiomyopathy (ARVC)* [22]: Assessment of RV size and function, myocardial fibrofatty infiltration, localized aneurysms. CMR has been shown to have a sensitivity of 96% and a specificity of 78% in detecting ARVC *Myocarditis* [23]: Assessed using the Modified Lake Louise Criteria, CMR assessment of T2-weighted imaging for myocardial edema, and LGE imaging for myocardial fibrosis (usually subepicardium and midmyocardium of the inferolateral walls). T2 mapping showed the most benefit in patients with chronic symptoms *Cardiac sarcoidosis* [24]: Assess ventricular function and LGE for scar/fibrosis (usually patchy involvement), presence of LGE has been associated with major arrhythmias and death, and guide endomyocardial biopsy (EMB) (particularly if septal LGE noted). Higher sensitivity in identifying cardiac sarcoidosis than the modified Japanese Ministry of Health guidelines *Cardiac amyloidosis:* Assess LV systolic function, presence of concentric increase in LV wall thickness, diffuse LGE of the LV (may involve the RV), and the amount of LGE has been associated with mortality *Other cardiomyopathies: Iron overload cardiomyopathy*, preserved systolic LV function in most cases, T2* technique for quantifying myocardial iron deposition (myocardial T2* <10 ms has highest risk of heart failure within 1 year). *Left ventricular noncompaction* [25], measuring diastolic noncompacted-to-compacted thickness ratio of >2.3, has been used to diagnose LV noncompaction

(continued)

Table 7.6 (continued)

Valvular heart disease [26]
In aortic valve disease, CMR can measure the aortic valve area by direct planimetry of the valve orifice. CMR phase-contrast imaging is used to quantify the regurgitant volume which is more reproducible than echocardiography [27]
Pericardial disease
Assessment of pericardial thickness (increased thickness with pericardial constriction), LGE imaging to assess for pericardial involvement → if present suggests active inflammation or pericardial fibrosis. Real-time cine *steady-state free precession* (SSFP) for the detection of cardiac constriction. Myocardial tagged (CSPAMM) imaging may be useful to identify any regional tethering caused by adhesions. CMR can help in differentiating constrictive pericarditis from restrictive cardiomyopathy
Congenital heart disease
Atrial septal defect: Presence of an atrial septal defect, suitability for transcatheter ASD closure, quantify right heart size and function, assess the pulmonary-to-systemic shunt ratio (Qp/Qs) *Ventricular septal defect:* Presence of a ventricular septal defect. Quantify ventricular size and function and Qp/Qs. LGE imaging may help to determine if a VSD developed as a complication of MI *Coarctation of the aorta:* Assess the aortic anatomy, the degree of obstruction, and aortic valvular dysfunction. LV size, LV function, and myocardial mass. Phase-contrast imaging can estimate pressure gradient across the coarctation and collateral formation *Tetralogy of Fallot:* Identifying pulmonary blood flow. Quantitation of the severity of infundibular or pulmonary stenosis, assessment of RV function, presence of an anomalous coronary artery. Post-surgery RV outflow aneurysm, pulmonary regurgitation, biventricular size and function, and residual shunt

Key Learning Points

- Multiple imaging options exist for the evaluation of cardiovascular disease. It is important to be aware of the wide array of choices available.
- Stress testing, whether exercise or pharmacologic, provides a functional assessment of ischemia.
- The addition of imaging (either echocardiogram or nuclear) increases the diagnostic accuracy of stress testing for the detection of CAD, particularly in women.
- Cardiac MRI has broad capabilities that are important across many specific cardiac disorders.
- A multimodality imaging approach to cardiac assessment can be particularly helpful in more complicated cases.

References

1. Johnson NP, Goldberger JJ. Prognostic value of late heart rate recovery after treadmill exercise. Am J Cardiol. 2012;110:45–9.
2. Weiss SA, Blumenthal RS, Sharrett AR, et al. Exercise blood pressure and future cardiovasculardeath in asymptomatic individuals. Circulation. 2010;121:2109–16.
3. Stein R, Nguyen P, Abella J, et al. Prevalence and prognostic significance of exercise-induced right bundle branch block. Am J Cardiol. 2010;105:677–80.
4. Marine JE, Shetty V, Chow GV, et al. Prevalence and prognostic significance of exercise induced nonsustained ventricular tachycardia in asymptomatic volunteers: BLSA (Baltimore Longitudinal Study of Aging). J Am Coll Cardiol. 2013;62:595–600.
5. Gibbons RJ, Balady GJ, Bricker JT, et al. ACC/AHA 2002 guideline update for exercise testing:summary article: a report of the American College of Cardiology/American Heart Association Task Force on Practice Guidelines (Committee to Update the 1997 Exercise Testing Guidelines). Circulation. 2002;106:1883–92.

6. Mieres JH, Gulati M, Bairey Merz N, et al. Role of noninvasive testing in the clinical evaluation of women with suspected ischemic heart disease: a consensus statement from the American Heart Association. Circulation. 2014;130:350–79.
7. Kiviniemi AM, Lepojarvi S, Kentta TV, et al. Exercise capacity and heart rate responses to exercise as predictors of short-term outcome among patients with stable coronary artery disease. Am J Cardiol. 2015;116:1495–501.
8. Fleisher LA, Fleischmann KE, Auerbach AD, et al. 2014 ACC/AHA guideline on perioperative cardiovascular evaluation and management of patients undergoing noncardiac surgery: a report of the American College of Cardiology/American Heart Association Task Force on practice guidelines. J Am Coll Cardiol. 2014;64:e77–e137.
9. Anderson JL, Halperin JL, Albert NM, et al. Management of patients with peripheral artery disease (compilation of 2005 and 2011 ACCF/AHA guideline recommendations): a report of the American College of Cardiology Foundation/American Heart Association Task Force on Practice Guidelines. Circulation. 2013;127:1425–43.
10. Marwick TH, Case C, Sawada S, et al. Prediction of mortality by exercise echocardiography: a strategy for combination with Duke treadmill score. Circulation. 2001;103:2566–71.
11. Cornel JH, Bax JJ, Ehendy A, et al. Biphasic response to dobutamine predicts improvement of global left ventricular dysfunction after surgical revascularization in patients with stable coronary artery disease: implications of time course of recovery on diagnostic accuracy. J Am Coll Cardiol. 1998;31:1002–10.
12. Holly TA, Abbott BG, Al-Mallah M, et al. ASNC imaging guidelines for nuclear cardiology procedures: single photonemission computed tomography. J Nucl Cardiol. 2010;17:941–73.
13. Schindler TH, Schelbert HR, Quercioli A, Dilsizian V. Cardiac PET imaging for the detection and monitoring of coronary artery disease and microvascular health. JACC Cardiovasc Imaging. 2010;3:623–40.
14. Amsterdam EA, Wenger NK, Brindis RG, et al. 2014 AHA/ACC guideline for the management of patients with non-ST-elevation acute coronary syndromes: a report of the American College of Cardiology/American Heart Association Task Force on Practice Guidelines. Circulation. 2014;130:e344–426.
15. Wolk MJ, Bailey SR, Doherty JU, et al. ACCF/AHA/ASE/ASNC/HFSA/ HRS/SCAI/SCCT/SCMR/ STS 2013 multimodality appropriate use criteria for the detection and risk assess-

ment of stable ischemic heart disease. A report of the American College of Cardiology Foundation Appropriate Use Criteria Task Force, American Heart Association, American Society of Echocardiography, American Society of Nuclear Cardiology, Heart Failure Society of America, Heart Rhythm Society, Society for Cardiovascular Angiography and Interventions, Society of Cardiovascular Computed Tomography, Society for Cardiovascular Magnetic Resonance, and Society of Thoracic Surgeons. J Am Coll Cardiol. 2014;63:380–406.

16. Patel MR, White RD, Abbara S, et al. 2013 ACCF/ACR/ASE/ASNC/SCCT/SCMR appropriate utilization of cardiovascular imaging in heart failure. A joint report of the American College of Radiology Appropriateness Criteria Committee and the American College of Cardiology Foundation Appropriate Use Criteria Task Force. J Am Coll Cardiol. 2013;61:2207–31.
17. Soman P, Udelson JE. Assessment of myocardial viability by nuclear imaging in coronary heart disease. UptoDate.
18. Fleisher LA, Fleischmann KE, Auerbach AD, et al. 2014 ACC/AHA guideline on perioperative cardiovascular evaluation and management of patients undergoing noncardiac surgery: executive summary. A report of the American College of Cardiology/American Heart Association Task Force on Practice Guidelines. Circulation. 2014;130:2215–45.
19. Heydari B, Juan YH, Liu H, et al. Stress perfusion cardiac magnetic resonance imaging effectively risk stratifies diabetic patients with suspected myocardial ischemia. Circ Cardiovasc Imaging. 2016;9:e004136.
20. Mordini FE, Haddad T, Hsu LY, et al. Diagnostic accuracy of stress perfusion CMR in comparison with quantitative coronary angiography: fully quantitative, semiquantitative, and qualitative assessment. JACC Cardiovasc Imaging. 2014;7:14–22.
21. Chan RH, Maron BJ, Olivotto I, et al. Prognostic value of quantitative contrast-enhanced cardiovascular magnetic resonance for the evaluation of sudden death risk in patients with hypertrophic cardiomyopathy. Circulation. 2014;130:484–95.
22. te Riele AS, Tandri H, Bluemke DA. Arrhythmogenic right ventricular cardiomyopathy (ARVC): cardiovascular magnetic resonance update. J Cardiovasc Magn Reson. 2014;16:50.
23. Radunski UK, Lund GK, Stehning C, et al. CMR in patients with severe myocarditis: diagnostic value of quantitative tissue markers including extracellular volume imaging. JACC Cardiovasc Imaging. 2014;7:667–75.

24. Murtagh G, Laffin LJ, Beshai JF, et al. Prognosis of myocardial damage in sarcoidosis patients with preserved left ventricular ejection fraction: risk stratification using cardiovascular magnetic resonance. Circ Cardiovasc Imaging. 2016;9:e003738.
25. Gati S, Rajani R, Carr-White GS, Chambers JB. Adult left ventricular noncompaction: reappraisal of current diagnostic imaging modalities. JACC Cardiovasc Imaging. 2014;7:1266–75.
26. Cawley PJ, Hamilton-Craig C, Owens DS, et al. Prospective comparison of valve regurgitation quantitation by cardiac magnetic resonance imaging and transthoracic echocardiography. Circ Cardiovasc Imaging. 2013;6:48–57.
27. Myerson SG, d'Arcy J, Mohiaddin R, et al. Aortic regurgitation quantification using cardiovascular magnetic resonance: association with clinical outcome. Circulation. 2012;126:1452–60.

Chapter 8
Coronary CTA and Calcium Scoring

Bruno B. Lima, Parth Patel, and Patrick Gleason

Abbreviations

ACS	Acute coronary syndromes
ASCVD	Atherosclerotic cardiovascular disease
CABG	Coronary artery bypass graft
CAC	Coronary artery calcium
CAD	Coronary artery disease
CAD-RADS	Coronary Artery Disease-Reporting and Data System
CCS	Coronary calcium score
cCTA	Coronary computed tomography angiography
CT	Computed tomography
ECG	Electrocardiogram
FFRCT	Fractional flow reserve derived from computed tomography
HU	Hounsfield units

B. B. Lima · P. Patel · P. Gleason (✉)
Department of Medicine, Division of Cardiology, Emory University School of Medicine, Atlanta, GA, USA
e-mail: Patrick.t.gleason@emory.edu

A. A. Bhargava et al. (eds.), *Handbook of Outpatient Cardiology*, https://doi.org/10.1007/978-3-030-88953-1_8

ICA	Invasive coronary angiography
LM	Left main
MACE	Major adverse cardiac events
MDCT	Multi-detector computed tomography

Cardiac Computed Tomography

Different uses of cardiac computed tomography (CT) include:

- Coronary artery calcium (CAC) scoring
- Coronary computed tomography angiography (cCTA)
- Structural heart and valve evaluation
- Cardiac function and chamber assessment
- Assessment of cardiac mass and thrombus

Coronary CT Angiography

- cCTA has a high negative predictive value and is particularly useful for the exclusion of obstructive coronary artery disease in native coronary arteries and bypass grafts.
- Patients suitable for cCTA should have reasonable clinical suspicion of nonacute ischemia or acute coronary syndromes (ACS) without definite objective evidence of ACS on EKG or myocardial necrosis by biomarkers [1] (Table 8.1).
- Alternative testing may be preferred in cases of allergic reaction to iodinated contrast, significantly impaired renal function, contraindications to beta-blockers, morbid obesity (BMI > 39 kg/m^2), or pregnancy.

Table 8.1 Summary of appropriate indications for coronary CT angiography

Detection of CAD in symptomatic patients without known heart disease			
Indication	**Appropriate use score**		
Nonacute symptoms possibly representing an ischemic equivalent	**Low pretest probability**	**Intermediate pretest probability**	**High pretest probability**
ECG interpretable *and* able to exercise	Uncertain	Appropriate	Inappropriate
ECG uninterpretable *or* unable to exercise	Appropriate	Appropriate	Uncertain
Acute symptoms with suspicion of ACS			
Normal ECG and cardiac biomarkers	Appropriate	Appropriate	Uncertain
ECG uninterpretable	Appropriate	Appropriate	Uncertain
Nondiagnostic ECG or equivocal cardiac biomarkers	Appropriate	Appropriate	Uncertain
Detection of CAD in other clinical scenarios			
Newly diagnosed heart failure without prior CAD			
Reduced left ventricular ejection fraction	Appropriate	Appropriate	Uncertain

(continued)

Table 8.1 (continued)

Detection of CAD in symptomatic patients without known heart disease			
Indication	**Appropriate use score**		
Nonacute symptoms possibly representing an ischemic equivalent	**Low pretest probability**	**Intermediate pretest probability**	**High pretest probability**
Preoperative assessment prior to noncardiac surgery			
Coronary evaluation before noncoronary cardiac surgery	Uncertain	Appropriate	Inappropriate
Adult congenital heart disease			
Assessment of anomalies of coronary arterial or other thoracic arteriovenous vessels	Appropriate		
Use of cCTA in the setting of prior test results			
Prior normal ECG exercise stress test with continued symptoms	Appropriate		
Prior ECG exercise testing	Uncertain	Appropriate	Inappropriate
Discordant ECG exercise and imaging results	Appropriate		

TABLE 8.1 (continued)

Detection of CAD in symptomatic patients without known heart disease			
Indication	**Appropriate use score**		
Nonacute symptoms possibly representing an ischemic equivalent	**Low pretest probability**	**Intermediate pretest probability**	**High pretest probability**
	Equivocal	*Mild*	*Moderate to severe*
Prior stress imaging procedure	Appropriate	Uncertain	Inappropriate
	CCS ≤ 400	*CCS 401–1000*	*CCS > 1000*
Impact of coronary calcium on the decision to perform coronary CTA in symptomatic patients	Appropriate	Uncertain	Uncertain
	Normal	*Abnormal*	
Evaluation of new or worsening symptoms in the setting of past stress imaging study	Appropriate	Uncertain	

Abbreviations: *ECG* electrocardiogram, *ACS* acute coronary syndromes, *CAD* coronary artery disease, *cCTA* coronary computed tomography angiography

Clinical Pearls
A major consideration for the selection of patients for coronary CTA is renal function with a goal GFR of >30 mL/min, as iodinated contrast can be nephrotoxic. Additional considerations relate to image quality and include body size and the ability to achieve a regular, low resting heart rate (ideally <70 bpm).

Brief Cardiac CT Technique Overview

- Multi-detector CT (MDCT) scanners use a rapidly rotating X-ray tube (sub-second rotation times) and several rows of detectors to generate images of the heart.
- Multiple gantry rotations are required to cover the cardiac length with small detector slice arrays, such as with a 64-slice MDCT (minimum required for cCTA), while scanners with more detectors (256–320 slices) can cover the whole heart in one rotation and one cardiac cycle.
- MDCT systems can operate in either prospectively triggered or retrospectively gated modes.
- Prospective ECG triggering only scans for a portion of the cardiac cycle (determined by the R-R interval) and uses less radiation. Retrospective gating scans for the entire R-R interval and generates images throughout the cardiac cycle at the cost of additional radiation to the patient.

Diagnostic Accuracy of cCTA for Obstructive CAD

- Native coronary arteries

  (a) Prior reports demonstrated the high diagnostic accuracy of cCTA with sensitivity (91–99%) and specificity (74–96%) in subjects without known CAD [2–4].

(b) cCTA provides a high negative predictive value (97–99%) in excluding obstructive CAD in symptomatic subjects without known CAD.

- Coronary artery stents

(a) cCTA is limited in the evaluation of coronary artery stents due to numerous limitations imposed by CT artifacts, including motion, beam hardening, and partial volume effects.
(b) Stent size is an important consideration for cCTA use. The ability to assess coronary stents is nonuniform across stents of different sizes.
(c) ACC Appropriate Use Criteria consider it appropriate to use cCTA for asymptomatic subjects who have undergone PCI with ≥3 mm stent or who underwent left main coronary artery PCI for evaluation of stent patency.

- Coronary artery bypass grafts (CABGs)

(a) Since CABGs are usually less affected by cardiac motion, larger than native coronary arteries, and less likely to possess calcified plaque components, cCTA is a robust test for evaluation of CABG patency.
(b) However, depending on the anatomy, the distal anastomosis can be challenging to examine, and the degree of stenosis tends to be overestimated.
(c) cCTA is also uniquely helpful in evaluating the position of prior CABGs and other retrosternal anatomies prior to reoperative chest or cardiac surgery.

Prognostic Utility of cCTA in Stable CAD

The prognostic value of CAD, as detected on cCTA, has been further supported by findings in large-scale clinical trials:

- The PROMISE study enrolled >10,000 symptomatic intermediate-risk patients for whom testing was recommended in the United States and Canada; there were no significant differences in outcomes between initial anatomic testing or functional testing strategy with respect to major adverse cardiac events (MACE) [5].

- The SCOT-HEART (Scottish Computed Tomography of the HEART) study was a large prospective multicenter trial of 4146 patients which showed that the use of cCTA in addition to standard care in patients with stable chest pain resulted in a significantly lower rate of MACE at 5 years than standard care alone, without resulting in higher rate of invasive coronary angiography (ICA) or revascularization [6].
- cCTA helps to appropriately allocate preventive therapies and to appropriately refer patients who will most benefit from ICA and revascularization based on SCOT-HEART trial data.
- Atherosclerotic plaque features derived from cCTA have been associated with increased risk of MACE and were shown to improve risk assessment, including [7]:

  (a) Positive remodeling (Fig. 8.1a)
  (b) Low attenuation plaque (Fig. 8.1b)
  (c) Spotty calcification (Fig. 8.1c)
  (d) Napkin ring sign (Fig. 8.1d)

- Fractional flow reserve derived from computed tomography (FFRCT) was developed from the application of computational fluid dynamic principles on cCTA and is currently under investigation with the goal of improving cCTA specificity for the identification of functionally significant lesions.

Prognostic Utility of cCTA in Acute Chest Pain

- cCTA has been shown to be a reliable diagnostic imaging tool for identifying low-risk individuals, shortening length of stay, and reducing expenditures related to the diagnostic pathway of patients presenting with undifferentiated chest pain to the emergency department.

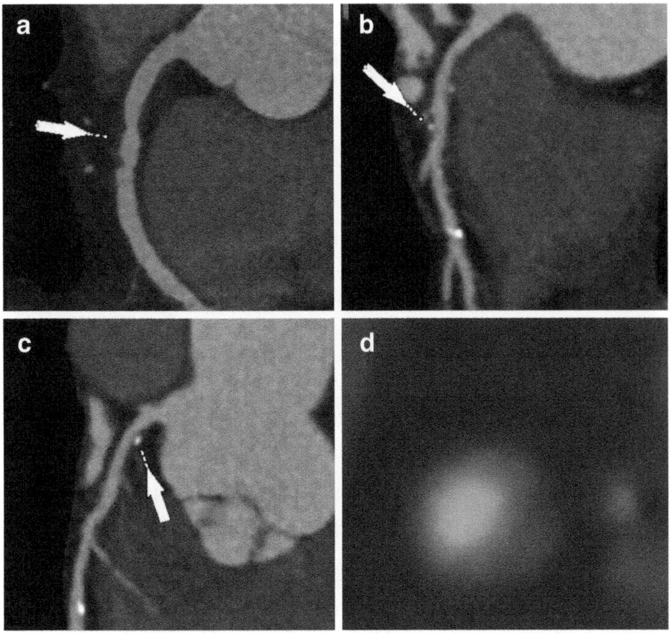

FIGURE 8.1 High-risk coronary plaque features: (**a**) non-calcified plaque with positive remodeling in the right coronary artery (RCA); (**b**) calcified and non-calcified low-attenuation plaque in the RCA; (**c**) partially calcified plaque in the mid RCA with spotty calcification; (**d**) napkin-ring sign plaque in the mid left anterior descending coronary artery

- Those results were corroborated by major clinical trials, including:
  (a) CT-STAT (Coronary Computed Tomography for Systemic Triage of Acute Chest Pain Patients to Treatment) [8]
  (b) ACRIN (CT Angiography for Safe Discharge of Patients With Possible Acute Coronary Syndromes) [9]
  (c) ROMICAT I & II (Rule Out Myocardial Ischemia/Infarction Using Computer Assisted Tomography) [10]

- With modern high sensitivity troponin assays, the impact of cCTA on length of stay is less pronounced.

Patient Preparation

- Thorough medical history with specific attention to age, renal function, allergies, and comorbidities.
- Establish peripheral IV with 18- or 20-gauge needles – above the wrist, ideally right antecubital vein.
  (a) Necessary for successful contrast enhancement.
  (b) The higher the contrast injection rate (4–6 cc/sec), the better the contrast opacification at the aortic root and coronary arteries.
- cCTA commonly requires the administration of chronotropic therapy and vasodilators.
  (a) Review ECG prior to scan.
  (b) Most imaging centers use beta-blockers for rate control that are typically administered orally (e.g., metoprolol in 25–50 mg oral increments 1 hour prior to the scan) and/or IV (e.g., metoprolol 5 mg in repeated doses) to achieve a resting heart rate of <70 bpm.
  (c) Alternatively, calcium channel blockers or ivabradine could also be used in certain circumstances.
  (d) Nitroglycerin (400–800 mcg sublingually) is typically administered just prior to cCTA to induce coronary vasodilation and optimize lumen and plaque visualization.

Clinical Pearls
Be cautious with the use of beta-blockers, calcium channel blockers, or ivabradine in setting of heart failure, aortic stenosis, hypotension, bradycardia, or conduction system disease.

Coronary Artery Disease Stenosis Grading

- The CAD-RADS classification system was proposed by the American College of Radiology in order to standardize cCTA reporting and decrease the potential discrepancies between physicians in the reporting of coronary stenosis [11] (Table 8.2).

Table 8.2 CAD-RADS classification system

	Maximal coronary stenosis	**Interpretation**	**Further cardiac testing**
CAD-RADS 0	0%	Absence of CAD	None
CAD-RADS 1	1–24% (or plaque without stenosis)	Minimal nonobstructive CAD	None
CAD-RADS 2	25–49%	Mild nonobstructive CAD	None
CAD-RADS 3	50–69%	Moderate stenosis	Consider functional assessment
CAD-RADS 4A	70–99% in 1 or 2 vessels	Severe stenosis	Consider ICA or functional assessment
CAD-RADS 4B	70–99% in 3 vessels or LM > 50%	Severe stenosis	ICA recommended
CAD-RADS 5	100%	Total coronary occlusion	Consider ICA and/or viability assessment

Abbreviations: *CAD* coronary artery disease, *CAD-RADS* Coronary Artery Disease-Reporting and Data System, *LM* left main, *ICA* invasive coronary angiography

Coronary Artery Calcium (CAC) Scoring

- Coronary calcium correlates strongly with the extent of atherosclerotic plaque burden and with the long-term occurrence of coronary events [12].
- The calcium burden of each coronary artery is quantified using the Agatston score which is calculated by the sum of coronary calcified plaque lesions with greater than or equal to the calcium density of 130 Hounsfield units (HU) having an area ≥1 mm^2.
- This lesion score is measured by the maximal CT number, with 1 for 130–199 HU, 2 for 200–299 HU, 3 for 300–399, and 4 for ≥400 HU. The total score is determined by the sum of each of these lesion scores (Fig. 8.2).
- CAC scoring has a weak correlation with the presence and severity of angiographic stenosis. A high CAC score in an asymptomatic patient does not mandate a coronary angiogram.

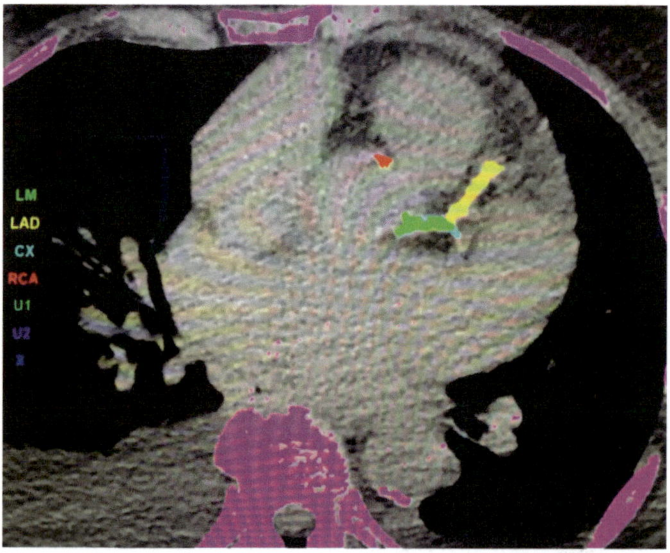

Figure 8.2 CT calcium scoring image showing calcified plaques in coronary vessel segments

Clinical Pearls
Individual plaques, including soft plaques particularly prone to rupture and eroded plaques, may not be calcified. Thus, the presence of calcium is not closely associated with the propensity of an individual plaque to rupture, and patients with ACS may not have any coronary calcium.

Prognostic Utility of CAC Scoring

The prognostic significance of CAC scoring has been derived from large, population-based observational studies with long-term follow-up, including:

- MESA (Multi-Ethnic Study of Atherosclerosis) was a prospective, multicenter study of 6814 individuals 45–84 years of age who underwent a baseline CAC score scan and were followed for the occurrence of major cardiac events which showed that CAC is a strong predictor of CAD in four racial and ethnic groups in the United States [13].
- EISNER (Early Identification of Subclinical Atherosclerosis by Noninvasive Imaging Research) was a prospective, randomized trial of 2137 volunteers that aimed at assessing the incremental impact of CAC scoring compared with conventional risk factor modification and found that it resulted in superior CAD risk factor control without an increase in downstream medical testing [14].
- The CAC consortium was a multicenter cohort study of 66,636 patients undergoing a clinically indicated CAC scoring between 1991 and 2010 with a mean follow-up of 12 years showing that CAC predicts adverse outcomes in all included race/ethnicity subgroups [15].

CAC Scoring in Clinical Practice

- For adults 40–75 years of age, clinicians should routinely assess traditional cardiovascular risk factors and calculated 10-year risk of atherosclerotic cardiovascular disease (ASCVD) events, employing commonly used pooled cohort equations [12].
- CAC scoring is most useful in asymptomatic patients with intermediate risk (5–20%). It is not appropriate for patients with a known history of CAD or for patients with symptoms.
- It is reasonable to utilize CAC score in the decision to withhold, postpone, or initiate statin therapy if there is uncertainty about ASCVD risk or if patient preference is to avoid statin therapy.
- CAC score can reclassify risk upward (when CAC is ≥100 or ≥ 75th age/sex/race percentile) or downward (if CAC score = 0).

  (a) If CAC = 0, treatment with statin may be withheld or delayed, as long as higher-risk conditions are absent (diabetes mellitus, heavy current cigarette smoking, or strong family history of premature ASCVD).
  (b) If CAC score is 1–99, statin therapy is favored, especially in those ≥55 years of age.
  (c) If CAC score is ≥100 or ≥75th percentile, then statin therapy is indicated.

Key Learning Points

- Patients suitable for cCTA should have reasonable clinical suspicion for ACS or nonacute ischemia, without objective evidence of ACS on EKG or myocardial necrosis by biomarkers.
- Impaired renal function may be a contraindication for pursuing a cCTA, as iodinated contrast can be nephrotoxic. Other limitations include body size and

the inability to tolerate chronotropic therapy or vasodilators.

- CAD-RADS calcification system was developed to standardize reporting of coronary stenosis on cCTA from CAD-RADS 0 (0% stenosis) to CAD-RADS 5 (100% stenosis).
- cCTAs have high diagnostic accuracy and can provide a high negative predictive value to exclude CAD in symptomatic patients without known CAD.
- Several studies (CT-STAT, ACRIN, ROMICAT I & II) have shown cCTA to be a reliable diagnostic imaging tool for identifying low-risk individuals, shortening length of stay, and reducing expenditures related to the diagnostic pathway of patients presenting with undifferentiated chest pain to the emergency department.
- Coronary calcium correlates strongly with the extent of atherosclerotic plaque burden and with the long-term occurrence of coronary events, but has weak correlation with the presence and severity of angiographic stenosis, since patients with plaque rupture or ACS may not have any coronary calcium.
- CAC scoring is most useful in asymptomatic patients with intermediate risk (5–20%) and is not appropriate for patients with a known history of CAD or for patients with symptoms. In particular, it is reasonable to utilize CAC score in the decision to withhold, postpone, or initiate statin therapy.

References

1. Taylor AJ, Cerqueira M, Hodgson JM, Mark D, Min J, O'Gara P, et al. ACCF/SCCT/ACR/AHA/ASE/ASNC/NASCI/SCAI/SCMR 2010 appropriate use criteria for cardiac computed tomography. A report of the American college of cardiology foundation appropriate use criteria task force, the society of

cardiovascular computed tomography, the American college of radiology, the American heart association, the American society of echocardiography, the American society of nuclear cardiology, the north American society for cardiovascular imaging, the society for cardiovascular angiography and interventions, and the society for cardiovascular magnetic resonance. J Am Coll Cardiol. 2010;56(22):1864–94. https://doi.org/10.1016/j.jacc.2010.07.005.
2. Budoff MJ, Dowe D, Jollis JG, Gitter M, Sutherland J, Halamert E, et al. Diagnostic performance of 64-multidetector row coronary computed tomographic angiography for evaluation of coronary artery stenosis in individuals without known coronary artery disease: results from the prospective multicenter ACCURACY (Assessment by Coronary Computed Tomographic Angiography of Individuals Undergoing Invasive Coronary Angiography) trial. J Am Coll Cardiol. 2008;52(21):1724–32. https://doi.org/10.1016/j.jacc.2008.07.031.
3. Meijboom WB, Meijs MF, Schuijf JD, Cramer MJ, Mollet NR, van Mieghem CA, et al. Diagnostic accuracy of 64-slice computed tomography coronary angiography: a prospective, multicenter, multivendor study. J Am Coll Cardiol. 2008;52(25):2135–44. https://doi.org/10.1016/j.jacc.2008.08.058.
4. Miller JM, Rochitte CE, Dewey M, Arbab-Zadeh A, Niinuma H, Gottlieb I, et al. Diagnostic performance of coronary angiography by 64-row CT. N Engl J Med. 2008;359(22):2324–36. https://doi.org/10.1056/NEJMoa0806576.
5. Douglas PS, Hoffmann U. Anatomical versus functional testing for coronary artery disease. N Engl J Med. 2015;373(1):91. https://doi.org/10.1056/NEJMc1505594.
6. Investigators S-H, Newby DE, Adamson PD, Berry C, Boon NA, Dweck MR, et al. Coronary CT angiography and 5-year risk of myocardial infarction. N Engl J Med. 2018;379(10):924–33. https://doi.org/10.1056/NEJMoa1805971.
7. Puchner SB, Liu T, Mayrhofer T, Truong QA, Lee H, Fleg JL, et al. High-risk plaque detected on coronary CT angiography predicts acute coronary syndromes independent of significant stenosis in acute chest pain: results from the ROMICAT-II trial. J Am Coll Cardiol. 2014;64(7):684–92. https://doi.org/10.1016/j.jacc.2014.05.039.
8. Goldstein JA, Chinnaiyan KM, Abidov A, Achenbach S, Berman DS, Hayes SW, et al. The CT-STAT (Coronary Computed Tomographic Angiography for Systematic Triage of Acute

Chest Pain Patients to Treatment) trial. J Am Coll Cardiol. 2011;58(14):1414–22. https://doi.org/10.1016/j.jacc.2011.03.068.
9. Litt HI, Gatsonis C, Snyder B, Singh H, Miller CD, Entrikin DW, et al. CT angiography for safe discharge of patients with possible acute coronary syndromes. N Engl J Med. 2012;366(15):1393–403. https://doi.org/10.1056/NEJMoa1201163.
10. Hoffmann U, Truong QA, Schoenfeld DA, Chou ET, Woodard PK, Nagurney JT, et al. Coronary CT angiography versus standard evaluation in acute chest pain. N Engl J Med. 2012;367(4):299–308. https://doi.org/10.1056/NEJMoa1201161.
11. Cury RC, Abbara S, Achenbach S, Agatston A, Berman DS, Budoff MJ, et al. CAD-RADS(TM) coronary artery disease - reporting and data system. An expert consensus document of the Society of Cardiovascular Computed Tomography (SCCT), the American College of Radiology (ACR) and the North American Society for Cardiovascular Imaging (NASCI). Endorsed by the American College of Cardiology. J Cardiovasc Comput Tomogr. 2016;10(4):269–81. https://doi.org/10.1016/j.jcct.2016.04.005.
12. Greenland P, Blaha MJ, Budoff MJ, Erbel R, Watson KE. Coronary calcium score and cardiovascular risk. J Am Coll Cardiol. 2018;72(4):434–47. https://doi.org/10.1016/j.jacc.2018.05.027.
13. Budoff MJ, Nasir K, McClelland RL, Detrano R, Wong N, Blumenthal RS, et al. Coronary calcium predicts events better with absolute calcium scores than age-sex-race/ethnicity percentiles: MESA (Multi-Ethnic Study of Atherosclerosis). J Am Coll Cardiol. 2009;53(4):345–52. https://doi.org/10.1016/j.jacc.2008.07.072.
14. Rozanski A, Gransar H, Shaw LJ, Kim J, Miranda-Peats L, Wong ND, et al. Impact of coronary artery calcium scanning on coronary risk factors and downstream testing the EISNER (Early Identification of Subclinical Atherosclerosis by Noninvasive Imaging Research) prospective randomized trial. J Am Coll Cardiol. 2011;57(15):1622–32. https://doi.org/10.1016/j.jacc.2011.01.019.
15. Peng AW, Mirbolouk M, Orimoloye OA, Osei AD, Dardari Z, Dzaye O, et al. Long-term all-cause and cause-specific mortality in asymptomatic patients with CAC >/=1,000: results from the CAC consortium. JACC Cardiovasc Imaging. 2020;13(1 Pt 1):83–93. https://doi.org/10.1016/j.jcmg.2019.02.005.

Chapter 9
Basics of Echocardiography

Merilyn Susan Varghese and Jordan B. Strom

Abbreviations

AHA	American Heart Association
ASD	Atrial septal defect
AV	Aortic valve
CW	Continuous wave
ECG	Electrocardiogram
LA	Left atrium
LV	Left ventricle
MAC	Monitored anesthesia care
ME	Mid-esophageal
MV	Mitral valve
PV	Pulmonic valve

M. S. Varghese
Department of Medicine, Division of Cardiology, Beth Israel Deaconess Medical Center, Harvard Medical School, Boston, MA, USA
e-mail: mvarghe1@bidmc.harvard.edu

J. B. Strom (✉)
Department of Medicine, Division of Cardiology, Beth Israel Deaconess Medical Center, Richard A. and Susan F. Smith Center for Outcomes Research in Cardiology, Harvard Medical School, Boston, MA, USA
e-mail: jstrom@bidmc.harvard.edu

A. A. Bhargava et al. (eds.), *Handbook of Outpatient Cardiology*, https://doi.org/10.1007/978-3-030-88953-1_9

PW	Pulsed wave
RV	Right ventricle
TEE	Transesophageal echocardiography
TTE	Transthoracic echocardiography
TV	Tricuspid valve
UEA	Ultrasound-enhancing agent

Introduction

Echocardiography utilizes reflections of ultrasound waves to elucidate cardiac structure and function and has revolutionized our understanding of cardiac diseases. The two major subtypes of echocardiography are transthoracic and transesophageal echocardiography. A simultaneous single-lead ECG tracing is recorded in order to correlate the phases of the cardiac cycle with imaging findings.

M-Mode

- An M ("Motion")-mode displays the reflections from a single ultrasound scan line versus time.
  - The intensity of ultrasound reflections is displayed as a function of depth of imaging on the *y*-axis and time on the *x*-axis, allowing for analysis of subtle cardiac motion and chamber dimensions due to high temporal resolution (Fig. 9.1).

Doppler

- Doppler ultrasound is based on the Doppler principle – there is a change in frequency of a moving structure (e.g., blood) depending on whether the structure is moving towards or away from the ultrasound source. Blood flow velocities can be visualized and calculated [1].

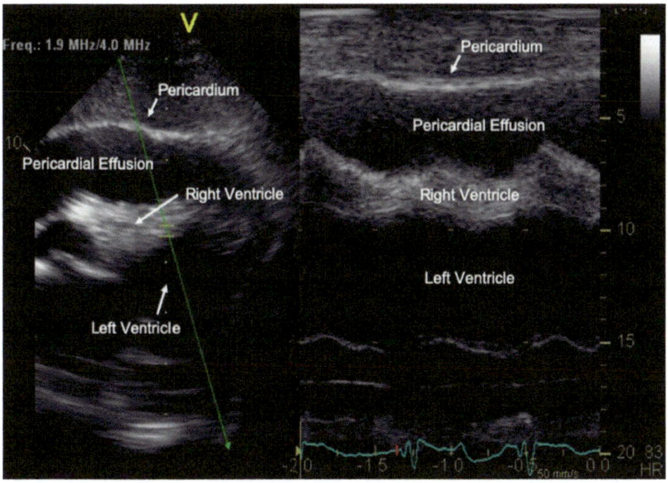

FIGURE 9.1 M-mode recording (green line on left side of image) through the right ventricular (RV) wall in a patient with a pericardial effusion. There is evidence of right ventricular diastolic collapse determined by correlation with the ECG lead recording

- By convention in color Doppler:
  - Blood moving towards the probe appears red.
  - Blood moving away from the probe appears blue.
- In continuous wave (CW) Doppler, a single ultrasound crystal sends and receives signals continuously. The peak velocity of moving structures (e.g., blood or myocardium) can thus be calculated. The magnitude of a CW signal is displayed on the *y*-axis vs. time on the *x*-axis. Signals moving towards the probe are displayed above baseline, and those moving away from the probe are displayed below.
- Pulsed-wave (PW) Doppler allows measurement of velocities in a specific location. It uses a sampling gate that filters the velocities received and displays only velocities from a given location and depth, which is determined by the time it takes to receive the signal.

Contrast Echocardiography

- Ultrasound contrast agents (also known as ultrasound-enhancing agents) are inert gases covered in lipid or protein shells that form microbubbles.
  - These agents are administered via IV and are small enough to pass through the pulmonary circulation into the left heart.
  - These microbubbles emit harmonic frequencies when exposed to low-frequency ultrasound that create contrast with myocardial tissue.
  - They can improve left ventricular opacification for evaluation of global and regional wall motion abnormalities, intracardiac masses, and aneurysms (Fig. 9.2).
- Contraindications to contrast agents include hypersensitivity to the agents themselves. UEAs are generally safe and cost-

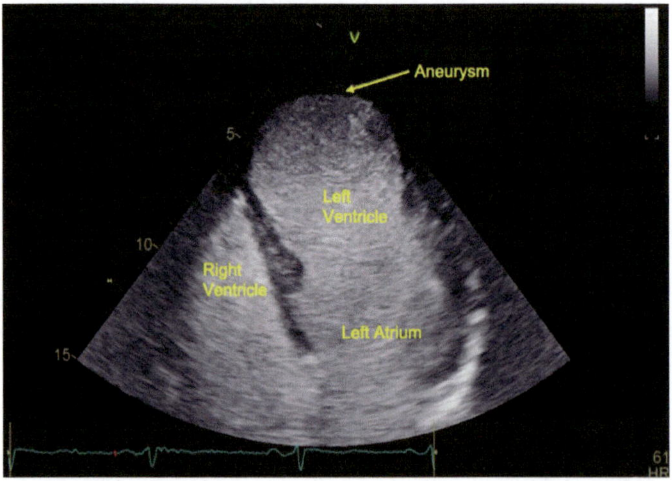

FIGURE 9.2 Contrast echocardiography study revealing an aneurysm at the left ventricular apex. Thinning of the left ventricular (LV) wall at the apex can be appreciated, indicating the presence of the aneurysm

effective, but associated with a 1:100,000 risk of an anaphylactoid response requiring therapy. Appropriate training and laboratory protocols are required to use them [2].

Three-Dimensional Echocardiography

- Standard echocardiography utilizes a scan sector that is roughly two-dimensional – the depth of the scan sector is assumed to be negligible. With the use of a multiarray transducer, a sector can be acquired in three dimensions. Images are acquired over several beats, and ECG-gating is used to reconstruct images [3].
- 3D echocardiography is an evolving technology, and applications include evaluating ventricular volumes and ejection fraction. However, 3D capable probes are not available at all sites.
- Lower spatial and temporal resolution of 3D echocardiography and need for ECG gating make it less accurate in certain circumstances (e.g., atrial fibrillation with substantially irregular R-R intervals).

Intracardiac Echocardiography

- Intracardiac echocardiography is an emerging modality and has procedural utility, such as with atrial septal defect (ASD) closures and arrhythmia ablations.
  - A transducer is placed on a catheter, which is advanced through a sheath placed in the femoral vein. The catheter is advanced to the heart, allowing for directed imaging of involved structures, often obviating the need for TEE [4].

Artifact

- The ultrasound assumes that the received signal is along the transmitted scan line with a depth proportional to the travel time of the signal. When these assumptions are not met, artifacts may occur, which can obscure images and mimic pathology.

> **Clinical Pearl:** When a possible pathologic finding is seen that is uncommon or unexpected, a thorough evaluation for artifact should ensue, including visualizing the pathology in two separate views.

  - Possible artifacts include reverberation, acoustic shadowing, mirror artifact, refraction artifact, side lobe artifact, beam width artifact, and near field clutter.
  - Reverberation artifact, for example, is a commonly observed artifact causing a step-ladder or comet-tail appearance, due to reflection of waves between highly reflective perpendicular structures [5].

Transthoracic Echocardiography

Indications

- Transthoracic echocardiography uses a surface probe applied to the thorax and has a variety of indications, including evaluation of:
  - Systolic and diastolic function
  - Valvular heart disease
  - Pericardial disease
  - Cardiac masses
- The American Society of Echocardiography has published Appropriate Use Criteria that define appropriate indications for TTE [6].

Views

- Standard views include:
  - Parasternal long axis
  - Parasternal short axis
  - Apical (two-, three-, and four-chamber views)
  - Subcostal
  - Suprasternal
- The parasternal long axis view is obtained at the left parasternal border (Fig. 9.3). Right ventricular (RV) inflow and outflow views, which evaluate the tricuspid valve (TV) and

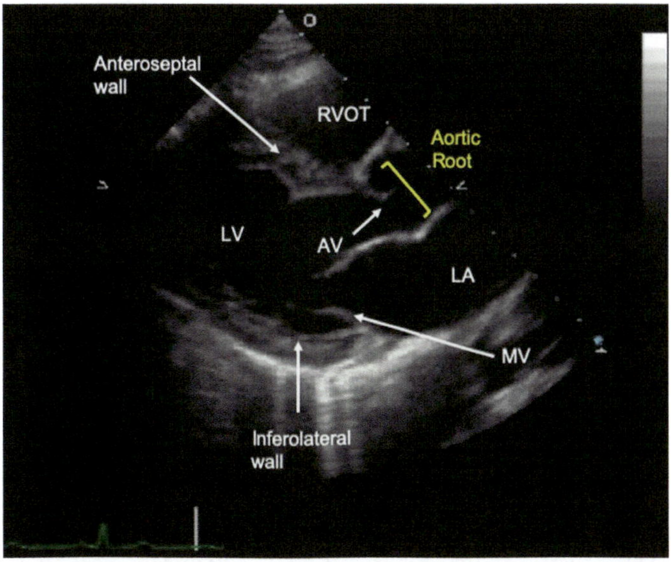

FIGURE 9.3 Parasternal long axis view: The right ventricular outflow tract (RVOT), left atrium (LA), mitral valve (MV), left ventricle (anteroseptal and inferolateral walls), aortic valve (AV), and the aortic root (in yellow) can be visualized. The proximal ascending aorta and coronary sinus can also be seen in this view in some patients

pulmonic valve (PV) respectively, are also obtained from the left parasternal border with angulation and tilting.

- Imaged perpendicular to the parasternal long axis view, the parasternal short axis view provides a "bread-loaf" view of the heart from the aortic valve to the apex. This view can be useful for evaluation of wall motion abnormalities and RV dysfunction (Fig. 9.4).
- Viewed from the left ventricular (LV) apex, the apical views include the two-chamber, three-chamber, and four-chamber views. The apical five-chamber view of the aortic valve (AV) and LV outflow tract can be seen with anterior angulation of the transducer probe (Fig. 9.5).
- The subcostal view is obtained from the subxiphoid approach (Fig. 9.6).
- The suprasternal view is acquired from the suprasternal notch and allows evaluation of the aortic arch to identify

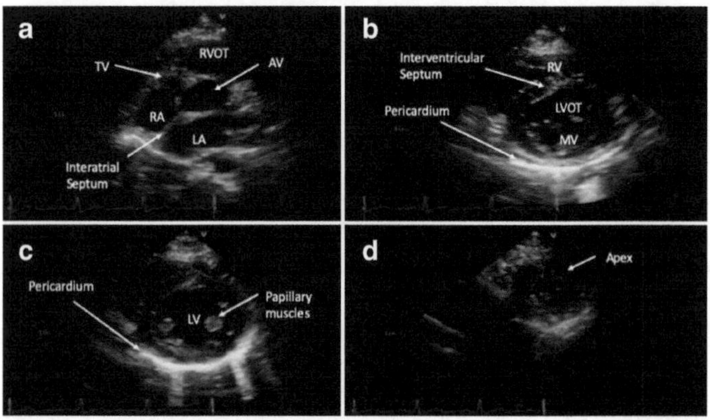

FIGURE 9.4 Parasternal short axis views: (**a**) Aortic valve (AV) view: AV is at the center. The interatrial septum (IAS), left atrium (LA), right atrium (RA), tricuspid valve (TV), and right ventricular outflow tract (RVOT) are seen. Sometimes, the pulmonic valve can be visualized to the right of the RVOT. (**b**) Mitral valve (MV view) – MV is in the center, with the left ventricular outflow tract (LVOT), right ventricle (RV), and bright pericardium also visualized. (**c**) Papillary muscle view: Left ventricle (LV) can also be seen. (**d**) Apex view: The LV apex is visualized centrally

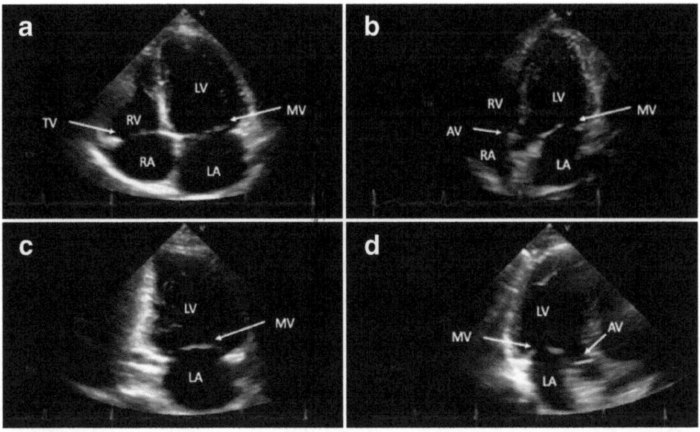

FIGURE 9.5 Apical views: (**a**) Apical four-chamber view: Right atrium (RA), tricuspid valve (TV), right ventricle (RV), left atrium (LA), mitral valve (MV), and left ventricle (LV) are visualized. The anterolateral wall and inferoseptal walls of the LV are seen in this view. (**b**) Apical five-chamber view: The aortic valve (AV) is also visualized in this view. (**c**) Apical two-chamber view: The inferior wall (on the left) and anterior wall (on the right) of the LV are seen. (**d**) Apical three-chamber view: The AV and MV are seen, as well as the inferolateral and anteroseptal walls of the LV

conditions such as aortic dissection, coarctation of the aorta, and patent ductus arteriosus (Fig. 9.7).

Left Ventricular Function

- Systolic function is evaluated by qualitative and quantitative means.
  - Qualitative assessment is dependent on the experience of the reader to assess thickening of the ventricular walls and inward motion. In the setting of tachycardia and bradycardia, visual assessment is more challenging as there is a tendency to overestimate or underestimate ventricular function, respectively.

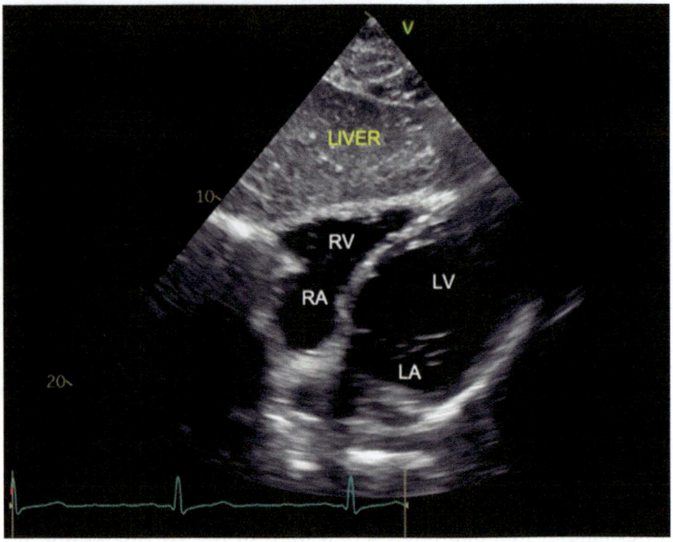

FIGURE 9.6 Subcostal view: The liver is the most anterior structure seen. All four chambers can be visualized – right atrium (RA), right ventricle (RV), left atrium (LA), and left ventricle (LV)

- Quantitative methods are numerous and include fractional shortening, Simpson's biplane ejection fraction, and global longitudinal strain.

  Fractional shortening is calculated using the percentage difference between the end-systolic and end-diastolic LV internal dimensions.
  Simpson's biplane method of disks subdivides the LV into discs of a fixed thickness and sums the volumes of these discs to produce volumetric measurements, which can be used to calculate ejection fraction.
  Global longitudinal strain is an emerging technology that uses "speckles" to evaluate tissue deformation and may be a sensitive marker of systolic dysfunction.

- Regional wall motion abnormalities can be discerned by absence of normal thickening of myocardial segments (according to the AHA 17-segment model) and are determined subjectively.

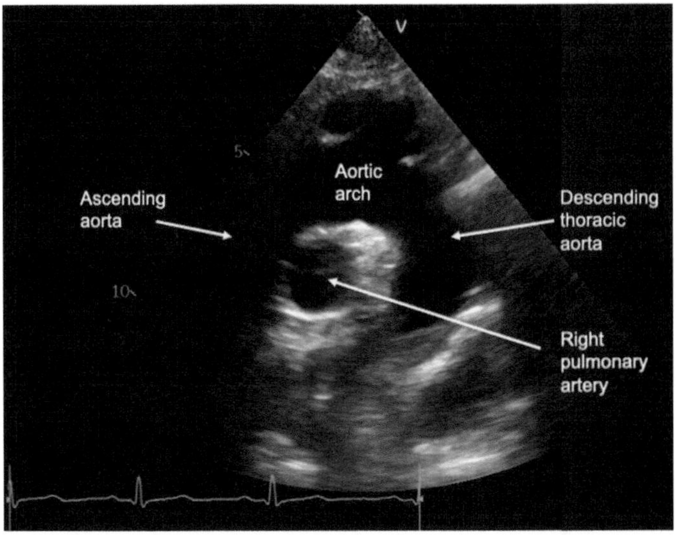

FIGURE 9.7 Suprasternal view: The proximal aorta, aortic arch, and descending aorta as well as the right pulmonary artery are seen. The left atrium can also sometimes be seen underneath and to the left of the right pulmonary artery

- Hypokinesis is defined as reduced (30–50%) myocardial thickening.
- Akinesis is defined as absent (>50%) myocardial thickening.
- Dyskinesis is defined as expansion (i.e., outward movement of the myocardium) during systole.

Right Ventricular Function

- RV function can be assessed visually and quantitatively.

Clinical Pearl: Due to its geometrically complex structure, evaluation of RV size and function is challenging.

- Several quantitative measurements have been developed:

- Tricuspid annular plane excursion (TAPSE)
- RV fractional area change
- 3D RV ejection fraction
- RV free wall strain

Valvular Disease

- The mitral, tricuspid, pulmonic, and aortic valves can be seen in multiple views. Valvular pathology such as masses (vegetations, thrombi, etc.), prolapse, stenosis, or rheumatic deformity can be assessed through visual inspection and quantitative measurements.
- Doppler echocardiography is essential to evaluating valvular regurgitation. In addition to qualitative visual inspection of the regurgitant jet, there are a number of quantitative techniques for defining regurgitant presence and severity:
  - The vena contracta refers to the width of the jet of color at its narrowest point (prior to dispersion in the receiving chamber).
  - Proximal isovolumic surface area (PISA) techniques can be used to calculate the volume of flow through the regurgitant orifice using Doppler information.
  - Other factors such as the shape and density of the regurgitant jet on Doppler profiling can support a diagnosis of significant regurgitation (Fig. 9.8).
- Doppler echocardiography is also standard of care for evaluating valvular stenosis, but the techniques used depend on the valve and circumstances evaluated.
  - For example, the MV area may be determined directly through planimetry of the short-axis area.
  - By contrast, the AV area is poorly assessed via planimetry (on TTE). Other techniques (e.g., the continuity equation) are used to determine the presence and extent of stenosis.

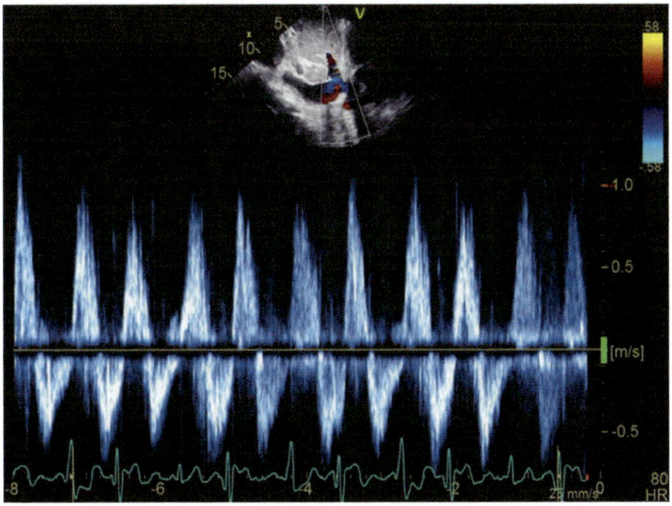

FIGURE 9.8 Pulsed wave Doppler through the hepatic vein on the subcostal view: Hepatic vein systolic flow reversal is seen with a positively directed peak along the *y*-axis after the QRS complex on the ECG tracing. Hepatic vein systolic flow reversal can be a marker of severe tricuspid regurgitation

Pericardium

- The pericardium is visualized and evaluated on multiple echocardiographic views.
- Feasibility of a safe pericardiocentesis is based on the amount of fluid visualized on the subcostal or apical views of a pericardial effusion.
- Pericardial masses and the presence of pericardial constriction can be suggested using TTE.

Aorta

- TTE can evaluate the aortic root, sinotubular junction, proximal ascending aorta, distal aortic arch, and portions of the descending and abdominal aorta.

- Potential findings include aortic dissection, aortic aneurysm, aortic dilation, aortic thrombus, or vasculitis.
- Though imaging the aorta may be challenging due to acoustic shadowing, anatomic assessment is possible, particularly for the proximal aorta.

Transesophageal Echocardiography

Indications

- There is a trade-off in ultrasound between depth of field and spatial resolution.
- Transthoracic probes use a lower frequency (4–5 MHz) to penetrate through the thorax to visualize cardiac structures. It cannot provide the same spatial resolution, particularly for posterior structures.
- A transesophageal probe is placed in the esophagus or stomach, directly adjacent to the heart, and uses a higher frequency (7–9 MHz).

Clinical Pearl: Due to its position in the esophagus, TEE is the optimal imaging modality to visualize posteriorly placed structures such as the left atrium, MV, pulmonary veins, and atrial appendages.

- Conversely, TTE may offer (dependent on habitus, etc.) a better view of anteriorly placed structures (e.g., RV, TV) due to its positioning on the chest wall.
- Some pathologies (e.g., AV replacement) may require both TTE and TEE to visualize all aspects of the pathology from different angles to avoid significant artifacts [7].

Procedure

- A TEE probe is inserted under sedation into the esophagus and stomach.
- The head of the probe is manipulated using operator controls that allow for flexion and extension of the probe, along with left and right angulation.
- The patient should have nothing by mouth for 6–8 hours before the procedure to reduce aspiration risk from sedation and probe insertion. Sedation may include conscious sedation, monitored anesthesia care (MAC), or general anesthesia, with the latter two administered by a consulting anesthesiologist.
- TEEs should generally be avoided in patients with:
  - An inability to cooperate
  - Respiratory difficulties that preclude sedation
  - Esophageal strictures or active upper GI bleeding
- After sedation has subsided and the gag reflex is no longer impaired, patients in the ambulatory setting can often be discharged home within a few hours.

Views

- During image acquisition, the probe is passed from the upper-esophagus to mid-esophagus and then through the gastroesophageal junction to obtain deep transgastric views. From each of these anatomical positions, there are multiple planes that can be evaluated (Fig. 9.9).

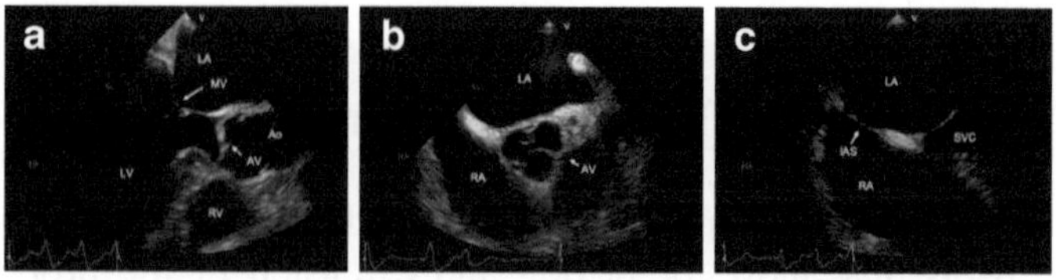

FIGURE 9.9 TEE views – there are 28 views that are included in a standard TEE examination, of which these are a few representative images. (**a**) Mid-esophageal (ME) long axis view: Left atrium (LA), mitral valve (MV), left ventricle (LV), aortic valve (AV), right ventricle (RV), and aorta (Ao) are seen. (**b**) ME AV short axis view: LA, RA, and AV are seen. (**c**) ME bicaval view: LA, interatrial septum (IAS), RA, and SVC (superior vena cava) are seen

Conclusion

- Echocardiography is a core imaging technology that provides essential anatomic and functional information. Findings must be interpreted within the contexts of a patient's presentation and imaging limitations.
- A cardiologist should be consulted if there is a question regarding optimal imaging modalities for a particular condition or abnormal findings that require review.

Key Learning Points

- Contrast agents improve left ventricular opacification and detection of regional wall motion abnormalities, intracardiac masses, and aneurysms.
- When a possible pathologic finding is seen that is uncommon or unexpected, a thorough evaluation for artifact should ensue.
- Transesophageal echocardiography, depending on the indication, may or may not provide additional information beyond transthoracic echocardiography.

References

1. Otto CM. Textbook of clinical echocardiography. Elsevier Health Sciences, Philadelphia, USA; 2013. 1 p.
2. Porter TR, Abdelmoneim S, Belcik JT, McCulloch ML, Mulvagh SL, Olson JJ, et al. Guidelines for the cardiac sonographer in the performance of contrast echocardiography: a focused update from the American Society of Echocardiography. J Am Soc Echocardiogr. 2014;27(8):797–810.
3. Lang RM, Badano LP, Mor-Avi V, Afilalo J, Armstrong A, Ernande L, et al. Recommendations for cardiac chamber quantification by echocardiography in adults: an update from the American Society of Echocardiography and the European Association of Cardiovascular Imaging. Eur Heart J Cardiovasc Imaging. 2015;16(3):233–70.
4. Enriquez A, Saenz LC, Rosso R, Silvestry FE, Callans D, Marchlinski FE, et al. Use of intracardiac echocardiography in interventional cardiology: working with the anatomy rather than fighting it. Circulation. 2018;137(21):2278–94.
5. Bertrand PB, Levine RA, Isselbacher EM, Vandervoort PM. Fact or artifact in two-dimensional echocardiography: avoiding misdiagnosis and missed diagnosis. J Am Soc Echocardiogr. 2016;29(5):381–91.
6. American College of Cardiology Foundation Appropriate Use Criteria Task Force, American Society of Echocardiography, American Heart Association, American Society of Nuclear Cardiology, Heart Failure Society of America, Heart Rhythm Society, et al. ACCF/ASE/AHA/ASNC/HFSA/HRS/SCAI/SCCM/SCCT/SCMR 2011 appropriate use criteria for echocardiography. A report of the American college of cardiology foundation appropriate use criteria task force, American society of echocardiography, American heart association, American society of nuclear cardiology, heart failure society of America, heart rhythm society, society for cardiovascular angiography and interventions, society of critical care medicine, society of cardiovascular computed tomography, society for cardiovascular magnetic resonance American college of chest physicians. J Am Soc Echocardiogr. 2011;24:229–67.
7. Hahn RT, Abraham T, Adams MS, Bruce CJ, Glas KE, Lang RM, et al. Guidelines for performing a comprehensive transesophageal echocardiographic examination: recommendations from the American Society of Echocardiography and the Society of Cardiovascular Anesthesiologists. J Am Soc Echocardiogr. 2013;26:921–64.

Part III
Cardiovascular Disease Risk Management

Chapter 10
Hypertension

Akanksha Agrawal and M. Carolina Gongora Nieto

Abbreviations

ABPM	Ambulatory blood pressure monitoring
ACE	Angiotensin-converting enzyme
ARB	Angiotensin receptor blockers
ASCVD	Atherosclerotic cardiovascular disease
CAD	Coronary artery disease
CCB	Calcium channel blockers
CKD	Chronic kidney disease
DASH	Dietary Approaches to Stop Hypertension
DBP	Diastolic blood pressure
HBPM	Home blood pressure monitoring
HELLP	Hemolysis, elevated liver enzymes, low platelet count
HFpEF	Heart failure with preserved ejection fraction
HFrEF	Heart failure with reduced ejection fraction
ICH	Intracranial hemorrhage
ICU	Intensive care unit
MRC	Medical Research Council

A. Agrawal (✉) · M. C. G. Nieto
Department of Medicine, Division of Cardiology, Emory University School of Medicine, Atlanta, GA, USA
e-mail: aagra30@emory.edu; mcgongora@emory.edu

A. A. Bhargava et al. (eds.), *Handbook of Outpatient Cardiology*, https://doi.org/10.1007/978-3-030-88953-1_10

NHANES	National Health and Nutrition Examination Survey
PAD	Peripheral artery disease
SAH	Subarachnoid hemorrhage
SBP	Systolic blood pressure
SHEP	The Systolic Hypertension in the Elderly Program
SPRINT	Systolic Pressure Intervention Trial
Syst-EUR	Systolic Hypertension in Europe

Epidemiology

- Important public health challenge affecting almost 45.4% of the adult population in the United States as per National Health and Nutrition Examination Survey (NHANES) data from 2017 to 2018 [1].
- NHANES 2017–2018 survey defines hypertension as systolic blood pressure (SBP) greater than or equal to 130 mmHg or diastolic blood pressure (DBP) greater than or equal to 80 mmHg or currently taking medication to lower high blood pressure [1].
- The prevalence of hypertension is higher among men (51.0%) than women (39.7%). Overall prevalence decreased from 47.0% in 1999–2000 to 41.7% in 2013–2014 and then increased to 45.4% in 2017–2018. The increase in prevalence may partly be attributed to the lowered blood pressure threshold from 140/90 to 130/80 [1].
- Prevalence increases with age: 22.4% (aged 18–39), 54.5% (40–59), and 74.5% (60 and over).
- Prevalence of hypertension varies across different races; highest among non-Hispanic black (57.1%), followed by non-Hispanic white (43.6%) and Hispanic (43.7%) [1].

Definition and Classification

The 2017 ACC/AHA guidelines define hypertension as SBP ≥130 mmHg or DBP ≥80 mmHg [2]. Blood pressure is classified as normal, elevated, stage 1, or stage 2 hypertension

(Table 10.1). The BP read is the average of ≥2 careful readings obtained on ≥2 separate occasions, measured with proper technique.

Primary Hypertension

Formerly called essential hypertension, primary hypertension is diagnosed when there is not an identifiable anatomic or screening laboratory finding that identifies a cause of hypertension. It corresponds to approximately 90% of patients with hypertension.

Secondary Hypertension

In approximately 10% of patients with hypertension, a specific, reversible cause of hypertension can be identified. Table 10.2 lists the common causes of secondary hypertension along with their screening and diagnostic tests.

Who to screen for secondary causes of hypertension?

- Difficult to control hypertension in adults (≥3 drugs)
- New onset or abrupt onset
- Age <30 years
- Target-organ damage such as cerebral vascular disease, retinopathy, left ventricular hypertrophy, heart failure with preserved ejection fraction (HFpEF); coronary artery disease (CAD); chronic kidney disease (CKD); peripheral artery disease (PAD); albuminuria

Table 10.1 Categories of BP in adults

BP			Hypertension	
category	Normal	Elevated	Stage 1	Stage 2
SBP	<120 mm Hg	120–129 mm Hg	130–139 mm Hg	≥140 mm Hg
	and	and	or	or
DBP	<80 mm Hg	<80 mm Hg	80–89 mm Hg	≥90 mm Hg

Table 10.2 Causes of secondary hypertension and their diagnostic screening tests and additional/confirmatory tests

Cause	Screening tests	Additional/confirmatory tests
Renal parenchymal disease	Renal ultrasound	Evaluate cause of renal disease
Renovascular disease	Renal duplex Doppler ultrasound; MRA; abdominal CTA	Bilateral selective renal intra-arterial angiography
Primary aldosteronism	Plasma aldosterone/renin ratio under standardized conditions	Oral sodium loading test (with 24-h urine aldosterone) or IV saline infusion test with plasma aldosterone at 4 h of infusion, adrenal CT scan, adrenal vein sampling
Obstructive sleep apnea	Berlin Questionnaire, Epworth Sleepiness Score, overnight oximetry	Polysomnography
Drug or alcohol induced	Urinary drug screen	Response to withdrawal of suspected agent
Pheochromocytoma/ paraganglioma	24-h urinary fractionated metanephrines or plasma metanephrines under standard conditions	CT or MRI scan of abdomen/pelvis
Cushing's syndrome	Overnight 1-mg dexamethasone suppression test	24-h urinary free cortisol excretion (preferably multiple); midnight salivary cortisol

Hypothyroidism	Thyroid-stimulating hormone; free thyroxine	None
Hyperthyroidism	Thyroid-stimulating hormone; free thyroxine	Radioactive iodine uptake and scan
Aortic coarctation (undiagnosed or repaired)	Echocardiogram	Thoracic and abdominal CT angiogram or MRA
Primary hyperparathyroidism	Serum calcium	Serum parathyroid hormone
Congenital adrenal hyperplasia	Hypertension and hypokalemia with low or normal aldosterone and renin	11-beta-OH; elevated deoxycorticosterone (DOC), 11-deoxycortisol, and androgens17-alpha-OH; decreased androgens and estrogen; elevated deoxycorticosterone and corticosterone
Mineralocorticoid excess syndromes other than primary aldosteronism	Low aldosterone and renin	Urinary cortisol metabolites; genetic testing
Acromegaly	Serum growth hormone ≥1 ng/mL during oral glucose load	Elevated age- and sex-matched IGF-1 level; MRI scan of the pituitary

- Onset of diastolic hypertension in older adults
- Unprovoked or excessive hypokalemia

White Coat Hypertension/Isolated Clinic Hypertension/Office Hypertension

White coat hypertension is defined as average BP readings in the office of ≥130/80 mmHg and out of office readings <130/80 mmHg determined by home measurements or ambulatory blood pressure monitoring (ABPM). Adults with untreated systolic BP between 130 and 160 mmHg or diastolic between 80 and 100 mmHg should be screened for the presence of white coat hypertension using either daytime ABPM or home blood pressure monitoring (HBPM).

Masked Hypertension

In contrast to white coat hypertension, masked hypertension is characterized by normal BP office readings but consistently elevated out-of-office or ABPM readings.

Adults with elevated office BP (120–129/<80 mmHg) but not meeting criteria for hypertension are reasonable candidates for screening for masked hypertension with daytime ABPM or HBPM.

Resistant Hypertension

Resistant hypertension = uncontrolled blood pressure while being on ≥3 different classes of antihypertensive agents, one of them being a diuretic OR blood pressure controlled with ≥3 medications.

Clinical Pearl

The term "refractory hypertension" has been defined as failure to control BP despite use of at least five antihypertensive agents of different classes, including a long-acting thiazide-type diuretic, such as chlorthalidone, and a mineralocorticoid receptor antagonist, such as spironolactone.

Management

Who to Treat?

Non-pharmacological interventions are recommended for all patients with hypertension. Threshold to start pharmacologic therapy is defined by the calculated atherosclerotic cardiovascular disease (ASCVD) risk level. Target blood pressure of <130/80 mm Hg is recommended. Use of BP-lowering medications is recommended in following scenarios:

- Adults with established cardiovascular disease and SBP ≥130 mmHg or DBP ≥80 mmHg
- Adults with SBP ≥130 mmHg or DBP ≥80 mmHg and estimated 10-year ASCVD risk of ≥10%
- Adults with SBP ≥140 mmHg or DBP ≥90 mmHg and estimated 10-year ASCVD risk <10% [2]

Non-pharmacological Management

- All patients with BP >120/80 mmHg should receive lifestyle modification counseling.
- Non-pharmacological interventions include:
  - Weight loss
  - DASH (Dietary Approaches to Stop Hypertension) diet

  - Sodium reduction
  - Potassium supplementation
  - Increased physical activity
  - Smoking cessation
  - Reduction in alcohol consumption.

- Lifestyle changes can reduce SBP by 4–5 mmHg and DBP by 2–4 mg. Low sodium and saturated fat diet with increased fruits, vegetables, and grains consumption may decrease SBP by approximately 11 mmHg.

Pharmacological Management

- First-line antihypertensive agents include thiazide diuretics, calcium channel blockers (CCBs), angiotensin-converting enzyme (ACE) inhibitors, or angiotensin receptor blockers (ARBs). The choice of one over the other is guided by patients' comorbidities such as chronic kidney disease, diabetes, heart failure (HF), albuminuria, and race. The commonly used medications, their dosing, and side effects have been listed in Table 10.3.
- As the initial agent, the thiazide-type diuretic chlorthalidone was superior to the CCB amlodipine and ACE inhibitor lisinopril in a large head-to-head comparison study [3]. For African American patients, ACE inhibitors showed less efficacy in preventing HF and strokes when compared to CCBs [4, 5].
- Non-dihydropyridine CCBs are not recommended for treating hypertension in patients with HFrEF.
- In adults with CKD stage 3 or higher, or CKD stage 1 and 2 with albuminuria (≥300 mg/d, or ≥300 mg/g albumin-to-creatinine ratio), an ACE inhibitor slowed kidney disease progression. When an ACE inhibitor is not tolerated, an ARB should be used instead [6].
- In African American adults with hypertension, but without HF or CKD, a first-line antihypertensive agent should include a thiazide-type diuretic or CCB.

TABLE 10.3 Initial choices for antihypertensive agents and their doses, mechanism of action, and side effects

Drug class and antihypertensive agents	Usual dose	Main mechanism of action	Indications	Side effects
Thiazide-type diuretics				
Chlorthalidone	12.5–25 mg once daily	Inhibit reabsorption of sodium (Na^+) and chloride (Cl^-) ions from the distal convoluted tubules in the kidneys	First-line agent or add-on as second/third agent	Hypokalemia, hyponatremia, orthostatic hypotension, hypovolemia
Hydrochlorothiazide	12.5–50 mg once daily			
Indapamide	1.25–2.5 mg once daily			
ACE inhibitors				

(continued)

Table 10.3 (continued)

Drug class and antihypertensive agents	Usual dose	Main mechanism of action	Indications	Side effects
Benazepril	5–80 mg/day, in one or two doses	Act on the renin-angiotensin-aldosterone system (RAAS), causing vasodilation by inhibiting the formation of angiotensin II	First-line agent or add-on as second/third agent, strong evidence for use in patients with CKD with albuminuria; congestive heart failure; and after myocardial infarction	Hyperkalemia, creatinine elevation (in patients with CKD or bilateral renal artery stenosis), angioedema. Not to be used in combination with ARB or direct renin inhibitor. Contraindicated in pregnancy
Fosinopril	10–80 mg/day, in one or two doses			
Lisinopril	5–40 mg/day once daily			
Moexipril	7.5–30 mg/day, in one or two doses			
Perindopril	4–16 mg/day, in one or two doses			
Quinapril	10–80 mg/day, in one or two doses			
Ramipril	2.5–20 mg/day, in one or two doses			
Trandolapril	2–8 mg/day, in one or two doses			
Captopril	25–150 mg every 8–12 hours			
Enalapril	10–40 mg/day, in one or two doses			

ARBs				
Azilsartan	40–80 mg once daily	Selectively block the angiotensin II type 1 (AT_1) receptor, antagonize angiotensin II-induced vasoconstriction, aldosterone release, catecholamine release, arginine vasopressin release, water intake, and hypertrophic response	First-line agent or add-on as second/third agent, strong evidence for use in patients with CKD with albuminuria; congestive heart failure; and after myocardial infarction. Alternative for patients with ACE inhibitor-associated cough	Hyperkalemia, creatinine elevation (in patients with CKD or bilateral renal artery stenosis), angioedema. Not to be used in combination with ACE inhibitor or direct renin inhibitor. Contraindicated in pregnancy
Candesartan	8–32 mg/day, in one or two doses			
Eprosartan	600 mg/day, in one or two doses			
Irbesartan	150–300 mg once daily			
Losartan	25–100 mg/day, in one or two doses			
Olmesartan	20–40 mg once daily			
Telmisartan	20–80 mg once daily			
Valsartan	80–320 mg once daily			
Calcium channel blockers				
Dihydropyridine type				

Table 10.3 (continued)

Drug class and antihypertensive agents	Usual dose	Main mechanism of action	Indications	Side effects
Amlodipine	2.5–10 mg once daily	Block the inward movement of calcium by binding to the L-type "long-acting" voltage-gated calcium channels in the vascular smooth muscles	First-line agent or ad-on as second/ third agent	Pedal edema, may worsen proteinuria, may worsen left ventricular outflow tract obstruction
Felodipine	2.5–10 mg once daily			
Isradipine	5–10 mg/day, in two doses			
Nicardipine	5–20 mg once daily			
Nifedipine	30–120 mg/day, in one or two doses			
Nisoldipine	17–34 mg once daily			
Nondihydropyridine type				
Diltiazem	180 to 420 mg/day (dosing slightly varies in different brands of diltiazem available)	Have inhibitory effects on the sinoatrial (SA) and atrioventricular (AV) nodes, resulting in slowing of cardiac conduction and contractility	Tachycardia, left ventricular outflow tract obstruction, hyperdynamic cardiac function, migraine prophylaxis	Constipation, can cause heart block when combined with beta-blockers
Verapamil	Immediate release: 80–320 mg every 12 hours Extended release: 180 to 360 mg/day			

Abbreviations: *ACE* angiotensin-converting enzyme, *ARB* angiotensin receptor blocker, *CKD* chronic kidney disease

- Choosing two first-line agents of different classes, either as separate agents or in a fixed dose combination, is recommended for adults with stage 2 hypertension and an average BP more than 20/10 mmHg above their BP target.

Clinical Pearl

A combination of non-pharmacological and pharmacological interventions is used to achieve a target blood pressure of <130/80 mm Hg.

Special Populations

Elderly

- Multiple randomized clinical trials including SHEP, Syst-EUR, and MRC have shown a clear benefit in treating hypertension in older adults including those over 80 years of age [7–9]. The aim of therapy in these trials was to either reduce SBP by 20 mmHg or below 160 mmHg.
- In the Systolic Pressure Intervention Trial (SPRINT), at 3.1 years, rates of both the primary cardiovascular endpoint and all-cause mortality were significantly lower among those assigned more intensive group (goal of <120 mmHg; mean achieved systolic blood pressure 123 mmHg) versus less intensive group (goal of <140 mmHg; mean achieved systolic blood pressure 135 mmHg) systolic blood pressure lowering (2.6 versus 3.8 percent and 1.8 versus 2.6 percent, respectively) [10].
- As per the most updated 2017 ACC/AHA guidelines, in noninstitutionalized ambulatory community-dwelling adults (≥65 years of age), a goal of SBP <130 mmHg is recommended [2].

Women and Pregnancy

- Per a large meta-analysis including 31 randomized controlled trials (RCTs), no significant differences in cardiovascular disease outcomes were observed between men and women with hypertension [11].
- Women with hypertension who become pregnant or are planning pregnancy should be transitioned to nifedipine and/or labetalol during pregnancy. Agents such as hydralazine and methyldopa are also acceptable.
- Beta-blockers should be continued in patients with concomitant HF, CAD, or other indications for beta-blockers. Atenolol should not be used as it can cross the utero-placental barrier and is associated with low birth weight.
- ACE inhibitors, ARBs, and direct renin inhibitors should not be used as antihypertensive agents during pregnancy (Class III – Harm).

Post-kidney Transplantation

- Patients with kidney transplant have a high incidence of hypertension due to preexisting kidney disease, immunosuppressive medication (calcineurin inhibitors), and presence of allograft pathology.
- Post-transplant, treatment of hypertension with CCB is recommended based on improved GFR and kidney survival [12].

Cerebrovascular Disease

- Management of BP in patients with stroke is complex and challenging due to its heterogenous causes and hemodynamic consequences. The stroke type, acuity, and therapeutic objectives guide the management of BP in a patient with stroke. Most of the management of BP in an acute stroke is performed in the inpatient setting. For the management of BP in the setting of acute intracerebral hemorrhage and acute ischemic stroke (within 72 hours of symptom onset), please refer to the Handbook of Inpatient Cardiology.

BP management after 72 hours in a patient with stroke: In patients with previously diagnosed or treated hypertension, the BP goal remains <130/80 mmHg. In patients with no previous history of hypertension, with established SBP ≥140 mmHg or DBP ≥90 mmHg, antihypertensive treatment should be initiated aiming for a BP goal of <130/80 mmHg. If SBP <140 mmHg and DBP <90 mmHg, the usefulness of starting antihypertensive treatment is not well established (Class IIb).

Hypertensive Crisis

- Hypertensive crisis is a sudden and severe elevation in blood pressure with or without associated target-organ dysfunction. Hypertensive crises are managed in the inpatient setting; however, it is important to recognize this entity in the outpatient setting for timely triaging and management.
- Hypertensive emergencies are characterized by BP >180/110 mm Hg with presence of target-organ dysfunction. Hypertensive urgencies on the other hand have similar elevation in BP but are not associated with target-organ dysfunction [13].
- Target-organ dysfunction can include neurologic (cerebral infarction, hypertensive encephalopathy, intracranial hemorrhage (ICH), or subarachnoid hemorrhage (SAH)), cardiovascular (acute pulmonary edema, acute coronary syndrome), renal (acute kidney injury), hepatic (liver enzyme elevation, hemolysis, low platelet count during pregnancy (HELLP syndrome)), ocular (retinal hemorrhage or exudate), and vascular manifestations (aortic dissection, eclampsia).
- Management of patients with hypertensive emergency requires admission to an intensive care unit (ICU) with continuous blood pressure monitoring and parenteral

administration of antihypertensive agents. For further details on management of hypertensive crisis, please refer to the Handbook of Inpatient Cardiology.

Clinical Pearl

Hypertensive crises are sudden, severe elevations in blood pressure with or without associated target-organ dysfunction. Management of patients with hypertensive emergency requires admission to intensive care unit for continuous blood pressure monitoring and parenteral administration of antihypertensive agent.

Key Learning Points

- Normal BP is defined as <120/<80 mm Hg; elevated BP 120–129/<80 mm Hg; hypertension stage 1 is 130–139 or 80–89 mm Hg, and hypertension stage 2 is ≥140 or ≥90 mm Hg.
- First-line antihypertensive agents include thiazide diuretics, calcium channel blockers (CCBs), angiotensin-converting enzyme (ACE) inhibitors, or angiotensin receptor blockers (ARBs). The choice of one over the other is guided by patients' comorbidities such as chronic kidney disease, diabetes, heart failure (HF), albuminuria, and race.

References

1. Ostchega Y, Fryar CD, Nwankwo T, Nguyen DT. Hypertension prevalence among adults aged 18 and over: United States, 2017–2018. NCHS Data Brief No. April 2020;364. https://www.cdc.gov/nchs/products/databriefs/db364.htm
2. Whelton PK, Carey RM, Aronow WS, Casey DE, Collins KJ, Himmelfarb CD, DePalma SM, Gidding S, Jamerson KA, Jones DW, MacLaughlin EJ, Muntner P, Ovbiagele B, Smith

SC, Spencer CC, Stafford RS, Taler SJ, Thomas RJ, Williams KA, Williamson JD, Wright JT. 2017 ACC/AHA/AAPA/ABC/ACPM/AGS/APhA/ASH/ASPC/NMA/PCNA guideline for the prevention, detection, evaluation, and management of high blood pressure in adults. J Am Coll Cardiol. 2018;71(19):e127–248. https://doi.org/10.1016/j.jacc.2017.11.006.

3. ALLHAT Officers and Coordinators for the ALLHAT Collaborative Research Group. Major outcomes in high-risk hypertensive patients randomized to angiotensin-converting enzyme inhibitor or calcium channel blocker vs diuretic: the Antihypertensive and Lipid-Lowering Treatment to Prevent Heart Attack Trial (ALLHAT). JAMA. 2002;288:2981–97.
4. Ogedegbe G, Shah NR, Phillips C, et al. Comparative effectiveness of angiotensin-converting enzyme inhibitor-based treatment on cardiovascular outcomes in hypertensive blacks versus whites. J Am Coll Cardiol. 2015;66:1224–33.
5. Leenen FHH, Nwachuku CE, Black HR, et al. Clinical events in high-risk hypertensive patients randomly assigned to calcium channel blocker versus angiotensin-converting enzyme inhibitor in the Antihypertensive and Lipid-Lowering Treatment to Prevent Heart Attack Trial. Hypertension. 2006;48:374–84.
6. Contreras G, Greene T, Agodoa LY, et al. Blood pressure control, drug therapy, and kidney disease. Hypertension. 2005;46:44–50.
7. Probstfield JL, Applegate WB, Borhani NO, David Curb J, Cutler JA, Davis BR, Furberg CD, Morton Hawkins C, Lakatos E, Page LB, Mitchell Perry H, Schron E, McFate Smith W. The systolic hypertension in the elderly program (SHEP): an intervention trial on isolated systolic hypertension, clinical and experimental hypertension. Part A: Theory Pract. 1989;11(5–6):973–89.
8. Staessen JA, Fagard R, Thijs L, Celis H, Arabidze GG, Birkenhager WH, Bulpitt CJ, de Leeuw PW, Dollery CT, Fletcher AE, Forette F, Leonetti G, Nachev C, ETO B, Rosenfeld J, Rodicio JL, Tuomilehto J, Zanchetti A. Systolic hypertension in Europe (Syst-Eur) trial investigators. Randomized double- blind comparison of placebo and active treatment for older patients with isolated systolic hypertension. Lancet. 1997;350(9080):757–64.
9. MRC Working Party. Medical research council trial of treatment of hypertension in older adults: principal results. BMJ. 1992;304(6824):405–12.
10. The SPRINT Research Group. A randomized trial of intensive versus standard blood- pressure control. N Engl J Med. 2015;373:2103–16.

11. Turnbull F, Woodward M, Neal B, et al. Do men and women respond differently to blood pressure-lowering treatment? Results of prospectively designed overviews of randomized trials. Eur Heart J. 2008;29:2669–80.
12. Cross NB, Webster AC, Masson P, et al. Antihypertensive treatment for kidney transplant recipients. Cochrane Database Syst Rev. 2009;2009(3):CD003598.
13. Benken ST, Hypertensive Emergencies. CCSAP 2018 Book 1, Medical Issues in the ICU.

Chapter 11
Dyslipidemia

Aneesha Thobani and Nanette K. Wenger

Abbreviations

ApoB	Apolipoprotein B
ASCVD	Atherosclerotic cardiovascular disease
CKD	Chronic kidney disease
DLD	Dyslipidemia
FH	Familial hypercholesterolemia
HDL-C	High-density lipoprotein-cholesterol
LDL-C	Low-density lipoprotein-cholesterol
Lp(a)	Lipoprotein(a)
SAMS	Statin-associated muscle symptoms
TC	Total cholesterol
TG	Triglycerides

Introduction and Definitions

- Dyslipidemia (DLD) is a metabolic derangement causing a persistent elevation in plasma cholesterol and/or triglycerides. The three manifestations of dyslipidemia are:

A. Thobani (✉) · N. K. Wenger
Department of Medicine, Division of Cardiology, Emory University School of Medicine, Atlanta, GA, USA
e-mail: aneesha.thobani@emory.edu; nwenger@emory.edu

A. A. Bhargava et al. (eds.), *Handbook of Outpatient Cardiology*, https://doi.org/10.1007/978-3-030-88953-1_11

  - Hypercholesterolemia
  - Hypertriglyceridemia
  - Mixed hyperlipidemia [1, 2]

- Common manifestations of DLD include:

  - High total cholesterol (TC)
  - High triglycerides (TG)
  - High low-density lipoprotein-cholesterol (LDL-C)
  - Low high-density lipoprotein-cholesterol (HDL-C)
  - Elevated non-high-density lipoprotein-cholesterol (non-HDL-C)
  - Altered lipoprotein compositions such as increased apolipoprotein B (apoB) and lipoprotein(a) [Lp(a)] [2, 3]

- Primary disorders of lipid metabolism include familial hypercholesterolemia (FH), familial combined hyperlipidemia, and familial dysbetalipoproteinemia [4].
- The most common primary disorder is FH, which affects ~1 in 200 individuals; most cases are due to a heterozygous mutation. Combined hyperlipidemia affects ~1 in 100 individuals [5, 6].
- Patients with phenotype for FH (LDL-C > 190 mg/dL) have a 20-fold increased risk for cardiovascular disease and accelerated atherosclerosis [7].
- Secondary dyslipidemia can be a consequence of obesity, diabetes mellitus type I or II, hypothyroidism, obstructive liver diseases, chronic kidney disease, and certain drugs (i.e., progestins, androgens, beta-blockers, anabolic steroids, retinoids, cyclosporine, and phenothiazines) [8].
- Table 11.1 shows reference values for TG, LDL-C, and HDL-C levels [8, 9] for patients without known atherosclerotic cardiovascular disease (ASCVD).

Dyslipidemia and Cardiovascular Disease

- ASCVD remains the leading cause of morbidity and mortality globally. In the United States, this results in an annual estimated cost of >$200 billion [9, 10].

TABLE 11.1 Low-density lipoprotein-cholesterol (LDL-C), low high-density lipoprotein-cholesterol (HDL-C)

Fasting triglyceride level	Normal: <150 mg/dL Mild hypertriglyceridemia: 150–175 mg/dL Moderate hypertriglyceridemia: 175–499 mg/dL Severe hypertriglyceridemia: >500 mg/dL
LDL-C level	Optimal: <100 mg/dL Near optimal: 100–129 mg/dL Borderline high: 130 to 159 mg/dL High: 160–189 mg/dL Very high: >190 mg/dL
HDL-C level	Low: <40 mg/dL High: >60 mg/dL

- It is crucial to screen, diagnose,and treat dyslipidemia in the general population due to the high attributable risk for atherosclerotic and non-atherosclerotic cardiovascular disease.
- Dyslipidemia increases atherosclerosis and ASCVD risk by accelerating the atherogenic process.

Therapeutic Agents

- Statin therapies have a proven substantial benefit in the primary and secondary prevention of ASCVD, and recent evidence reveals that this benefit far outweighs potential risks [9].
- Other lipid-lowering therapies include:
  - LDL-C-lowering agents:

    Ezetimibe
    Bile acid sequestrants
    Proprotein convertase subtilisin/kexin type 9 (PCSK9) inhibitors

  - Triglyceride-lowering agents:

Fibrates
Niacin
Icosapent ethyl (a pure omega-3 fatty acid derivative of EPA) [9]

- Statins remain the cornerstone of treatment. Table 11.2 outlines the currently available statins with intensity levels [9].
- High-intensity statins have a ≥50% reduction of LDL-C, moderate-intensity statins result in 30–49% reduction of LDL-C, and low intensity confers a <30% reduction of LDL-C [9].
- Statins interact with several medications. Risk mitigation strategies should be used when co-prescribing with one of these medications (either limiting the dose, avoiding co-administration, or using an alternative statin which does not have a direct effect). Table 11.3 lists common medications [9].

TABLE 11.2 Intensity of statin therapy with current available statins

	High intensity	**Moderate intensity**	**Low intensity**
Statins	Atorvastatin 40 mg, 80 mg Rosuvastatin 20 mg, 40 mg	Atorvastatin 10–20 mg Rosuvastatin 5–10 mg Simvastatin 20–40 mg	Simvastatin 10 mg
	–	Pravastatin 40–80 mg Lovastatin 40 mg Fluvastatin 80 mg Pitavastatin 1–4 mg	Pravastatin 10–20 mg Lovastatin 20 mg Fluvastatin 20–40 mg

Table 11.3 Adapted from 2019 cholesterol guidelines[6] Statins requiring a risk mitigation approach

Amiodarone	Darunavir plus ritonavir	Nefazodone
Amlodipine	Diltiazem	Nelfinavir
Atazanavir plus ritonavir	Dronedarone	Niacin
Boceprevir	Erythromycin	Posaconazole
Clarithromycin	Fenofibrate/ fenofibric acid	Ranolazine
Cobicistat-containing products	Fluconazole	Rifampin
Colchicine	Fosamprenavir	Saquinavir plus ritonavir
Cyclosporine	Gemfibrozil[a]	Telaprevir
Danazol	Itraconazole	Telithromycin
	Ketoconazole	Tipranavir plus ritonavir
	Lomitapide	Verapamil
	Lopinavir plus ritonavir	Voriconazole
		Warfarin

[a]Absolutely do not use with any statin

Guidelines

- The American College of Cardiology/American Heart Association (ACC/AHA) 2019 combined cholesterol guidelines emphasize the importance of a heart-healthy lifestyle throughout the lifetime.
- In patients with clinical ASCVD, high-risk ASCVD, severe primary hypercholesterolemia, and populations with diabetes mellitus, statin therapy is recommended as first line. Table 11.4 highlights primary and Table 11.5 highlights secondary prevention strategies.

Clinical Pearl

In patients (age 40–75 years) without known ASCVD, the first step is to use the pooled cohort equation (PCE) calculator to calculate an individual's ASCVD risk score which is divided into low risk (<5%), borderline risk (5 to <7.5%), intermediate risk (≥7.5 to <20%), and high risk (≥20%). In patients with low and intermediate categories, the risk-enhancing factors (outlined in Table 11.6) should be considered.

Table 11.4 Primary prevention guidelines from ACC/AHA 2019 for initiating statin therapy in patients without prior ASCVD

Risk	Recommendation
Low risk (<5%)	Lifestyle to reduce risk factors (Class I)
Borderline risk (5 to <7.5%)	If risk enhancers present, consider moderate-intensity statin (Class IIb)
Intermediate risk (≥7.5 to <20%)	If risk estimate + risk enhancers present, initiate moderate-intensity statin to reduce LDL-C by 30–49% (Class I) If risk uncertain, obtain calcium score (CAC). If CAC = 0, no statin. CAC 1–99, favor statin. CAC 100+, initiate statin therapy
High risk (≥20%)	Initiate statin to reduce LDL-C ≥ 50% (Class I)
LDL-C ≥190 mg/dL	No risk assessment; high-intensity statin (Class I)
Diabetes mellitus (age 40–75 y)	At least moderate-intensity statin (Class I) Additional risk-enhancing factors present = consider high intensity
Age >75 y	Clinical assessment, risk discussion (shared decision-making)

LDL-C low-density lipoprotein-cholesterol

TABLE 11.5 Secondary prevention guidelines for known clinical ASCVD as per ACC/AHA guidelines, statin as first line after healthy lifestyle emphasis

Very high risk[a] ASCVD	**ASCVD not at very high risk**
Initiate high-intensity or maximally tolerated statin (Class I)	Initiate high-intensity statin with goal LDL-C reduction of ≥50% (Class I) If high-intensity statin not tolerated, use moderate intensity (Class I)
If on maximal statin and LDL-C ≥70 mg/dL, add ezetimibe (Class IIa)	If on maximal statin and LDL-C ≥70 mg/dL, add ezetimibe (Class IIb)
If on maximal statin + ezetimibe and LDL-C ≥70 mg/dL, add PCSK9-I (Class IIb)	

Clinical ASCVD is acute coronary syndrome, history of myocardial infarction, stable or unstable angina, coronary or other arterial revascularizations, stroke, transient ischemic attack, or peripheral artery disease, all of atherosclerotic origin. In age >75 y, okay to initiate and/or continue moderate- or high-intensity statin for secondary prevention (Class IIa)

[a]Very high risk = multiple major ASCVD events or 1 major ASCVD event and multiple high-risk conditions. Low-density lipoprotein-cholesterol (LDL-C), proprotein convertase subtilisin/kexin type 9 inhibitors (PCSK9-I)

Monitoring

- Monitoring response to LDL-C lowering agents is recommended and should be undertaken after initiation of agents or addition of agents.

Clinical Pearl

- Effects should be assessed by measuring fasting or non-fasting lipid levels 4–12 weeks after starting statin therapy or after a dose adjustment. After that, consider measuring every 3–12 months based on need to assess adherence or safety [9].

Table 11.6 Risk enhancers as outlined by ACC/AHA Guidelines which confer additional ASCVD risk

Risk enhancers
Family history of premature ASCVD
Persistently elevated LDL-C ≥160 mg/dL
Chronic kidney disease
Metabolic syndrome
Conditions specific to women
Preeclampsia
Premature menopause
Inflammatory diseases
Rheumatoid arthritis
Psoriasis
HIV
Ethnicity
South Asian Ancestry
Lipid/biomarkers:
Persistently elevated triglycerides (≥175 mg/dL)
In select individuals if measured:
Hs-CRP ≥2.0 mg/L
Lp(a) >50 mg/dL
ApoB ≥130 mg/dL
Ankle-brachial index (ABI) <0.9

ApoB Apolipoprotein B, *LDL-C* low-density lipoprotein-cholesterol, *hs-CRP* high-sensitivity C-reactive protein, *(Lp(a))* lipoprotein (a)

Special Populations

- Special consideration should be given to the following:
  - Elderly (age >75 years) patients
  - Racial/ethnic backgrounds
  - Women
  - Adults with HIV
  - Adults with CKD
- See Table 11.7 for a summary of these populations.

TABLE 11.7 Special populations to consider for lipid-lowering agents, based on ACC/AHA 2019 guidelines

Population	Recommendation
Elderly (age >75 y)	1. If LDL-C 70–189 mg/dL, reasonable to start moderate-intensity statin 2. Stop statin if functional decline, frailty, or reduced life expectancy 3. Adults 76–80, reasonable to measure CAC to reclassify risk
Specific ethnic/racial backgrounds	1. Reasonable to review race/ethnic features that influence ASCVD risk 2. Heightened risk of ASCVD in South Asians 3. Increased sensitivity to statins in East Asians 4. Increased prevalence of hypertension in Blacks 5. High rates of risk factors for ASCVD in Native Americans/Alaskan natives
Women	1. Consider conditions specific to women such as premature menopause (age < 40 y), history of pregnancy-associated disorders (hypertension, preeclampsia, gestation diabetes mellitus, small for gestational age infants, preterm deliveries 2. Women of childbearing age on statin therapy must be counseled to use contraception 3. Women who plan to become pregnant and are on statin should stop the agent 1–2 months before pregnancy is attempted or stop statin as soon as pregnancy is identified
Patients with HIV	1. Inflammatory conditions, especially HIV is risk enhancing. Start statin if ASCVD score >7.5% 2. Obtain baseline lipid panel for all patients with HIV
Patients with CKD	1. Adults 40–75 y with LDL-C 70–189 mg/dL with ASCVD score >7.5%, start moderate-intensity statin (if not on dialysis or kidney transplantation) 2. Moderate-intensity statin can be combined with ezetimibe

LDL-C low-density lipoprotein-cholesterol, *CAC* coronary artery calcium, *HIV* human immunodeficiency virus, *CKD* chronic kidney disease

Triglyceride-Lowering Therapy

- Hypertriglyceridemia (HTG) is a distinct lipid abnormality, and certain triglyceride-lowering agents have been found to reduce either ASCVD risk or the risk of pancreatitis. These include prescription strength omega-3 fatty acids and fibrates such as fenofibrate and gemfibrozil, which are peroxisome proliferator-activated receptor-α (PPAR-α) agonists.
- Recent trials have shown benefit with icosapent ethyl (a pure omega-3 fatty acid derivative of EPA). REDUCE-IT showed a 25% reduction in the risk of ischemic events and CVD death with 4 grams of icosapent ethyl superimposed on use of moderate- to high-intensity statins in high-risk patients with either ASCVD or diabetes mellitus with elevated fasting triglyceride levels of 135–499 mg/dL [11]. However, guidelines have yet to endorse its use, and it should be considered on a case-by-case basis.
- Statins remain the first-line therapy for TG lowering. See Table 11.8 for the most recent recommendations from the American Heart Association.
- Fibric acid derivatives (fenofibrate and gemfibrozil) are renally excreted, and the safety of these needs to be considered with possible dose adjustments, particularly in those on statin therapy.

Clinical Pearl

- The National Kidney Foundation and National Lipid Association recommend dose adjustment of fibrates based on estimated glomerular filtration rate (eGFR).
- Fenofibrate is the preferred fibrate to use with statin therapy; gemfibrozil inhibits the glucuronidation of statins which increases the blood level of the statin and therefore increases the risk of myopathy and rhabdomyolysis. Gemfibrozil should not be combined with statin therapy [12, 13].

Table 11.8 Highlights the treatment for moderate and severe hypertriglyceridemia as outlined by the most recent ACC/AHA guidelines [6]

Recommendations for hypertriglyceridemia	
Moderate hypertriglyceridemia (fasting or non-fasting TG 175–499 mg/dL)	Age >20 y: treat lifestyle factors (obesity, metabolic syndrome) and secondary factors Age 40–75 y: If ASCVD risk >7.5%, favor initiation of statin with lifestyle modification
Severe hypertriglyceridemia (fasting or non-fasting TG ≥500 mg/dL)	Age 40–75 y: Address reversible causes, initiate or intensify statin therapy If TG >1000 mg/dL: implement very low-fat diet, avoid refined carbohydrates and consumption of omega-3 fatty acids, and fibrate therapy can be considered

Addressing Side Effects

- Statin therapy is safe and generally well tolerated. Statin-associated side effects may be present in a few patients [9].
- Statin-associated muscle symptoms (SAMS) are the most common side effect and include myalgias (observationally reported in 5–20% of patients).
- The rarer SAMS:
  - Myositis/myopathy with elevated creatine kinase (CK)
  - Rhabdomyolysis (CK >10x upper limit of normal [ULN])
  - Statin-associated autoimmune myopathy (only in case reports)
- Statins have also been associated with new-onset diabetes mellitus in predisposed individuals with BMI > 30, fasting glucose >100, metabolic syndrome, and prediabetes [9].
- Observational studies report transaminase elevation >3× ULN and rarely hepatic failure, but these are rare to infrequent occurrences [9].

- To address SAMS, a statin rechallenge should be considered with an alternative statin, or a dose reduction with or without decrease in frequency of administration.
- It is crucial to have a clinician-patient risk discussion (CPRD) regarding potential adverse effects, drug-drug interactions, ASCVD risk reduction benefit, and patient preferences to promote a shared decision-making (SDM) process before prescribing therapy.

Emerging Lipid-Lowering Agents

- Several newer lipid-lowering agents are on the horizon. Several new therapies target atherogenic lipids (LDL-C, Lp(a), non-HDL-C, remnants) using a variety of different mechanisms [14].
- These newer agents are promising and may prove beneficial for patients, highlighted in Table 11.9.

Key Learning Points

1. Dyslipidemia (DLD) is a metabolic derangement causing a persistent elevation in plasma cholesterol and/or triglycerides. The three manifestations of dyslipidemia are hypercholesterolemia, hypertriglyceridemia, and mixed hyperlipidemia.
2. It is crucial to screen, diagnose, and treat dyslipidemia in the general population due to the high attributable risk for cardiovascular disease. Dyslipidemia increases atherosclerosis and ASCVD risk by accelerating the atherogenic process.
3. Statin therapies have a substantial benefit in the primary and secondary prevention of ASCVD, and recent evidence reveals that this benefit far outweighs potential risks.

TABLE 11.9 Current and new lipid-lowering therapeutics

Therapeutic drug	Major effect on plasma lipids/proteins
Statins	↓ LDL ↓ TC
Fibrates	↓ TG
Omega-3 fatty acids	↓ TG
PCSK9 inhibitors	↓ LDL ↓ Lp(a)
Bempedoic acid	↓ LDL ↓ non-HDL
Inclisiran	↓ PCSK9
AKACEA-APO(a)-LRx	↓ Lp(a)
Evinacumab	↓ TG
Volanesorsen	↓ TG

LDL low-density lipoprotein, *TC* total cholesterol, *TG* triglyceride, *PCSK9* proprotein convertase subtilisin/kexin type 9, *(Lp(a))* lipoprotein(a)

References

1. Adhyaru BB, Jacobson TA. Safety and efficacy of statin therapy. Nat Rev Cardiol. 2018;15(12):757–69. https://doi.org/10.1038/s41569-018-0098-5.
2. Jacobson TA, Maki KC, Orringer CE, Jones PH, Kris-Etherton P, Sikand G, et al. National lipid association recommendations for patient-centered management of dyslipidemia: part 2. J Clin Lipidol. 2015;9(6 Suppl):S1–122.e1. https://doi.org/10.1016/j.jacl.2015.09.002.
3. Wilson DP, Jacobson TA, Jones PH, Koschinsky ML, McNeal CJ, Nordestgaard BG, et al. Use of lipoprotein(a) in clinical practice: a biomarker whose time has come. A scientific statement from the National Lipid Association. J Clin Lipidol. 2019;13(3):374–92. https://doi.org/10.1016/j.jacl.2019.04.010.
4. Fredrickson DS. An international classification of hyperlipidemias and hyperlipoproteinemias. Ann Intern Med. 1971;75(3):471–2. https://doi.org/10.7326/0003-4819-75-3-471.
5. Nordestgaard BG, Chapman MJ, Humphries SE, Ginsberg HN, Masana L, Descamps OS, et al. Familial hypercholesterolaemia is underdiagnosed and undertreated in the general population:

guidance for clinicians to prevent coronary heart disease: consensus statement of the European Atherosclerosis Society. Eur Heart J. 2013;34(45):3478–90a. https://doi.org/10.1093/eurheartj/eht273.

6. Benjamin EJ, Muntner P, Alonso A, Bittencourt MS, Callaway CW, Carson AP, et al. Heart disease and stroke statistics-2019 update: a report from the American heart association. Circulation. 2019;139(10):e56–e528. https://doi.org/10.1161/CIR.0000000000000659.
7. Goldberg AC, Hopkins PN, Toth PP, Ballantyne CM, Rader DJ, Robinson JG, et al. Familial hypercholesterolemia: screening, diagnosis and management of pediatric and adult patients: clinical guidance from the National Lipid Association Expert Panel on Familial Hypercholesterolemia. J Clin Lipidol. 2011;5(3 Suppl):S1–8. https://doi.org/10.1016/j.jacl.2011.04.003.
8. Expert Panel on Detection Ea, and Treatment of High Blood Cholesterol in Adults. Executive summary of the third report of the national cholesterol education program (NCEP) expert panel on detection, evaluation, and treatment of high blood cholesterol in adults (adult treatment panel III). JAMA. 2001;285(19):2486–97. https://doi.org/10.1001/jama.285.19.2486.
9. Grundy SM, Stone NJ, Bailey AL, Beam C, Birtcher KK, Blumenthal RS, et al. 2018 AHA/ACC/AACVPR/AAPA/ABC/ACPM/ADA/AGS/APhA/ASPC/NLA/PCNA guideline on the management of blood cholesterol: executive summary: a report of the American College of Cardiology/American Heart Association Task Force on Clinical Practice Guidelines. J Am Coll Cardiol. 2019;73(24):3168–209. https://doi.org/10.1016/j.jacc.2018.11.002.
10. Jialal I, Devaraj S. AHA/ACC/Multisociety cholesterol guidelines: highlights. Ther Adv Cardiovasc Dis. 2019;13:1753944719881579. https://doi.org/10.1177/1753944719881579.
11. Bhatt DL, Steg PG, Miller M, Brinton EA, Jacobson TA, Ketchum SB, et al. Cardiovascular risk reduction with icosapent ethyl for hypertriglyceridemia. N Engl J Med. 2019;380(1):11–22. https://doi.org/10.1056/NEJMoa1812792.
12. Group KDOQIKD. K/DOQI clinical practice guidelines for management of dyslipidemias in patients with kidney disease. Am J Kidney Dis. 2003;41(4 Suppl 3):I–IV, S1-91.

13. Jacobson TA, Ito MK, Maki KC, Orringer CE, Bays HE, Jones PH, et al. National lipid association recommendations for patient-centered management of dyslipidemia: part 1--full report. J Clin Lipidol. 2015;9(2):129–69. https://doi.org/10.1016/j.jacl.2015.02.003.
14. Agarwala A, Shapiro MD. Emerging strategies for the management of atherogenic dyslipidaemia. Eur Cardiol. 2020;15:1–3. https://doi.org/10.15420/ecr.2019.16.

Chapter 12
Hypoglycemic Therapies and Reducing CVD Risk

Inbar Raber and Eli V. Gelfand

Abbreviations

ADA	American Diabetes Association
ASCVD	Atherosclerotic cardiovascular disease
BMI	Body mass index
CV	Cardiovascular
DKA	Diabetic ketoacidosis
DPP-4	Dipeptidyl peptidase-4
ESRD	End-stage renal disease
FDA	Food and Drug Administration
GLP-1R	Glucagon-like peptide-1 receptor
GFR	Glomerular filtration rate
HF	Heart failure
HFrEF	Heart failure with reduced ejection fraction
MACE	Major adverse cardiovascular events
MEN2	Multiple endocrine neoplasia type 2
MI	Myocardial infarction
NYHA	New York Heart Association
SGLT2	Sodium glucose co-transporter 2

I. Raber (✉) · E. V. Gelfand
Department of Medicine, Division of Cardiology, Beth Israel Deaconess Medical Center, Harvard Medical School, Boston, MA, USA
e-mail: iraber@bidmc.harvard.edu; egelfand@bidmc.harvard.edu

A. A. Bhargava et al. (eds.), *Handbook of Outpatient Cardiology*, https://doi.org/10.1007/978-3-030-88953-1_12

T2DM	Type 2 diabetes mellitus
UKPDS	United Kingdom Prospective Diabetes Study

Introduction

Cardiovascular disease is a major cause of morbidity and mortality among patients with type 2 diabetes mellitus. Cardiovascular preventive strategies should first emphasize lifestyle modifications, blood pressure control, and lipid-lowering therapies. In addition, certain hypoglycemic therapies have emerged as having cardioprotective properties for diabetic patients. Metformin, sodium glucose co-transporter 2 (SGLT2) inhibitors, and glucagon-like peptide 1 receptor (GLP-1R) agonists are currently known to confer cardiovascular benefits to patients with diabetes (Fig. 12.1). More recently, randomized control trials demonstrated that for SGLT2 inhibitors these cardiovascular benefits extend to patients with HFrEF, regardless of diabetic status.

Clinical Pearl
Consider metformin, SGLT2 inhibitors, and GLP-1R agonists to reduce the risk of cardiovascular events in patients with type 2 diabetes mellitus.

Metformin

Metformin lowers blood glucose by decreasing hepatic glucose production and intestinal absorption of glucose. Observational and clinical trial evidence have suggested metformin has potential cardiovascular benefits in diabetic patients [1]. The American Diabetes Association (ADA) currently recommends metformin as the preferred initial pharmacologic treatment for all T2DM patients with GFR > 30 based on strong evidence of its long-term safety and efficacy [2].

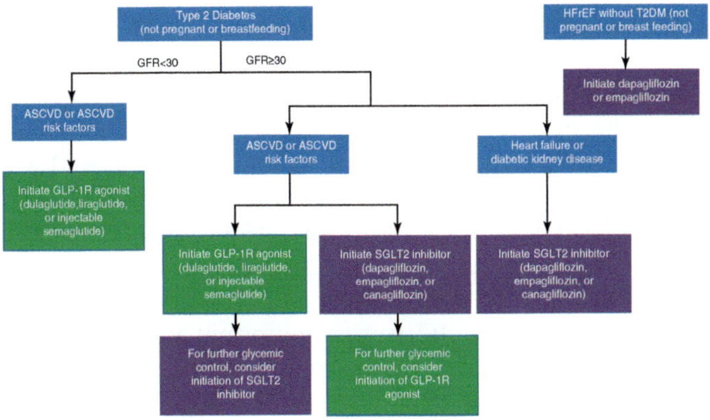

FIGURE 12.1 Algorithm for GLP-1R agonist and SGLT2 inhibitor prescribing in patients with known CVD or CVD risk factors

However, the most recent European Society of Cardiology (ESC) guidelines endorse initiation of monotherapy with SGLT2 inhibitors or GLP-1R agonists in drug-naive patients with ASCVD or high CV risk. In patients without ASCVD or CV risk, the ESC guidelines continue to recommend metformin monotherapy as the initial hypoglycemic agent [3].

Reduction of Cardiovascular Events in Patients with T2DM

An analysis of patients included in the United Kingdom Prospective Diabetes Study (UKPDS) found that overweight patients with T2DM randomized to metformin therapy rather than conventional dietary therapy had a reduced rate of MI by 33% and death from any cause by 27% over a median follow-up of 10 years [4]. A systematic review and meta-analysis of two randomized control trials and three observational studies found that metformin had a greater reduction in cardiovascular mortality compared to sulfonylureas [1].

Contraindications and Precautions

Metformin is contraindicated in patients with hypersensitivity to the drug, GFR <30, and acute or chronic metabolic acidosis. Long-term use of metformin can be associated with B12 deficiency, and surveillance of B12 levels should be considered for patients on metformin. Metformin has a pregnancy category B designation and should not be used during pregnancy unless strongly indicated. The most commonly experienced adverse effects with metformin are gastrointestinal including nausea, vomiting, and diarrhea [2].

Sodium Glucose Co-transporter 2 (SGLT2) Inhibitors

SGLT2 inhibitors exert their hypoglycemic effect by blocking glucose reabsorption in the proximal renal tubule and thus promoting glucosuria. While the cardioprotective mechanisms of SGLT2 inhibitors are not fully elucidated, certain favorable cardiovascular effects of SGLT2 inhibitors have been demonstrated, including improvements in ventricular loading conditions, changes in myocardial metabolism, and reduction in myocardial fibrosis [2, 5, 6].

Reduction of Cardiovascular Events in Patients with T2DM

Multiple randomized control trials have demonstrated that SGLT2 inhibitors reduce cardiovascular morbidity in diabetic patients (Table 12.1):

- *Empagliflozin*: The EMPA-REG OUTCOME (Empagliflozin CV Outcome Event Trial in T2D Patients) trial randomized patients with T2DM to empagliflozin or placebo. Empagliflozin was associated with a 15% reduction in the incidence of major adverse cardiovascular events,

TABLE 12.1 SGLT2 inhibitors with cardiovascular benefit

	Canagliflozin	**Dapagliflozin**	**Empagliflozin**
Dose for cardiovascular benefit	100 mg daily	10 mg daily	10 mg daily
FDA indications for cardiovascular benefits	1. Glycemic control 2. Reduction in MI, stroke, CV death in adults with T2DM and CV disease (CANVAS) 3. Reduction in HF hospitalizations, ESRD, and worsening kidney function in patients with T2DM and diabetic kidney disease (CREDENCE)	1. Glycemic control 2. Reduction in HF hospitalization in adults with T2DM and CV disease or CV risk factors (DECLARE) 3. Reduction in CV death and HF hospitalization for adults with HFrEF, with or without T2DM (DAPA-HF)	1. Glycemic control 2. Reduction in CV death in adults with T2DM and CV disease (EMPA-REG) 3. Reduction in CV death and HF hospitalization for adults with HFrEF, with or without T2DM (EMPEROR-reduced)

(continued)

TABLE 12.1 (continued)

	Canagliflozin	Dapagliflozin	Empagliflozin
Contraindications	1. Hypersensitivity 2. Pregnancy/breastfeeding 3. ESRD on dialysis 4. Initiation is not recommended for low GFR (GFR <30 for canagliflozin, GFR<20 for empagliflozin for heart failure and GFR<30 for empagliflozin for glycemic control and GFR <25 for dapagliflozin for cardiovascular benefit and GFR <45 for dapagliflozin for glycemic control		
Precautions	*Intravascular volume depletion*: Consider empiric decrease in diuretic dose *Hypoglycemia*: Consider empiric decrease in insulin and decrease or discontinue insulin secretagogues *DKA (including euglycemic DKA)*: Monitor for ketoacidosis and discontinue 3 days prior to surgery to prevent postoperative ketoacidosis *Amputation risk*: Use with caution with patients with lower limb amputation, PVD, soft tissue infection, neuropathy, and foot ulcers *Infections*: Monitor for genital mycotic infections, urinary tract infections, soft tissue infections, and lower limb ulcerations *Bone fractures*: Monitor for bone fracture (canagliflozin)		

Ongoing areas of investigation	Heart failure with reduced or preserved ejection fraction (CHIEF-HF)	Acute myocardial infarction (DAPA-MI), heart failure with preserved ejection fraction (DELIVER, PRESERVED-HF)	Acute myocardial infarction (EMPACT-MI)

Adapted and updated from Das et al. JACC 2020 Expert Consensus Decision Pathway on Novel Therapies for Cardiovascular Risk Reduction in Patients with Type 2 Diabetes [5]. CHIEF-HF, A Study on Impact of Canagliflozin on Health Status, Quality of Life, and Functional Status in Heart Failure (NCT04252287); DAPA-MI, Dapagliflozin Effects on Cardiovascular Events in Patients With an Acute Heart Attack (NCT04564742); DELIVER, Dapagliflozin Evaluation to Improve the LIVEs of Patients With PReserved Ejection Fraction Heart Failure (NCT03619213); PRESERVED-HF, Dapagliflozin in PRESERVED Ejection Fraction Heart Failure (NCT03030235); EMPACT-MI, A Study to Test Whether Empagliflozin Can Lower the Risk of Heart Failure and Death in People Who Had a Heart Attack (Myocardial Infarction) (NCT04509674) driven largely by a 38% reduction in cardiovascular death [7]. Empagliflozin subsequently received FDA approval to reduce the risk of CV death in adults with T2DM with CV disease.

- *Dapagliflozin*: The DECLARE-TIMI 58 (Multicenter Trial to Evaluate the Effect of Dapagliflozin on the Incidence of CV Events-Thrombolysis in Myocardial Infarction 58) trial showed a 17% reduction in CV death or HF hospitalizations among patients taking dapagliflozin, compared with placebo, largely driven by a 27% reduction in HF hospitalizations [8]. In this trial, the overall incidence of MACE was not reduced. Dapagliflozin was approved by the FDA to reduce the risk of HF hospitalization in patients with T2DM and ASCVD or ASCVD risk factors.
- *Canagliflozin*: In an integrated analysis of the CANVAS (Canagliflozin Cardiovascular Assessment Study) and CANVAS-Renal trials, canagliflozin was found to reduce MACE among diabetic patients by approximately 14%. The CREDENCE (Evaluation of the Effects of Canagliflozin on Renal and CV Outcomes in Participants With Diabetic Nephropathy) trial showed that patients taking canagliflozin had a 30% reduction in a composite of ESRD, a doubling of the serum creatinine level, or death from renal or cardiovascular causes [9]. The risk of HF hospitalization was also reduced by 39% in the canagliflozin group, compared with placebo. Canagliflozin received FDA approval to reduce the risk of MACE in patients with CVD and to decrease the risk of ESRD, worsening kidney function, and HF hospitalizations in patients with diabetic kidney disease.

Reduction of Cardiovascular Events in Patients with HFrEF

Recent randomized control trials have demonstrated that the cardiovascular benefits of SGLT2 inhibitors extend to patients with HFrEF regardless of the presence of T2DM.

- *Dapagliflozin*: DAPA-HF (Dapagliflozin and Prevention of Adverse Outcomes in Heart Failure) included HFrEF patients with and without T2DM and found that dapagliflozin reduced CV death and HF hospitalizations by 25% [10]. Dapagliflozin's FDA approval was subsequently expanded to reduce CV death and HF hospitalization in patients with NYHA class II–IV HFrEF, both with or without T2DM.
- *Empagliflozin*: The EMPEROR-Reduced (Empagliflozin Outcome Trial in Patients with Chronic Heart Failure with Reduced Ejection Fraction) similarly included HFrEF patients with and without T2DM and demonstrated that empagliflozin decreases CV death and HF hospitalizations by 25% [11]. As of 2021, empagliflozin received FDA approval for HFrEF patients regardless of T2DM status. The EMPEROR-Preserved (Empagliflozin outcome trial in Patients With chronic heart Failure With Preserved Ejection Fraction) included patients with HFpEF with and without T2DM and showed a 21% decrease in CV death and heart failure hospitalizations in the patients randomized to empagliflozin [12].

Contraindications and Precautions

Contraindications for all SGLT2 inhibitors include hypersensitivity to the drug, pregnancy or breast feeding, and ESRD on dialysis. SGLT2 inhibitors are not intended for the treatment of T1DM or DKA and should not be used in these patients. Initiation of canagliflozin is not recommended for patients with GFR <30. Initiation of empagliflozin is not recommended in patients with GFR<20 for heart failure and with GFR<30 for glycemic control. Initiation of dapagliflozin for cardiovascular benefit is not recommended for GFR <25 and for glycemic control is not recommended for GFR <45.

Adverse events associated with SGLT2 inhibitors include an increased risk of genital mycotic infections which have been demonstrated in randomized control trials and urinary tract infections which were described in post-marketing reports [5, 7–9]. Patients on SGLT2 inhibitors are also at risk for developing DKA, including euglycemic DKA. While initial randomized control trials had suggested that canagliflozin has a higher rate of lower limb amputations, subsequent clinical trial data demonstrated lower rates of amputations than previously reported, and the FDA black box warning for amputation risk was removed [2, 5, 6]. Higher amputation rates were not observed in clinical trials of dapagliflozin or empagliflozin [7, 8]. An increase in bone fractures was observed among patients taking canagliflozin in the CANVAS trial [9]. Expert consensus suggests cautious use of SGLT2 inhibitors in patients with lower limb amputations, peripheral vascular disease, soft tissue infections, neuropathy, and diabetic foot ulcers and recommends regular foot exams and careful attention to perineal hygiene for patients on SGLT2 inhibitors [5].

Clinical Pearls

- Consider empirically reducing the insulin dose for patients starting SGLT2 inhibitors and for CV risk reduction, especially in patients that are normoglycemic at baseline.
- SGLT2 inhibitors are contraindicated in patients who are pregnant, are breastfeeding, or have ESRD on dialysis and not recommended in patients with low GFR (GFR <30 for canagliflozin, GFR<20 for empagliflozin for heart failure and GFR<30 for empagliflozin for glycemic control, and GFR <25 for dapagliflozin for cardiovascular benefit and GFR <45 for dapagliflozin for glycemic control).

While the diuretic and anti-glycemic effects of SGLT2 inhibitors are modest, physicians can consider an empiric reduction in diuretic dose and insulin/insulin secretagogue doses in patients who are starting SGLT2 inhibitors to prevent volume depletion and hypoglycemia, respectively [5].

Glucagon-like Peptide 1 Receptor Agonists (GLP-1R Agonists)

GLP-1R agonists are incretin mimetics that stimulate insulin secretion from the pancreas, suppress glucagon release, and slow gastric emptying. There are currently three GLP-1R agonists available in the United States which have demonstrated a reduction in MACE among diabetic patients with ASCVD or ASCVD risk factors: dulaglutide, liraglutide, and injectable semaglutide (Table 12.2).

Cardiovascular Benefits

- *Liraglutide*: The LEADER (Liraglutide Effect and Action in Diabetes: Evaluation of CV Outcome Results) trial enrolled a majority of diabetic patients with cardiovascular disease at baseline (81.3%) or cardiovascular risk factors. The LEADER trial found that in patients with diabetes, liraglutide was associated with a 13% decreased rate of MACE compared with placebo [13]. The SCALE (Satiety and Clinical Adiposity – Liraglutide Evidence in Nondiabetic and Diabetic Individuals) trial randomized nondiabetic patients with elevated body mass index (BMI) to liraglutide 3.0 mg daily versus placebo. Patients receiving liraglutide lost 5.6 kilograms more than those in the placebo group at 56 weeks [14]. Liraglutide was subsequently approved by the FDA to reduce the risk of MACE in patients with T2DM and for weight loss in nondiabetic patients with elevated BMI.
- *Semaglutide*: SUSTAIN-6 (Trial to Evaluate CV and Other Long term Outcomes With Semaglutide in Subjects With Type 2 Diabetes) similarly enrolled a large proportion of diabetic patients with baseline cardiovascular disease (83.0%) and found that subcutaneous semaglutide was

Table 12.2 GLP-1R agonists with cardiovascular benefit

	Dulaglutide	**Liraglutide**	**Semaglutide**
Initial dose	0.75 mg SC weekly	0.6 mg SC daily	0.25 mg SC weekly
Up-titration and target dose for CV benefit	Can increase to target 1.5 mg SC weekly	Increase by 0.6 mg every week until 1.8 mg SC daily	Double dose every 4 weeks until target 1 mg SC weekly
FDA indications for cardiovascular benefits	1. Glycemic control 2. Reduction MACE in adults with T2DM and ASCVD or ASCVD risk factors (REWIND) 3. 3.0–4.5 mg weekly for weight loss in patients with T2DM (AWARD-11)	1. Glycemic control 2. Reduction in MI, stroke, or CV death in adults with T2DM and ASCVD (LEADER) 3. Weight loss at 3.0 mg daily (SCALE)	1. Glycemic control 2. Reduction in MI, stroke, or CV death in adults with T2DM and ASCVD (SUSTAIN-6) 3. Weight loss at 2.4 mg weekly (STEP 1)
Contraindications	1. Hypersensitivity to drug 2. Pregnancy or breastfeeding 3. Personal or family history of medullary thyroid cancer or multiple endocrine neoplasia type 2 (MEN2) 4. Not recommended for patients with severe gastrointestinal disease		

Precautions	*Nausea*: Monitor for nausea and vomiting. Start at low-dose and up-titrate gradually *Hypoglycemia*: Consider empiric decrease in insulin and decrease or discontinuation of insulin secretagogues. Discontinue DPP-4 inhibitor before starting GLP-1R agonist. Monitor for hypoglycemia *Gastric emptying*: Use with caution in patients with prior gastric surgery, not recommended for patients with gastroparesis *Diabetic retinopathy*: (reported with semaglutide) advise guideline-directed eye examinations *Pancreatitis*: Monitor for pancreatitis and discontinue medication indefinitely if pancreatitis is diagnosed		
Ongoing areas of investigation	Non-alcoholic steatohepatitis (REALIST)	Overweight/obesity with comorbidities (NCT04487743)	Peripheral artery disease (STRIDE)

Adapted and updated from Das et al. JACC 2020 Expert Consensus Decision Pathway on Novel Therapies for Cardiovascular Risk Reduction in Patients with Type 2 Diabetes [5]; REALIST, Researching an Effect of GLP-1 Agonist on Liver Steatosis (NCT03648554); Efficacy and Safety of Liraglutide on Body Weight in Obese Subjects or Overweight Subjects With Co-morbidities (NCT04487743); STRIDE, A Research Study to Compare a Medicine Called Semaglutide Against Placebo in People With Peripheral Arterial Disease and Type 2 Diabetes (NCT04560998) associated with a 26% decrease in the rate of MACE, mostly driven by a decrease in nonfatal stroke [15]. STEP 1 (Semaglutide Treatment Effect in People with obesity) randomized nondiabetic patients with elevated BMI to semaglutide 2.4 mg weekly versus placebo. Patients receiving semaglutide lost 12.7 kilograms more than those in the placebo group at 68 weeks [16]. The FDA approved subcutaneous semaglutide to reduce the risk of MACE in patients with T2DM and approved the higher dose of 2.4 mg weekly semaglutide for weight loss in adults with obesity or overweight with at least one weight-related condition.

- *Dulaglutide*: The REWIND (Researching Cardiovascular Events with a Weekly Incretin in Diabetes) trial had the largest proportion of patients without prior CVD compared to the other GLP-1R agonist trials, with 31.5% of participants reporting a baseline history of CVD [17]. Dulaglutide was associated with a 12% decrease in MACE compared with placebo, again driven by a decrease in nonfatal stroke. The AWARD-11 (Assessment of Weekly AdministRation of LY2189265 in Diabetes) trial randomized patients with T2DM on metformin to 3.0 or 4.5 mg versus 1.5 mg dulaglutide weekly, and found patients randomized to the 4.5 mg dose had 1.6 kg more weight loss at 36 weeks compared to the 1.5 mg dose [18]. Dulaglutide is approved by the FDA to reduce MACE in diabetic patients both with and without baseline ASCVD and the 3.0–4.5 mg doses have been approved for weight loss in patients with T2DM.

Contraindications and Precautions

Contraindications for GLP-1R agonists include hypersensitivity to the drug, pregnancy or breast feeding, and a personal or family history of medullary thyroid cancer or multiple endocrine neoplasia type 2 (MEN2). Similar to SGLT2 inhibitors, GLP-1R agonists are not intended for the treatment of T1DM or DKA [2, 5, 6].

When initiating GLP-1R agonists in patients with reasonably controlled diabetes, expert consensus suggests empirically reducing insulin dose (when present as a baseline medication) and decreasing the dose or discontinuing insulin secretagogues (e.g., glyburide, glipizide, glimepiride) to avoid precipitating hypoglycemia [5]. Dipeptidyl peptidase-4 (DPP-4) inhibitors should be discontinued before starting GLP-1R agonists. Nausea and vomiting are the most common side effects experienced upon initiation of GLP-1R agonists, and these drug effects can be mitigated by starting at low doses and up-titrating gradually [2, 5, 6, 19]. GLP-1R agonists cause delayed gastric emptying and thus should be used with caution in patients with prior gastric surgery. They are not recommended for use in patients with symptomatic gastroparesis or severe gastrointestinal disease [2, 5, 6, 19]. Diabetic retinopathy has been reported with semaglutide, and guideline-directed eye exams are advised for patients initiated on semaglutide [15]. Pancreatitis has been described in post-marketing reports of GLP-1R agonists, though was not observed in the randomized control trials [19]. Patients who experience an episode of pancreatitis should have their GLP-1R agonists discontinued indefinitely [5].

Clinical Pearls

- Consider empirically reducing the insulin dose for patients starting GLP-1R agonists for CV risk reduction, especially in patients that are normoglycemic at baseline.
- Contraindications for GLP-1R agonists include hypersensitivity to drug, pregnancy or breast feeding, and a personal or family history of medullary thyroid cancer or multiple endocrine neoplasia type 2 (MEN2).
- DPP-4 inhibitors should be discontinued before starting GLP-1R agonists.

Key Learning Points

- Three GLP-1R agonists – dulaglutide, liraglutide, and injectable semaglutide – have been shown to reduce MACE in patients with T2DM and ASCVD. Dulaglutide has also been shown to reduce MACE in patients with T2DM and ASCVD risk factors. GLP-1R agonists have also been shown to promote weight loss in patients with elevated BMI.

- Three SGLT2 inhibitors – canagliflozin, dapagliflozin, and empagliflozin – have been shown to reduce cardiovascular events including heart failure hospitalizations and CV mortality in patients with T2DM and ASCVD or ASCVD risk factors. Additionally, dapagliflozin and empagliflozin have been shown to reduce HF hospitalizations and CV mortality in HFrEF patients regardless of T2DM status.
- Metformin is contraindicated in patients with hypersensitivity to the drug, GFR <30, and acute or chronic metabolic acidosis.
- Pregnancy, breastfeeding, and ESRD on dialysis are contraindications for all SGLT2 inhibitors. Initiation of SLGT2 inhibitors is not recommended for low GFR (GFR <30 for canagliflozin, GFR<20 for empagliflozin for heart failure and GFR<30 for empagliflozin for glycemic control, and GFR <25 for dapagliflozin for cardiovascular benefit and GFR <45 for dapagliflozin for glycemic control).
- Contraindications for GLP-1R agonists include hypersensitivity to drug, pregnancy or breast feeding, and a personal or family history of medullary thyroid cancer or multiple endocrine neoplasia type 2 (MEN2).
- In patients starting SGLT2 inhibitors, reported adverse effects include diabetic ketoacidosis (DKA; including euglycemic DKA), genital mycotic infections, urinary tract infections, soft tissue infections, and lower limb ulcerations.
- In patients starting GLP-1R agonists, reported adverse effects include nausea, vomiting, delayed gastric emptying, and pancreatitis.

References

1. UK Prospective Diabetes Study (UKPDS) Group. Effect of intensive blood-glucose control with metformin on complications in overweight patients with type 2 diabetes (UKPDS 34). Lancet (London, England). 1998;352(9131):854–65.
2. American Diabetes A. Standards of medical care in diabetes-2019 abridged for primary care providers. Clin Diabetes. 2019;37(1):11–34.
3. Cosentino F, Grant PJ, Aboyans V, Bailey CJ, Ceriello A, Delgado V, et al. 2019 ESC Guidelines on diabetes, pre-diabetes, and cardiovascular diseases developed in collaboration with the EASD: The Task Force for diabetes, pre-diabetes, and cardiovascular diseases of the European Society of Cardiology (ESC) and the European Association for the Study of Diabetes (EASD). Eur Heart J. 2020;41(2):255–323.
4. Holman RR, Paul SK, Bethel MA, Matthews DR, Neil HAW. 10-year follow-up of intensive glucose control in type 2 diabetes. N Engl J Med. 2008;359(15):1577–89.
5. Das SR, Everett BM, Birtcher KK, Brown JM, Januzzi JL, Kalyani RR, et al. 2020 expert consensus decision pathway on novel therapies for cardiovascular risk reduction in patients with type 2 diabetes. A report of the american college of cardiology solution set oversight committee. J Am Coll Cardiol. 2020;76(9):1117–45.
6. Cosentino F, Grant PJ, Aboyans V, Bailey CJ, Ceriello A, Delgado V, et al. 2019 ESC Guidelines on diabetes, pre-diabetes, and cardiovascular diseases developed in collaboration with the EASD: The Task Force for diabetes, pre-diabetes, and cardiovascular diseases of the European Society of Cardiology (ESC) and the European Association for the Study of Diabetes (EASD). Eur Heart J. 2019;41(2):255–323.
7. Zinman B, Wanner C, Lachin JM, Fitchett D, Bluhmki E, Hantel S, et al. Empagliflozin, cardiovascular outcomes, and mortality in type 2 diabetes. N Engl J Med. 2015;373(22):2117–28.
8. Wiviott SD, Raz I, Bonaca MP, Mosenzon O, Kato ET, Cahn A, et al. Dapagliflozin and cardiovascular outcomes in type 2 diabetes. N Engl J Med. 2018;380(4):347–57.
9. Perkovic V, Jardine MJ, Neal B, Bompoint S, Heerspink HJL, Charytan DM, et al. Canagliflozin and renal outcomes in type 2 diabetes and nephropathy. N Engl J Med. 2019;380(24):2295–306.

10. McMurray JJV, Solomon SD, Inzucchi SE, Køber L, Kosiborod MN, Martinez FA, et al. Dapagliflozin in patients with heart failure and reduced ejection fraction. N Engl J Med. 2019;381(21):1995–2008.
11. Packer M, Anker SD, Butler J, Filippatos G, Pocock SJ, Carson P, et al. Cardiovascular and renal outcomes with empagliflozin in heart failure. N Engl J Med. 2020;383(15):1413–24.
12. Anker SD, Butler J, Filippatos G, et al. Empagliflozin in Heart Failure with a Preserved Ejection Fraction. New England Journal of Medicine. 2021;385(16):1451–61.
13. Marso SP, Daniels GH, Brown-Frandsen K, Kristensen P, Mann JFE, Nauck MA, et al. Liraglutide and cardiovascular outcomes in type 2 diabetes. N Engl J Med. 2016;375(4):311–22.
14. Pi-Sunyer X, Astrup A, Fujioka K, Greenway F, Halpern A, Krempf M, et al. A randomized, controlled trial of 3.0 mg of liraglutide in weight management. N Engl J Med. 2015;373(1):11–22.
15. Marso SP, Bain SC, Consoli A, Eliaschewitz FG, Jódar E, Leiter LA, et al. Semaglutide and cardiovascular outcomes in patients with type 2 diabetes. N Engl J Med. 2016;375(19):1834–44.
16. Wilding JPH, Batterham RL, Calanna S, Davies M, Van Gaal LF, Lingvay I, et al. Once-weekly semaglutide in adults with overweight or obesity. N Engl J Med. 2021;384(11):989–1002.
17. Gerstein HC, Colhoun HM, Dagenais GR, Diaz R, Lakshmanan M, Pais P, et al. Dulaglutide and cardiovascular outcomes in type 2 diabetes (REWIND): a double-blind, randomised placebo-controlled trial. Lancet. 2019;394(10193):121–30.
18. Frias JP, Bonora E, Nevarez Ruiz L, et al. Efficacy and Safety of Dulaglutide 3.0 mg and 4.5 mg Versus Dulaglutide 1.5 mg in Metformin-Treated Patients With Type 2 Diabetes in a Randomized Controlled Trial (AWARD-11). Diabetes Care. 2021;44(3):765–73.
19. Honigberg MC, Chang LS, McGuire DK, Plutzky J, Aroda VR, Vaduganathan M. Use of glucagon-like peptide-1 receptor agonists in patients with type 2 diabetes and cardiovascular disease: a review. JAMA Cardiol. 2020;5(10):1182–90.

Part IV
Coronary Disease

Chapter 13
Stable Ischemic Heart Disease

Daniel Katz and Michael C. Gavin

Abbreviations

ACS	Acute coronary syndrome
BMI	Body mass index
BNP	B-type natriuretic peptide
BP	Blood pressure
CABG	Coronary artery bypass graft
CAD	Coronary artery disease
CBC	Complete blood count
CCTA	Coronary computed tomography angiography
CK	Creatinine kinase
CMP	Complete metabolic panel
CMR	Cardiac magnetic resonance imaging
CV	Cardiovascular
ECG	Electrocardiogram
EF	Ejection fraction
GDMT	Guideline directed medical therapy
GI	Gastrointestinal

D. Katz (✉) · M. C. Gavin
Department of Medicine, Division of Cardiology, Beth Israel Deaconess Medical Center, Harvard Medical School, Boston, MA, USA
e-mail: dkatz@bidmc.harvard.edu; mgavin2@bidmc.harvard.edu

A. A. Bhargava et al. (eds.), *Handbook of Outpatient Cardiology*, https://doi.org/10.1007/978-3-030-88953-1_13

HbA1c	Hemoglobin A1c
HMG-CoA	3-hydroxy-3-methyl-glutaryl-CoA reductase
LDL-C	Low density lipoprotein cholesterol
MI	Myocardial infarction
NEJM	New England Journal of Medicine
NNT	Number needed to treat
PCI	Percutaneous Coronary Intervention
PCSK9	Proprotein convertase subtilisin/kexin type 9
PDE5	Phosphodiesterase type 5
SARS-Cov-2	Severe acute respiratory syndrome coronavirus 2
SGLT2	Sodium-glucose co-transporter-2
SIHD	Stable ischemic heart disease
SPECT	Single photon Emission Computed Tomography
UA	Unstable angina

Diagnosis and Clinical Assessment

Key Definitions

- Coronary artery disease (CAD): any atheromatous plaque in the coronary arteries, regardless of effect on blood flow.
- Stable ischemic heart disease (SIHD): a clinical syndrome marked by *stable* symptoms. Symptoms are usually angina: pain or pressure brought on reliably by exertion or emotion and relieved by rest or nitroglycerine.
  - CAD is one possible cause of SIHD.
- *Unstable* angina (UA): the symptomatic manifestation of an acute coronary syndrome (ACS).
  - These symptoms (possibly similar to SIHD) are either brought on with less provocation or with no provocation at all, i.e., at rest.

- ACS results from an acute imbalance in myocardial oxygen supply and demand, often from an acute reduction in coronary blood flow.
  - ACS ranges from UA alone to myocardial infarction (MI).
  - ACS requires inpatient management.

- **Clinical Pearl:** Do not confuse a *new* diagnosis of SIHD with ACS!
  - The first presentation of "new" angina does not necessarily mean it is unstable.

History

- Whether seeing a patient with SIHD for the first time or in follow-up, establish details of their symptoms.
  - What symptoms do they typically experience (typical angina, dyspnea, or other atypical symptoms)?
  - What level of stress elicits their symptoms?
  - What do they do when they experience those symptoms (rest, take nitroglycerin, etc.)?
  - Have the symptoms changed or evolved? *Evolution of symptoms should prompt additional workup and management.*
- Assess other vascular beds.
  - Claudication
  - Transient neurologic symptoms
- Watch for *new red flag* symptoms.
  - Previous or new anginal symptoms now occurring at rest
  - Syncope/periodic dizziness/palpitations suggesting arrhythmia
  - New lower extremity edema

Physical Exam

- The physical examination is often normal or nonspecific in patients with SIHD, but it is useful to look for other associated findings that suggest non-coronary atherosclerotic vascular disease [1].
- New or worsening symptoms should prompt more detailed examination:
  - Syncope → auscultation of new murmurs
  - Claudication → peripheral pulses/ankle-brachial index
  - Neurologic symptoms → Neuro exam
  - Lower extremity edema → jugular venous pulsation, point of maximal impulse, auscultation for S3, lung auscultation for rales

Routine Workup in SIHD

- *Labs*
  - Lab work in SIHD focuses on comorbidities: CBC, CMP, lipid panel, HbA1c, BNP, and baseline CK especially upon diagnosis of CAD.
  - If symptoms are progressing, consider repeating lab work.
- *Electrocardiogram*
  - All patients with suspected SIHD should have a resting electrocardiogram (ECG) at initial diagnosis and with new or evolving symptoms [2].
  - ECG is typically normal; pathologic Q waves indicate a prior MI.
  - ECG abnormalities also guide stress test selection (see below and Chap. 7).
- *Rest echocardiography*
  - Not needed routinely
  - Consider if:

Heart failure/valvular disease signs/symptoms
Known prior MI or a pathologic Q-wave on the ECG
Evidence of ventricular arrhythmias, suggesting underlying cardiomyopathy [2]

Advanced Noninvasive Testing: Who and when to Test

- Outpatient noninvasive testing is typically indicated in two groups:
  - Patients with new symptoms suspicious for SIHD.
  - Patients with known SIHD who have new or worsening symptoms.
  - As above, new SIHD and ACS are *distinct clinical syndromes* – new SIHD can be assessed with outpatient testing, whereas ACS requires inpatient management.
- Noninvasive testing can identify patients with CAD and estimate prognosis.
- Most valuable when cause of new chest pain is truly uncertain (i.e., pretest probability 20–80%).
  - When probability of CAD is low (Fig. 13.1 and Table 13.1), additional testing is generally not indicated and risks a false positive [3].

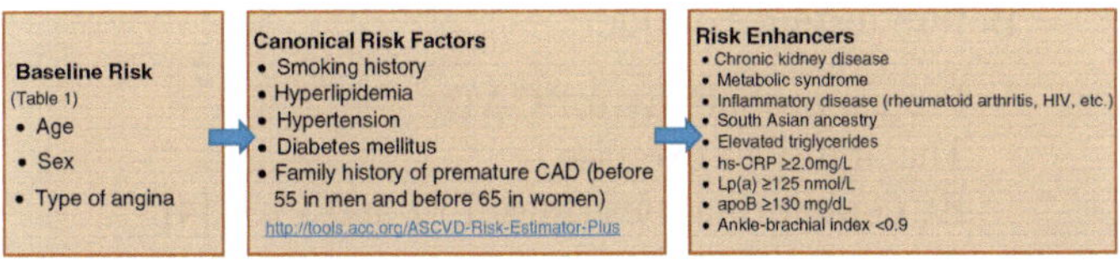

FIGURE 13.1 Approach to CAD risk assessment. Begin with baseline risk and modify using canonical risk factors, utilizing the risk calculator available online. Further risk stratification can be achieved with risk enhancers

TABLE 13.1 Pretest likelihood of coronary artery disease with ≥70% obstruction in symptomatic patients according to age and sex[a]

Age, y	Nonangina chest pain, %		Atypical angina, %		Typical angina, %	
	Men	Women	Men	Women	Men	Women
40–49	0 (0.0–8.4)		5 (2.5–7.9)		10 (2.1–26.5)	
50–59	5 (1.7–11.9)	2 (0.2–6.7)	7 (5.1–8.9)	3 (1.9–4.3)	9 (4.3–15.7)	0 (0.0–3.6)
60–69	6 (1.7–15.0)	3 (0.6–7.9)	11 (8.6–14.3)	4 (2.9–6.0)	19 (11.4–29.4)	1 (0.0–5.4)
≥70	5 (0.1–26.0)	8 (1.7–21.9)	13 (7.9–18.9)	6 (3.5–9.3)	40 (21.1–61.3)	8 (2.2–19.2)

[a]Adapted from Ref. [3]

FIGURE 13.2 Features of an uninterpretable ECG

Uninterpretable ECG for Stress
- Left ventricular hypertrophy with associated repolarization abnormalities
- Left bundle branch block
- Ventricular pacing
- Digitalis effect
- Wolf Parkinson White
- ≥1mm resting ST segment depression

– Before testing, consider:

Pretest probability for CAD
The ability to exercise
ECG abnormalities (Figs. 13.2 and 13.3) [4]

Types of Testing

- Stress (functional) testing (see Table 13.2).
  - Most common form of noninvasive testing.

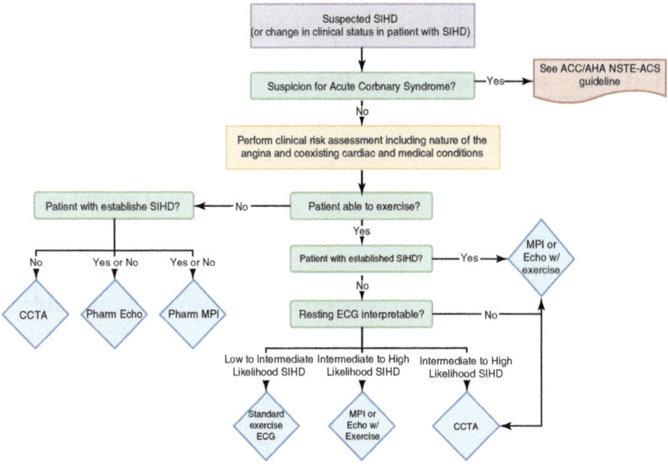

FIGURE 13.3 Choice of noninvasive study for the evaluation of newly suspected SIHD or a change in clinical status in a patient with SIHD. SIHD stable ischemic heart disease, ACC/AHA NSTE-ACS American College of Cardiology/American Heart Association Non-ST segment elevation acute coronary syndrome, MPI myocardial perfusion imaging, Pharm pharmacologic, ECG electrocardiogram, echo echocardiogram, CCTA coronary computed tomography angiogram. (Reproduced with permission from Katz and Gavin. *Ann Intern Med*, 2019 [34])

- Select the stressor.

  Exercise
  Pharmacologic

- Select the modality to assess ischemia.

  ECG
  Echocardiography
  Single-photon emission computed tomography [SPECT]
  And less often, positron emission tomography [PET] or cardiac MRI [CMR]

TABLE 13.2 Summary of CAD testing options

Test	Preferred stress modalities	Pros	Cons
ECG without imaging	Exercise	Low cost	Lowest sensitivity (61%) Limited by ECG suitability
Stress echo	Exercise, dobutamine	Highly sensitive Also obtain valvular data and filling pressures No radiation	Less interpretable in LBBB or paced hearts Poor image quality can occur in very thin or very obese individuals
SPECT	Exercise, vasodilator (regadenoson, dipyridamole)	Highly sensitive Works well in overweight individuals	Radiation More expensive
PET	Exercise, vasodilator (regadenoson, dipyridamole)	Extremely sensitive Works well in overweight individuals Can provide microvascular dysfunction data	Radiation More expensive Not widely available
MRI	Vasodilator (regadenoson, dipyridamole)	Extremely sensitive Works well in overweight individuals Can provide viability data	Radiation More expensive Not widely available

Table 13.2 (continued)

Test	Preferred stress modalities	Pros	Cons
CCTA	N/A	No exercise required Only noninvasive anatomic test, giving data on coronary anomalies Less radiation than SPECT	Requires iodinated contrast Some radiation Images limited in irregular rhythms or high heart rates

ECG electrocardiogram, *LBBB* left bundle branch block, *echo* echocardiogram, *CCTA* coronary computed tomography angiogram, *SPECT* single-photon emission computed tomography, *PET* positron emission tomography, *MRI* magnetic resonance imaging

- Anatomical testing with coronary computed tomography angiography (CCTA)
  - Increasingly utilized for evaluation of chest pain.
  - The European Society of Cardiology and the National Institute for Health and Care Excellence in the United Kingdom recommend CCTA as the initial test for the evaluation of chest pain in patients without known CAD [5, 6].
  - Key advantages:

    High negative predictive value (avoids unnecessary cardiac catheterization)
    Identifies nonobstructive coronary disease and coronary congenital anomalies
    Does not require exercise

  - Recent key trials:

    PROMISE, NEJM 2015 – *CCTA compared to functional testing as the initial diagnostic test among intermediate-risk patients with symptomatic SIHD: no difference in adverse cardiovascular events* [7].

SCOT-HEART, NEJM 2018 – *CCTA + standard care in SIHD = lowered rates of combined primary endpoint of death from CHD or non-fatal MI* [8].

- Invasive coronary angiography.
  - Not typically indicated for initial evaluation of SIHD.
  - In patients with very high likelihood of disease (i.e., >90%), noninvasive testing provides little additional information, so angiography is used when it will affect therapy.

Test Selection Pearls

- In intermediate-risk patients that can exercise and have an interpretable ECG (Fig. 13.3), exercise with ECG alone carries a Class IA indication [2].
  - Sensitivity of exercise without imaging is limited at 61% (i.e., 39% false-negative rate) and worse for women [2].

  - **Clinical Pearl:** In practice, it is often preferred to add imaging to exercise to improve sensitivity. Use of imaging for this indication carries a Class IIa indication in the guidelines [2].

  - It is essential to add imaging if the ECG is uninterpretable.
- CCTA is an appropriate first-line test for the evaluation of chest pain among patients at intermediate pretest probability regardless of the ability to exercise [9].
- Pharmacologic stress with imaging can be used for patients who [1] cannot exercise or [2] cannot exercise strenuously enough to generate a valid test result.
  - For echocardiography and MRI, dobutamine is used as stressor.
  - For SPECT and PET, vasodilators (regadenoson or dipyridamole).

- To choose between imaging modalities, *consider the resources and technical expertise at your institution* [2].
- Echocardiography has no radiation and provides information on valvular function and filling pressures.

> - **Clinical Pearl:** In patients with left bundle branch block or ventricular pacing, avoid stress echo.
>   - The abnormal electrical activation of the heart impairs evaluation of ischemia in the interventricular septum (LAD territory).

- CCTA, SPECT, or PET imaging are less susceptible to poor image quality related to body habitus.
- When CAD/SIHD is already known, evolving or ongoing symptoms on anti-anginal therapy are ideally assessed by functional testing with imaging to localize and quantify ischemia to inform decisions on revascularization [10].
  - CCTA/non-functional imaging is less valuable in this setting.

SIHD Without Obstructive CAD

- Approximately 30% of patients presenting with angina have no obstructive CAD.
- Angina without obstructive coronary disease is more common among women [11].
- Risk of ischemic events is still increased, and medical therapy is still indicated [12, 13]!
- CCTA is the best test for diagnosing nonobstructive CAD.
- Among patients with angina and nonobstructive CAD, 50–65% are believed to have coronary microvascular dysfunction.
  - Assessment of microvascular function can be done with CMR and PET perfusion [14].

When to Refer to a Cardiologist

- When testing approach is unclear
- Uncertain diagnosis after noninvasive testing, to consider coronary angiography [10]
- Suspected microvascular dysfunction or variant (Prinzmetal's) angina

Treatment

Goals of Treatment

- Prevention of ischemic events (cerebral, coronary, and peripheral) (Fig. 13.4).
- Reducing anginal symptoms.
- These goals are independent!

Behavior Modification

- *Smoking cessation:* Smoking increases cardiovascular disease mortality by 50%.
- *Physical activity:* Current guidelines recommend 150 minutes of at least moderate activity or 75 minutes of vigorous activity per week [15]. Patients with SIHD and those post-MI should participate in a cardiac rehabilitation program [2].
- *Dietary modification:* Emphasize intake of vegetables, fruits, whole grains, legumes, healthy protein sources (low-fat dairy, low-fat poultry, fish/seafood, and nuts), and non-tropical vegetable oils. The intake of sweets, sugar-sweetened beverages, and red meats should be limited [16].
- *Alcohol moderation:* One drink per day, no harm and possible benefit; beyond two drinks per day, no benefit and likely harm [17]. Heavy drinking worsens hypertension and may precipitate ischemia in SIHD and should be avoided [18].

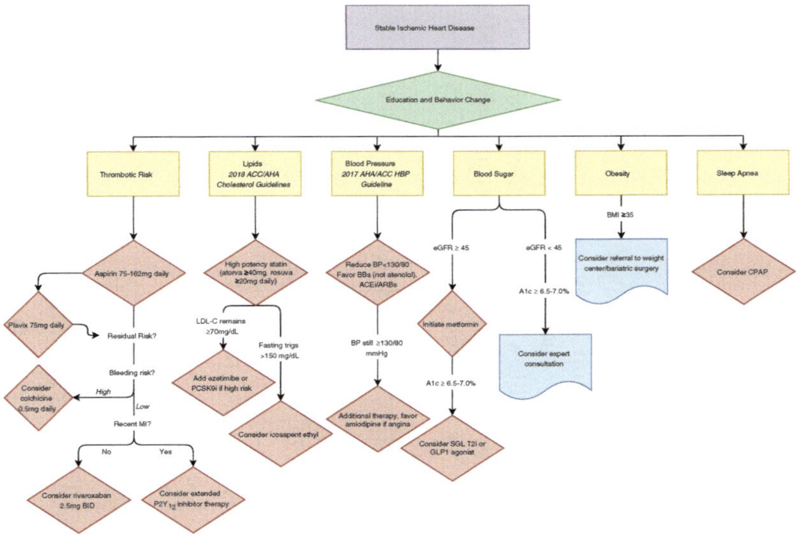

FIGURE 13.4 Guideline-directed medical therapy for patients with stable ischemic heart disease. A1c hemoglobin A1c, ACC American College of Cardiology, ACEi angiotensin-converting enzyme inhibitor, AHA American Heart Association, ARB angiotensin receptor blocker, BBs beta-blockers, BID twice daily, BMI body mass index, CPAP continuous positive airway pressure, eGFR estimated glomerular filtration rate, GLP1 glucagon-like peptide 1, HBP high blood pressure, LDL-C low-density lipoprotein cholesterol, MI myocardial infarction, SGLT2i sodium-glucose cotransporter 2 inhibitor. (Reproduced with permission from Katz and Gavin. *Ann Intern Med*, 2019 [34])

- *Psychological well-being:* Interventions to reduce psychological stress may improve clinical outcomes in patients with SIHD [19].

Pharmacologic Therapy for Specific Risk Factors/ Comorbidities

Lipids

- HMG-COA reductase inhibitors (*statins*) are the mainstay of lipid management.
- In SIHD patients: < 75 years, high potency statin (atorvastatin 80 mg or rosuvastatin 20–40 mg) is recommended; >75 years reasonable to reduce potency.
- Target LDL-C < 70 mg/dL with addition of *ezetimibe and PCKS9 inhibitors in sequence* in patients at high risk [16]. High risk = multiple previous CV events or CV event + multiple risk factors.
- *Niacin is no longer recommended* for the lowering of LDL-C [16].
- *Fish oil*: Over-the-counter formulations have not shown consistent benefit [20], but *icosapent ethyl* reduced cardiovascular events 25% on top of high-dose statins and aspirin in patients with SIHD and elevated triglycerides (REDUCE-IT, NEJM 2019) [21].

Hypertension

- Guidelines: goal BP of <130/80 mmHg in SIHD [22].
  - Recent trial: SPRINT, NEJM 2015 – in SIHD patients over 50, targeting lower BP (121 vs 136 mmHg) decreased CV events by 31%, NNT = 44 [23].
- Agent of choice depends on comorbidities and other targets (i.e., angina, congestive heart failure, chronic kidney disease, or diabetes).

Diabetes

- Start with metformin when possible [24, 25].
- For SIHD patients with HbA1c still >6.5–7%, consider SGLT2 inhibitors (e.g., *empagliflozin, canagliflozin, dapagliflozin*) and/or GLP-1 receptor agonists (e.g., *liraglutide, semaglutide*). Both have been shown to reduce CV events [24].

Obesity

- Lifestyle change is critical.
- If BMI >35, consider weight loss surgery.
  - In patients with type 2 diabetes, Roux-en-Y gastric bypass has been shown to reduce CV events [26].

Pharmacologic Therapy to Prevent MI or Death in SIHD Independent of Risk Factors

Antiplatelet Therapy

- If any atherosclerotic cardiovascular disease (CAD, SIHD, peripheral arterial disease, etc.), treat with medium-dose *aspirin*, usually 81 mg [15].
- When aspirin is contraindicated (e.g., allergy), patients can be treated with *clopidogrel* 75 mg daily.

Anticoagulation

- Anticoagulation reduces ischemic events but raises bleeding events! Consider risk/benefit with a cardiologist.
  - Recent trial: COMPASS, NEJM 2017 – *Rivaroxaban* at a very reduced dose of 2.5 mg twice daily reduced cardiovascular mortality in SIHD at the expense of increased bleeding [27].

Anti-inflammatory Therapy

- *Colchicine* 0.5 mg daily was shown in the LoDoCo2 trial (NEJM 2020) to reduce cardiovascular events in patients with chronic coronary disease [28].

Other Therapies

- Patients with SIHD should receive an annual influenza vaccine [2, 29].
- Patients with SIHD are at increased risk for complications from SARS-CoV-2 and vaccination is recommended [30].

Medications that Treat Angina

- β-Blockers,
  - Initial therapy for prolonged relief of symptoms. Typically start here!

  - **Clinical Pearl:** All beta-blockers reduce symptoms, though in patients with peripheral arterial disease, drugs with additional alpha blockade, such as *carvedilol or labetalol*, may prevent vasoconstriction mediated by unopposed alpha agonism [2].

  - In patients with reduced EF, carvedilol, metoprolol succinate, and bisoprolol should be favored per guidelines [31].
  - Contraindicated in severe bronchospastic lung disease.
- *Calcium channel blockers*
  - *Amlodipine*: the preferred option, a dihydropyridine calcium channel blocker
  - *Diltiazem and verapamil*: non-dihydropyridine calcium channel blockers

    Useful if beta-blockers produce side effects
    Should be avoided in patients with reduced ejection fraction given their negative inotropic effects

- *Nitrates*
  - *Short-acting nitrates*: in the form of *sublingual nitroglycerin or nitroglycerin spray* are ideal for immediate relief of angina.

    Patients can administer one dose every 5 minutes for up to three doses.
  - *Long-acting nitrates*:

    Three times daily isosorbide dinitrate
    Once (sometimes twice) daily isosorbide mononitrate
    Nitropaste
  - Warn patients about the interaction between nitrates and PDE5 inhibitors leading to hypotension.
- *Ranolazine* is an anti-anginal that appears to reduce angina through its effect on the late sodium current.
  - It prolongs QTc and therefore should be used with caution if a patient is on other QT-prolonging medications.
  - Side effects are primarily GI upset.
  - Usually a fourth-line agent.

Revascularization in SIHD

- Revascularization (either by PCI or CABG) is indicated in patients with ischemic symptoms that are *progressive or refractory to maximal medical management* (*Class 1A recommendation*) [2].
- In the ISCHEMIA trial (NEJM 2020), *revascularization did not reduce ischemic cardiovascular events or death* in SIHD patients with moderate or severe ischemia. However revascularization did improve symptoms.
- Based on observational data, treatment of symptomatic patients with proximal left anterior descending artery disease or multivessel disease with an initial strategy of

revascularization plus GDMT may be considered [32, 33]. Discuss with a cardiologist.

Key Learning Points

- In patients presenting with new symptoms: differentiate new SIHD and ACS, and consider baseline risk based on demographics and comorbidities.
- Consider noninvasive functional (exercise or pharmacologic stress test with ECG, echo, or nuclear imaging) or anatomic (CCTA) assessment for CAD in patients with new SIHD evaluation. CCTA is increasingly being recommended as a first-line test.
- The goals of treatment are to minimize adverse cardiovascular outcomes and death and reduce symptoms. These goals are often achieved with different pharmacotherapy. Therapy should be guideline based.
- Consider angiography/revascularization in conjunction with a cardiologist, particularly for patients with severe proximal disease when there are persistent symptoms despite GDMT.

Adapted with permission from Ref. [3]

References

1. Pryor DB, Shaw L, Harrell FE, Lee KL, Hlatky MA, Mark DB, et al. Estimating the likelihood of severe coronary artery disease. Am J Med. 1991;90(5):553–62.
2. Fihn SD, Gardin JM, Abrams J, Berra K, Blankenship JC, Dallas AP, et al. 2012 ACCF/AHA/ACP/AATS/PCNA/SCAI/STS guideline for the diagnosis and management of patients with stable ischemic heart disease. J Am Coll Cardiol. 2012;60(24):e44–164.

3. Foldyna B, Udelson JE, Karády J, Banerji D, Lu MT, Mayrhofer T, et al. Pretest probability for patients with suspected obstructive coronary artery disease: re-evaluating Diamond-Forrester for the contemporary era and clinical implications: insights from the PROMISE trial. Eur Heart J Cardiovasc Imaging. 2019;20(5):574–81.
4. Genders TSS, Steyerberg EW, Alkadhi H, Leschka S, Desbiolles L, Nieman K, et al. A clinical prediction rule for the diagnosis of coronary artery disease: validation, updating, and extension. Eur Heart J. 2011;32(11):1316–30.
5. Knuuti J, Wijns W, Saraste A, Capodanno D, Barbato E, Funck-Brentano C, et al. 2019 ESC Guidelines for the diagnosis and management of chronic coronary syndromes. Eur Heart J. 2020;41(3):407–77.
6. Moss AJ, Williams MC, Newby DE, Nicol ED. The updated NICE guidelines: cardiac CT as the first-line test for coronary artery disease. Curr Cardiovasc Imaging Rep [Internet]. 2017 [cited 2021 Jan 30];10(5). Available from: https://www.ncbi.nlm.nih.gov/pmc/articles/PMC5368205/.
7. Douglas PS, Hoffmann U, Patel MR, Mark DB, Al-Khalidi HR, Cavanaugh B, et al. Outcomes of anatomical versus functional testing for coronary artery disease. N Engl J Med. 2015;372(14):1291–300.
8. Investigators SCOT-HEART, Newby DE, Adamson PD, Berry C, Boon NA, Dweck MR, et al. Coronary CT angiography and 5-year risk of myocardial infarction. N Engl J Med. 2018;379(10):924–33.
9. Ferraro R, Latina JM, Alfaddagh A, Michos ED, Blaha MJ, Jones SR, et al. Evaluation and management of patients with stable angina: beyond the ischemia paradigm: JACC state-of-the-art review. J Am Coll Cardiol. 2020;76(19):2252–66.
10. Fihn SD, Blankenship JC, Alexander KP, Bittl JA, Byrne JG, Fletcher BJ, et al. 2014 ACC/AHA/AATS/PCNA/SCAI/STS focused update of the guideline for the diagnosis and management of patients with stable ischemic heart disease: a report of the American College of Cardiology/American Heart Association Task Force on Practice Guidelines, and the American Association for Thoracic Surgery, Preventive Cardiovascular Nurses Association, Society for Cardiovascular Angiography and Interventions, and Society of Thoracic Surgeons. J Am Coll Cardiol. 2014;64(18):1929–49.

11. Gulati M, Shaw LJ, Bairey Merz CN. Myocardial ischemia in women: lessons from the NHLBI WISE study. Clin Cardiol. 2012;35(3):141–8.
12. Hoffmann U, Ferencik M, Udelson JE, Picard MH, Truong QA, Patel MR, et al. Prognostic value of noninvasive cardiovascular testing in patients with stable chest pain: insights from the PROMISE trial (prospective multicenter imaging study for evaluation of chest pain). Circulation. 2017;135(24):2320–32.
13. Chow BJW, Small G, Yam Y, Chen L, McPherson R, Achenbach S, et al. Prognostic and therapeutic implications of statin and aspirin therapy in individuals with nonobstructive coronary artery disease: results from the CONFIRM (COronary CT Angiography EvaluatioN For Clinical Outcomes: An InteRnational Multicenter registry) registry. Arterioscler Thromb Vasc Biol. 2015;35(4):981–9.
14. Marinescu MA, Löffler AI, Ouellette M, Smith L, Kramer CM, Bourque JM. Coronary microvascular dysfunction, microvascular angina, and treatment strategies. JACC Cardiovasc Imaging. 2015;8(2):210–20.
15. Arnett DK, Blumenthal RS, Albert MA, Buroker AB, Goldberger ZD, Hahn EJ, et al. 2019 ACC/AHA guideline on the primary prevention of cardiovascular disease. Circulation. 2019;13:E157–98.
16. Grundy SM, Stone NJ, Bailey AL, Beam C, Birtcher KK, Blumenthal RS, et al. AHA/ACC/AACVPR/AAPA/ABC/ACPM/ADA/AGS/APhA/ASPC/NLA/PCNA guideline on the management of blood cholesterol: a report of the American college of cardiology/American heart association task force on clinical practice guidelines. J Am Coll Cardiol. 2018;2018:25709.
17. McClelland RL, Bild DE, Burke GL, Mukamal KJ, Lima JA, Kronmal RA. Alcohol and coronary artery calcium prevalence, incidence and progression: results from the Multi-Ethnic Study of Atherosclerosis (MESA). Am J Clin Nutr. 2008;88(6):1593–601.
18. Rossinen J, Partanen J, Koskinen P, Toivonen L, Kupari M, Nieminen MS. Acute heavy alcohol intake increases silent myocardial ischaemia in patients with stable angina pectoris. Heart Br Card Soc. 1996;75(6):563–7.
19. Dimsdale JE. Psychological stress and cardiovascular disease. J Am Coll Cardiol. 2008;51(13):1237–46.
20. Abdelhamid AS, Brown TJ, Brainard JS, Biswas P, Thorpe GC, Moore HJ, et al. Omega-3 fatty acids for the primary and second-

ary prevention of cardiovascular disease. Cochrane Database Syst Rev. 2018;7:CD003177.

21. Bhatt DL, Steg PG, Miller M, Brinton EA, Jacobson TA, Ketchum SB, et al. Cardiovascular risk reduction with icosapent ethyl for hypertriglyceridemia. N Engl J Med. 2019;380(1):11–22.
22. Whelton PK, Carey RM, Aronow WS, Casey DE, Collins KJ, Himmelfarb CD, et al. 2017 ACC/AHA/AAPA/ABC/ACPM/AGS/APhA/ASH/ASPC/NMA/PCNA guideline for the prevention, detection, evaluation, and management of high blood pressure in adults: a report of the American college of cardiology/American heart association task force on clinical practice guidelines. J Am Coll Cardiol. 2018;71(19):e127–248.
23. The SPRINT Research Group. A randomized trial of intensive versus standard blood-pressure control. N Engl J Med. 2015;373(22):2103–16.
24. Association, American Medical. Cardiovascular benefits of SGLT2 inhibitors and GLP-1 receptor agonists in type 2 diabetes. JAMA J Am Med Assoc. 2019;321(17):1720–1.
25. American Diabetes Association. Pharmacologic approaches to glycemic treatment: standards of medical care in diabetes-2019. Diabetes Care. 2019;42(Suppl 1):S90–102.
26. Fisher DP, Johnson E, Haneuse S, Arterburn D, Coleman KJ, O'Connor PJ, et al. Association between bariatric surgery and macrovascular disease outcomes in patients with type 2 diabetes and severe obesity. JAMA. 2018;320(15):1570–82.
27. Eikelboom JW, Connolly SJ, Bosch J, Dagenais GR, Hart RG, Shestakovska O, et al. Rivaroxaban with or without aspirin in stable cardiovascular disease. N Engl J Med. 2017;377(14):1319–30.
28. Nidorf SM, Fiolet ATL, Mosterd A, Eikelboom JW, Schut A, Opstal TSJ, et al. Colchicine in patients with chronic coronary disease. N Engl J Med. 2020;383(19):1838–47.
29. de Diego C, Vila-Córcoles A, Ochoa O, Rodriguez-Blanco T, Salsench E, Hospital I, et al. Effects of annual influenza vaccination on winter mortality in elderly people with chronic heart disease. Eur Heart J. 2009;30(2):209–16.
30. CDC. COVID-19 and Your Health [Internet]. Centers for Disease Control and Prevention. 2020 [cited 2021 Jan 30]. Available from: https://www.cdc.gov/coronavirus/2019-ncov/need-extra-precautions/people-with-medical-conditions.html.
31. Yancy CW, Jessup M, Bozkurt B, Butler J, Casey DE, Colvin MM, et al. 2017 ACC/AHA/HFSA Focused Update of the

2013 ACCF/AHA guideline for the management of heart failure: a report of the American college of cardiology/American heart association task force on clinical practice guidelines and the heart failure society of America. J Am Coll Cardiol. 2017;70(6):776–803.
32. Hachamovitch R, Hayes SW, Friedman JD, Cohen I, Berman DS. Comparison of the short-term survival benefit associated with revascularization compared with medical therapy in patients with no prior coronary artery disease undergoing stress myocardial perfusion single photon emission computed tomography. Circulation. 2003;107(23):2900–7.
33. Windecker S, Stortecky S, Stefanini GG, da Costa BR, Rutjes AW, et al. Revascularisation versus medical treatment in patients with stable coronary artery disease: network meta-analysis. BMJ. 2014;348(8):g3859.
34. Katz D, Gavin MC. Stable ischemic heart disease. Ann Intern Med. 2019;171(3):ITC17.

Chapter 14
Post-myocardial Infarction Evaluation and Management

Mariem A. Sawan and Michael McDaniel

Abbreviations

ACEI	Angiotensin-converting enzyme inhibitor
ARB	Angiotensin receptor blocker
ASA	Aspirin
AV fistula	Arteriovenous fistula
BMS	Bare metal stent
CABG	Coronary artery bypass graft surgery
CAD	Coronary artery disease
CKD	Chronic kidney disease
DES	Drug-eluting stent
DM	Diabetes mellitus
ICD	Implantable cardioverter defibrillator
LV	Left ventricle
MI	Myocardial infarction
NSTEMI	Non-ST-elevation myocardial infarction
PCI	Percutaneous coronary intervention

M. A. Sawan (✉) · M. McDaniel
Department of Medicine, Division of Cardiology, Emory University School of Medicine, Atlanta, GA, USA
e-mail: Mariem.sawan@emory.edu

A. A. Bhargava et al. (eds.), *Handbook of Outpatient Cardiology*, https://doi.org/10.1007/978-3-030-88953-1_14

PHQ-2	Patient health questionnaire-2
STEMI	ST-elevation myocardial infarction
TTE	Transthoracic echocardiography

During the first outpatient visit, it is extremely important to establish rapport and gauge patients' understanding of present medical condition(s) and overall health literacy. Address potential obstacles to regular follow-up visits or access to medications in addition to screening for depression.

Evaluation

Conduct a thorough review of patient's hospital admission: did the patient have a NSTEMI or STEMI and receive conservative management vs fibrinolytic therapy (STEMI) vs PCI vs CABG? In the case of PCI, "was balloon angioplasty and/or stent placed?", type of stent (BMS vs DES), and "was revascularization successful?". Know degree of coronary artery disease before and after revascularization, in-hospital TTE results, and whether the patient had any acute post-MI complications.

History important positives and negatives include symptoms related to ongoing ischemia, late MI complications, procedure-related complications, and medication side effects.

- Symptoms of CAD: angina or anginal equivalent, e.g., shortness of breath. Gradual increase in severity or frequency of angina after successful PCI and despite optimal medical therapy is concerning for in-stent restenosis.
- Heart failure symptoms: dyspnea on exertion, orthopnea, paroxysmal nocturnal dyspnea, bilateral lower extremity edema, weight gain, early satiety, bloating.
- Pericarditis: sharp substernal chest pain, fever.

- Arrhythmias: palpitations described as irregular-fluttering sensation, flip-flop sensation, skipped beat, pause, or forceful contraction.
- PCI-related complications: pain or hematoma at access site (AV fistula, pseudoaneurysm, subcutaneous hematoma). Oliguria, skin changes, postprandial abdominal pain (cholesterol emboli syndrome).
- CABG-related complications: fever, sternotomy wound dehiscence. Complications related to vein graft: wound dehiscence, ulcer, cellulitis.
- Post-lytic therapy: symptoms of new focal neurological deficits
- Screen for any bleeding diathesis especially in elderly patients and patients on triple therapy.
- Medication side effects: rhinosinusitis (aspirin allergy), dry hacking cough (ACEI or ARB).
- Medication compliance especially if on twice daily drug, e.g., ticagrelor.
- Social history: illicit drug use, alcohol or tobacco abuse.
- Screen for depression using PHQ-2.

Physical exam Full physical and detailed cardiovascular exam should be conducted. Make sure to include the following:

- Patients managed by PCI (especially with femoral access): check access site and distal pulses. Look for signs of pseudoaneurysm: pain on palpation, expansile mass, systolic bruit. Signs of AV fistula: continuous bruit near access site.
- Patients' s/p CABG: assess sternotomy wound and site of vein graft.
- Bleeding diathesis: pallor, bruising, ecchymosis.

Clinical Pearls

1. An effective outpatient visit should include a thorough review of symptoms, activity limitations, medication reconciliation, cardiovascular risk assessment, screening for depression, and referral to cardiac rehabilitation if not already done.
2. Make sure to ask and examine for symptoms and signs (respectively) related to ongoing ischemia, late MI complications, procedure-related complications, and medication side effects.
3. Gradual increase in severity or frequency of angina after successful PCI and despite optimal medical therapy is concerning for in-stent restenosis.

Electrocardiogram keep an eye out for:

- New arrhythmia
- Contraindications to BB therapy: PR interval >0.24, second- and third-degree AV block
- Signs of pericarditis: diffuse ST segment elevation and PR depression (except in aVR: ST depression and PR elevation)
- Sign of LV aneurysm: persistent ST segment elevation

Transthoracic echocardiography (TTE) repeat TTE if TTE prior to hospital discharge was evident for reduced LVEF, or if the patient is presenting with new signs and/or symptoms concerning heart failure, late MI complications, or new murmur. Examples of TTE findings that impact management:

- Reduction or improvement in LVEF.
- Large anterior wall dyskinesia might warrant anticoagulation therapy.
- LV thrombus.
- LV aneurysm or pseudoaneurysm.

Clinical Pearl
A repeat TTE is indicated if a post-MI patient is presenting with symptoms and/or signs of new or worsening heart failure, late MI complications, or new murmur. Recent MI alone (with normal TTE result during admission) is not an indication for repeat TTE.

Long-term Medical Management: [1, 2] Table 14.1

- Aspirin 81 mg po QD indefinitely or clopidogrel 75 mg po QD indefinitely if aspirin intolerance.
- $P2Y_{12}$ inhibitor therapy (see Fig. 14.1 for indication and duration of therapy): use one of the following:
  - Clopidogrel (Plavix) 75 mg po QD (unique adverse effect: upper respiratory tract infection, flulike syndrome, arthralgia)
  - Ticagrelor 90 mg po BID (unique adverse effect: dyspnea)
  - Prasugrel 10 mg po QD (contraindicated if history of TIA or stroke. Reduce dose to 5 mg po QD in patients ≥75 years of age or weight <60 kg due to increased risk of bleeding)
- Beta-adrenergic blockers (BB): if EF ≤40%. Use sustained-release metoprolol succinate, carvedilol, or bisoprolol. Up-titrate gradually (e.g., doubling the dose every >2 weeks) to maximally tolerated dose while closely monitoring for signs and symptoms of heart failure.
- ACEI: lifelong in all post-MI patients with HF, EF ≤0.40, HTN, DM, stable CKD, or post anterior MI. Use ARB if ACEI intolerant.

Table 14.1 Medications used post-myocardial infarction and their adverse effects. See indications under long-term medication management

Class, starting dose	Target dose	Common adverse effects	Contraindications
BB Bisoprolol 1.25 mg QD Carvedilol 3.125 mg BID Metoprolol XL 12.5 mg QD	Bisoprolol 10 mg QD Carvedilol 25 mg BID Metoprolol XL 25 mg BID	Dizziness, headache, fatigue, hypotension, broncho-constriction	PR interval ≥0.24 seconds, second- and third-degree heart blocks, severe sinus bradycardia (HR < 45 bpm), sick sinus syndrome (unless patient has functioning pacemaker) Cardiogenic shock, overt heart failure Active asthma
ACEI Enalapril 2.5 mg BID Lisinopril 5 mg QD	Enalapril 10 mg BID Lisinopril 20–35 QD	Dizziness, hypotension, cough (dry hacking)	History of ACEI-induced angioedema, hereditary or idiopathic angioedema Coadministration of neprilysin inhibitors Coadministration with aliskiren in diabetic patients or patient with renal impairment (GFR <60 ml/min/1.73 m^2) Pregnancy
ARB Candesartan 4 mg QD Losartan 50 mg QD Valsartan 20 mg BID	Candesartan 32 mg QD Losartan 150 mg QD Valsartan 240 mg BID	Dizziness, hypotension, fatigue, cough (dry hacking)	Coadministration with aliskiren in diabetic patients or patient with renal impairment (GFR <60 ml/min/1.73 m^2) Severe hepatic impairment (candesartan) Pregnancy

Table 14.1 (continued)

Class, starting dose	Target dose	Common adverse effects	Contraindications
Aldosterone antagonists Spironolactone 25 mg QD Eplerenone 25 mg QD	Spironolactone 50 mg QD Eplerenone 50 mg QD	Gynecomastia, hyperkalemia, decreased libido, gastritis	Serum potassium >5.5 mEq/L at initiation CrCl ≤30 ml/min Concomitant use of strong CYP3A4 inhibitors (e.g., ketoconazole) Conditions associated with hyperkalemia (e.g., Addison disease) Pregnancy The following contraindications apply to patients with hypertension: Type 2 diabetes mellitus (noninsulin dependent) with microalbuminuria; serum creatinine >2.0 mg/dL in males or >1.8 mg/dL in females; CrCl <50 mL/minute; concomitant use with potassium supplements or potassium-sparing diuretics

BB beta-adrenergic blocker, *ACEI* angiotensin-converting enzyme inhibitor, *ARB* angiotensin receptor blocker, *BID* twice daily, *CrCl* creatinine clearance, *GFR* glomerular filtration rate, *HR* heart rate, *QD* once daily

- Aldosterone: is recommended in patients post-MI who are already receiving therapeutic doses of BB and ACEI who have an EF ≤0.4 and either symptomatic HF or DM.
- Statins: lifelong high-intensity statin therapy (atorvastatin 40–80 mg po QD or rosuvastatin 20–40 mg po QD) regardless of baseline low-density lipoprotein (LDL) cholesterol.

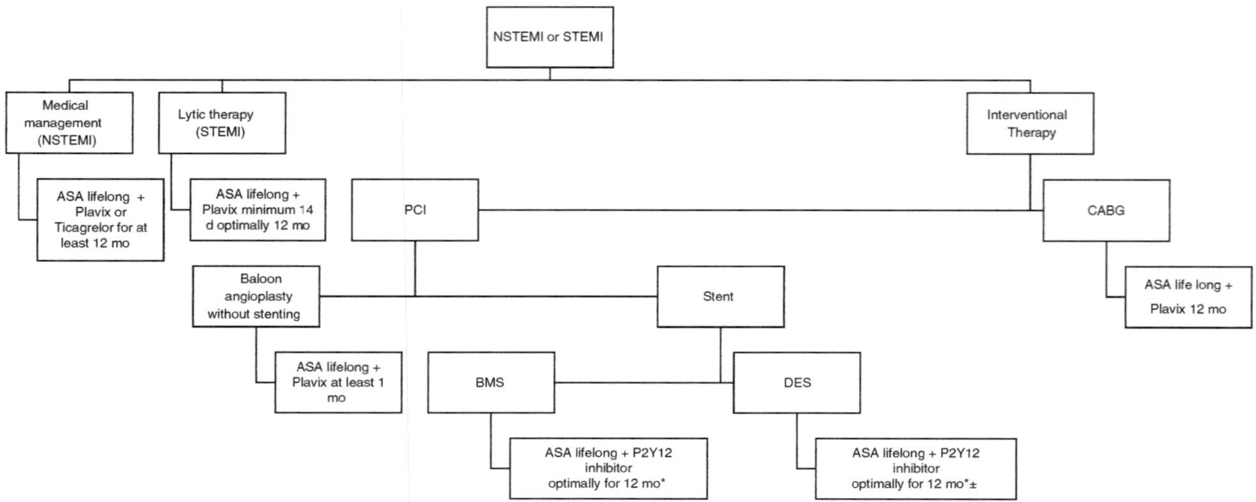

FIGURE 14.1 Treatment algorithm and duration of $P2Y_{12}$ inhibitor therapy post-myocardial infarction [3]. *Consider indefinite Plavix in PCI patients with DES or BMS if at risk for catastrophic consequences from stent thrombosis (i.e., left main or proximal LAD stent). ±Recent trials recommend 3 months of DAPT, followed by 9 months of $P2Y_{12}$ inhibitor monotherapy (refer to references [4–11] for more details); this recommendation is not part of the AHA/ACC guidelines at time of publication. *BMS* bare metal stent, *CABG* coronary artery bypass graft surgery, *DES* drug-eluting stent, *lytic* fibrinolytic therapy, *NSTEMI* non-ST-elevation myocardial infarction, *PCI* percutaneous coronary intervention, *STEMI* ST-elevation myocardial infarction

Anti-anginal medications:

- Calcium channel blockers (CCB): non-dihydropyridine calcium antagonists (e.g., verapamil or diltiazem) are recommended, in the absence of LV dysfunction, for ischemic symptoms when beta-blockers are not successful, are contraindicated, or cause unacceptable side effects.
- Sublingual nitroglycerin: 0.3–0.4 mg per dose. Instruct patient to take one dose (when experiencing acute anginal attack) every 5 minutes for up to three doses before calling 911 to access emergency medical services.
  - Nitroglycerin tablets are heat and light sensitive. Patients should be instructed to keep bottles tightly capped and refrigerated with only a small supply carried by the patient. Discard opened bottles after 12 months.
  - Nitroglycerin is contraindicated in patients who have taken sildenafil or vardenafil within 24 hours or tadalafil within 48 hours.
- Ranolazine: 500 mg po BID may increase to 1000 po twice daily as needed. Indicated for treatment of chronic angina.

Triple antithrombotic therapy: warfarin +ASA + $P2Y_{12}$ inhibitor therapy.

- If warfarin is needed for atrial fibrillation, LV thrombus, mechanical valve, deep venous thromboembolism after stent placement, consider stopping ASA after 1 month.
- Proton pump inhibitors (PPI): add PPI if patient has a history of gastrointestinal bleeding. Consider PPI in patients at risk for gastrointestinal bleeding: elderly, patients on triple antithrombotic therapy, chronic steroid or NSAID use, *H. pylori* infection.

Implantable cardioverter defibrillator (ICD) for prevention of sudden cardiac death in post-MI patient with

- Ischemic cardiomyopathy with LVEF ≤35% and NYHA functional class II or III
- Ischemic cardiomyopathy with LVEF ≤30% and NYHA functional class I

In both cases, patients should be ≥40 days post-MI, more than 3 months after revascularization and on guideline-directed medical therapy.

Secondary prevention comprehensive risk factor management reduces recurrent events and improves survival and quality of life.

- Smoking cessation: encourage complete cessation. Refer patient to a smoking cessation program.
- Strict glycemic control: target A1C ≤7. Metformin is an effective first-line drug if not contraindicated. SLGT2 inhibitors (empagliflozin, dapagliflozin) and liraglutide are preferred given cardiovascular disease benefit. Avoid rosiglitazone if HF.
- Blood pressure management: goal <130/80 per 2017 ACC/AHA guidelines
- Lipid management: goal LDL <70 mg/dl. Use high-intensity statins. Add ezetimibe if goal not achieved.
- Weight management: target BMI 18.5–24.9 kg/m^2. Waist circumference < 40 inches in men, <35 inches in women.
- Exercise: 30–60 min moderate-intensity aerobic exercise 5–7 times/week
- Influenza and *S. pneumoniae* vaccines
- Cardiac rehabilitation: all eligible outpatients with diagnosis of acute coronary syndrome, s/p CABG or PCI within the past year should be referred to a comprehensive outpatient cardiovascular rehabilitation program.
- Diet: encourage Mediterranean diet.

- Avoid illicit drug use especially cocaine. Limit alcohol intake: 1 drink/day for women, 1–2 drinks/day for men.
- Sexual activity can be safely resumed once patient is able to achieve 4–5 METs (walking ~4 mph on flat ground); patients should wait 3–4 weeks after MI.

Key Learning Points

1. An effective outpatient visit should include a thorough review of symptoms, activity limitations, medication reconciliation, cardiovascular risk assessment, and referral to cardiac rehabilitation if not already done.
2. Make sure to ask and examine for symptoms and signs (respectively) related to ongoing ischemia, late MI complications, procedure-related complications, and medication side effects.
3. Gradual increase in severity or frequency of angina after successful PCI and despite optimal medical therapy is concerning for in-stent restenosis.
4. A repeat TTE is indicated if a post-MI patient is presenting with symptoms and/or signs of new or worsening heart failure, late MI complications, or new murmur. Recent MI alone (with normal TTE result during admission) is not an indication for repeat TTE.
5. All post-MI patients should be on aspirin indefinitely or clopidogrel if aspirin intolerant.
6. If warfarin is needed for atrial fibrillation, LV thrombus, mechanical valve, and deep venous thromboembolism after stent placement, consider stopping ASA after 1 month.
7. Assess every patient's eligibility for ICD. Candidates for ICD should be ≥40 days post-MI, more than 3 months after revascularization and on guideline-directed medical therapy.
8. Post-discharge optimization of secondary prevention measures has been shown to improve long-term outcomes and therefore should be reassessed at each follow-up visit.

References

1. O'Gara PT, Kushner FG, Ascheim DD, Casey DE Jr, Chung MK, de Lemos JA, et al. 2013 ACCF/AHA guideline for the management of ST-elevation myocardial infarction: a report of the American College of Cardiology Foundation/American Heart Association Task Force on Practice Guidelines. Circulation. 2013;127(4):e362–425.
2. Amsterdam EA, Wenger NK, Brindis RG, Casey DE Jr, Ganiats TG, Holmes DR Jr, et al. 2014 AHA/ACC guideline for the management of patients with non-ST-elevation acute coronary syndromes: a report of the American college of cardiology/American heart association task force on practice guidelines. J Am Coll Cardiol. 2014;64(24):e139–228.
3. Levine GN, Bates ER, Bittl JA, Brindis RG, Fihn SD, Fleisher LA, et al. 2016 ACC/AHA guideline focused update on duration of dual antiplatelet therapy in patients with coronary artery disease: a report of the American college of cardiology/American heart association task force on clinical practice guidelines: an update of the 2011 ACCF/AHA/SCAI guideline for percutaneous coronary intervention, 2011 ACCF/AHA guideline for coronary artery bypass graft surgery, 2012 ACC/AHA/ACP/AATS/PCNA/SCAI/STS guideline for the diagnosis and management of patients with stable ischemic heart disease, 2013 ACCF/AHA guideline for the management of ST-elevation myocardial infarction, 2014 AHA/ACC guideline for the management of patients with non-ST-elevation acute coronary syndromes, and 2014 ACC/AHA guideline on perioperative cardiovascular evaluation and management of patients undergoing noncardiac surgery. Circulation. 2016;134(10):e123–55.
4. Hahn JY, Song YB, Oh JH, Chun WJ, Park YH, Jang WJ, et al. Effect of P2Y12 inhibitor monotherapy vs dual antiplatelet therapy on cardiovascular events in patients undergoing percutaneous coronary intervention: the SMART-CHOICE randomized clinical trial. JAMA. 2019;321(24):2428–37.
5. Kim BK, Hong SJ, Cho YH, Yun KH, Kim YH, Suh Y, et al. Effect of ticagrelor monotherapy vs ticagrelor with aspirin on major bleeding and cardiovascular events in patients with acute coronary syndrome: the TICO randomized clinical trial. JAMA. 2020;323(23):2407–16.

6. Kim C, Hong SJ, Shin DH, Kim BK, Ahn CM, Kim JS, et al. Randomized evaluation of ticagrelor monotherapy after 3-month dual-antiplatelet therapy in patients with acute coronary syndrome treated with new-generation sirolimus-eluting stents: TICO trial rationale and design. Am Heart J. 2019;212:45–52.
7. Mehran R, Baber U, Sharma SK, Cohen DJ, Angiolillo DJ, Briguori C, et al. Ticagrelor with or without aspirin in high-risk patients after PCI. N Engl J Med. 2019;381(21):2032–42.
8. Tomaniak M, Chichareon P, Modolo R, Takahashi K, Chang CC, Kogame N, et al. Ticagrelor monotherapy beyond one month after PCI in ACS or stable CAD in elderly patients: a pre-specified analysis of the GLOBAL LEADERS trial. EuroIntervention. 2020;15(18):e1605–e14.
9. Tomaniak M, Chichareon P, Onuma Y, Deliargyris EN, Takahashi K, Kogame N, et al. Benefit and risks of aspirin in addition to ticagrelor in acute coronary syndromes: a post hoc analysis of the randomized GLOBAL LEADERS trial. JAMA Cardiol. 2019;4(11):1092–101.
10. Watanabe H, Domei T, Morimoto T, Natsuaki M, Shiomi H, Toyota T, et al. Effect of 1-month dual antiplatelet therapy followed by clopidogrel vs 12-month dual antiplatelet therapy on cardiovascular and bleeding events in patients receiving PCI: the STOPDAPT-2 randomized clinical trial. JAMA. 2019;321(24):2414–27.
11. Smith SC Jr, Benjamin EJ, Bonow RO, Braun LT, Creager MA, Franklin BA, et al. AHA/ACCF secondary prevention and risk reduction therapy for patients with coronary and other atherosclerotic vascular disease: 2011 update: a guideline from the American heart association and American college of cardiology foundation. Circulation. 2011;124(22):2458–73.

Part V
Heart Failure

Chapter 15
Heart Failure with Reduced Ejection Fraction

Prashant Rao and Marwa A. Sabe

Abbreviations

ACE	Angiotensin-converting enzyme
ARB	Angiotensin II receptor
ARNI	Angiotensin receptor-neprilysin inhibitors
BNP	B-type natriuretic peptide
CRT	Cardiac resynchronization therapy
eGFR	Estimated glomerular filtration rate
FDG-PET	Fluorodeoxyglucose-positron emission tomography
GDMT	Guideline-directed medical therapy
HF	Heart failure
HFpEF	Heart failure with preserved ejection fraction
HFrEF	Heart failure with reduced ejection fraction
ICD	Implantable cardiac defibrillator

P. Rao · M. A. Sabe (✉)
Department of Medicine, Division of Cardiology, Beth Israel Deaconess Medical Center, Harvard Medical School, Boston, MA, USA
e-mail: msabe@bidmc.harvard.edu

A. A. Bhargava et al. (eds.), *Handbook of Outpatient Cardiology*, https://doi.org/10.1007/978-3-030-88953-1_15

MRA	Mineralocorticoid receptor antagonist
NT-proBNP	N-terminal pro-B-type natriuretic peptide
NYHA	New York Heart Association
RAAS	Renin-angiotensin-aldosterone system
SGLT2	Sodium-glucose cotransporter 2

Background and Epidemiology

- Heart failure (HF) is a rising epidemic with an estimated prevalence of >6 million Americans, projected to rise to >8 million by 2030 [1, 2].
- HF is characterized by dyspnea or exercise intolerance due to impaired ventricular filling, ejection of blood, or a combination of both.

Clinical Pearl
North American guidelines categorize HF into HF with preserved ejection fraction (HFpEF) (LVEF ≥50%), heart failure with mildly reduced ejection fraction (LVEF 41–49%), and heart failure with reduced ejection fraction (HFrEF) (LVEF is ≤40%) [3]. HF with a recovered EF (HFrecovEF) is defined as a reduced EF in the past but with improved ejection fraction to ≥50%.

Signs and Symptoms

Clinical Pearl
Patients with HFrEF typically present with symptoms of dyspnea and fatigue, as well as orthopnea, paroxysmal nocturnal dyspnea, ankle/abdominal swelling, and weight gain. Bendopnea (shortness of breath when leaning forward) may also indicate the presence of heart failure. The New York Heart Association (NYHA) classification is used to grade the severity of heart failure by functional class (Table 15.1).

Table 15.1 New York heart association classification

Class I: No limitation in normal physical activity
Class II: Mild symptoms only during normal activity
Class III: Marked symptoms during daily activity, comfortable at rest
Class IV: Marked symptoms during minimal activity and even at rest

- On examination, patients may have evidence of left and/or right heart congestion including bibasilar crackles, elevated jugular venous pressure, positive hepatojugular reflux, ascites, and peripheral edema. An S3 may be present (suggestive of ventricular stiffness and elevated ventricular diastolic pressure), and the presence of cool peripheries is suggestive of a low cardiac output state.
- The physical examination may provide clues as to the etiology and chronicity of heart failure through the presence of murmurs of valvular regurgitation or stenosis, arrhythmias, or a laterally displaced apical impulse.

Diagnostic Evaluation

- While the diagnosis of heart failure is based on clinical evaluation, initial testing includes measurement of natriuretic peptides B-type natriuretic peptide (BNP) and its precursor N-terminal pro-B-type natriuretic peptide (NT-proBNP), electrocardiogram, chest radiograph, and transthoracic echocardiogram.

Clinical Pearl

Once a diagnosis of HFrEF is confirmed, the etiology should be ascertained, beginning with an evaluation for coronary artery disease. A coronary angiogram is performed in the majority of patients, although patient-specific factors such as age, comorbidities, and candidacy for revascularization should be considered. Alternatively, a coronary CT angiogram may be a reasonable option for those with a low pre-test probability of coronary artery disease. Other imaging modalities may be helpful to determine etiology of HFrEF including cardiac magnetic resonance imaging (e.g., myocarditis), fluorodeoxyglucose-positron emission tomography (FDG-PET) (e.g., sarcoidosis), and ^{99m}technetium pyrophosphate scan (e.g., transthyretin cardiac amyloidosis).

Medical Therapy

- There have been several developments in the past decade pertaining to medical therapy in HFrEF. These therapies either improve symptoms, mortality, or both.
- Until recently, the combination of renin-angiotensin-aldosterone system (RAAS) inhibitors, β-blockers, and mineralocorticoid receptor antagonists (MRA) formed the foundation of triple therapy for HFrEF. Each of these agents provides clear benefit on mortality and morbidity in patients with HFrEF, and they collectively came to be termed guideline-directed medical therapy (GDMT).

Clinical Pearl
There are now four pillars of pharmacologic therapy to improve outcomes for patients with HFrEF. These are angiotensin receptor-neprilysin inhibitors (ARNI), β-blockers, MRAs, and sodium-glucose cotransporter 2 (SGLT2) inhibitors.

- Despite their proven benefit, many eligible patients are either not prescribed these medications or prescribed doses below target levels [4].
- Although doses of GDMT are currently the same for men and women, recent data suggest that women may require lower doses [5].

Angiotensin-Converting Enzyme (ACE) Inhibitor, Angiotensin II Receptor Blocker (ARB), and ARNI

- HFrEF causes upregulation of RAAS leading to fluid retention and peripheral arterial vasoconstriction. RAAS has also been implicated in cardiac fibrosis and pathological cardiac remodeling.
- Several randomized controlled trials demonstrate mortality and morbidity benefit with ACE inhibitors or ARBs (SOLVD, NEJM 1992 [6], CONSENSUS, NEJM 1987 [7], CHARM, Lancet 2003 [8])
- PARADIGM-HF (Prospective Comparison of ARNI With ACE-i to Determine Impact on Global Mortality and Morbidity in Heart Failure) demonstrated substantial improvements in survival and reduced heart failure hospitalizations with the angiotensin receptor-neprilysin inhibitor sacubitril-valsartan above and beyond the benefits provided by the angiotensin-converting enzyme inhibitor enalapril (PARADIGM-HF, NEJM 2014 [9])
- ARNIs should be started in patients with LVEF ≤40% and Class II–IV symptoms (although limited data pertain to patients with Class IV symptoms); ARNIs have recently been approved for use in patients with symptomatic heart failure and LVEF <60%.
- Those already on an ACE-i require a washout period of 36 hours before transitioning to ARNI to avoid angioedema. Recent data suggest it is likely safe to start ARNI de novo in patients naïve to ACE-i/ARB [10].
- Following initiation of ARNI, patients should be monitored for symptomatic hypotension, worsening renal function, hyperkalemia, and angioedema.
- Dose reduction should be considered if there is a >30% decrease in eGFR or the patient develops hyperkalemia, but also consider that a decrease in eGFR may be due to overdiuresis (ARNIs have a natriuretic effect) and may require a reduction in diuretics rather than ARNI.
- There is data to suggest that ARNIs may be safely used in patients with HFrEF and ESRD on HD [11].

β-Blockers

- β-blockers reduce all-cause and cardiovascular mortality, sudden cardiac death, and heart failure hospitalizations in patients with HFrEF (bisoprolol, CIBIS-II, Lancet 1999 [12]; metoprolol succinate, MERIT-HF, JAMA 2000 [13]; carvedilol, U.S Carvedilol HF Study Group, NEJM 1996 [14])
- Avoid initiation of β-blockers in patients who are in a low cardiac output state (may be peripherally cool on exam or confirmed low cardiac output using pulmonary artery catheter); with acute HF symptoms or decompensated HF until compensated; or with symptomatic bradycardia or high-grade atrioventricular block (unless or until the patient has a permanent pacemaker). Use with caution in those with second-degree AV block.
- Patients should not be prescribed a new β-blocker without diuretics if they are currently volume overloaded. Once diuresed to euvolemia, a beta-blocker may be initiated.
- Patients should be monitored for symptomatic hypotension, fatigue, worsening HF and fluid retention, as well as bradycardia and heart block.

Mineralocorticoid Receptor Antagonists

- Spironolactone and eplerenone act via RAAS blockade and have been shown to reduce all-cause mortality and HF hospitalizations in randomized controlled trials (RALES, NEJM 1999 [15], EMPHASIS-HF, NEJM 2010 [16]).
- MRAs should be initiated in patients with LVEF $\leq$35% and NYHA Class II to IV.
- MRAs should be avoided in patients with chronic kidney disease and baseline serum creatinine level above 2.5 mg/dL in men and 2 mg/dL in women (or estimated glomerular filtration rate <30 mL/min/1.73m^2) or hyperkalemia ($K \geq 5$).
- Following initiation of MRA, patients should be monitored for worsening renal function and hyperkalemia.

SGLT2 Inhibitors

- While early data provided evidence that SGLT2-i may prevent incident HF in patients with type 2 diabetes mellitus, recent studies demonstrate substantial benefits in outcomes in addition to triple therapy for patients with chronic HFrEF (DAPA-HF, NEJM 2019 [17], EMPORER-REDUCED, NEJM 2020 [18]). These benefits hold true for patients with and without diabetes mellitus. As a result, SGLT2-i have been included in the ACC Expert Consensus Decision Pathway for Optimization of Heart Failure Treatment [19].
- Dapagliflozin and empagliflozin should be avoided in patients with eGFR <30 ml/min/1.73 m^2 and eGFR <20 ml/min/1.73 m^2, respectively [19]. Importantly, SGLT2-i are generally not limited by hypotension. In DAPA-HF, while older patients developed more adverse events and drug intolerance, these rates were similar in both the dapagliflozin and placebo groups.

Diuretics

- Loop diuretics (furosemide, bumetanide, torsemide) are often used to prevent fluid retention in patients with HFrEF, but do not improve mortality. Thiazide-like diuretics (oral metolazone) may supplement fluid removal in patients demonstrating resistance to high doses of loop diuretics.
- Patients with HFrEF should record their weight regularly and may be directed to increase diuretic dosing regimen if their dry weight increases >3 lbs in 24–48 hours or >5 lbs in 1 week.
- Patients should be monitored for acute kidney injury, hypotension, and electrolyte abnormalities.
- Caution should be used when increasing diuretic doses in patients with suspected restrictive physiology and/or similar right atrial and pulmonary capillary wedge pressure.

Other Medical Therapies

- Ivabradine may be used for patients with HFrEF and NYHA Class II–III on a maximally tolerated β-blocker in sinus rhythm with a heart rate of ≥70/min or greater (SHIFT, Lancet 2010) [20].
- Among African-Americans with HFrEF, isosorbide dinitrate and hydralazine should be considered if patients have NYHA Class III to IV symptoms despite target or maximally tolerated doses of other guideline-directed medical therapy (A-HeFT, NEJM 2004) [21]. Although there are no compelling data for the use of isosorbide dinitrate and hydralazine in non-African-Americans with HFrEF, this combination therapy may be an additional option to treat hypertension in patients with HFrEF if already on maximally tolerated doses of ACE/ARB/ARNi (Table 15.2).

Device Therapy

Implantable Cardiac Defibrillator (ICD)

- Implantation of an ICD reduces all-cause mortality in patients with both infarct-mediated and non-infarct-mediated HFrEF (SCD-HeFT, NEJM 2005).
- For patients with infarct-mediated cardiomyopathy, ICD implantation should be considered among those with LVEF ≤35%, NYHA Class II–III symptoms, and > 1 year survival, who are at least >40 days post-MI [22], if not revascularized. In patients who have been revascularized, ICD implantation should be considered only after 90 days post-revascularization. In addition, ICD implantation is recommended in patients with asymptomatic infarct-mediated HF who are at least 40 days post-MI, have an LVEF ≤30%, and on GDMT (Class I for Stage C HF, Class IIa for Stage B HF) [22].
- For patients with non-infarct-mediated cardiomyopathy, primary prevention ICDs should also be considered among

Table 15.2 Practical information for initiation and uptitration of the main therapies used as GDMT

Drug	Indications	Target doses	Monitor for	Avoid
ACE-i/ ARB/ ARNI	LVEF is ≤40% and Class II–IV symptoms	*ARNI* Sacubitril/valsartan 97/103 mg twice daily *ACE-i* Captopril 50 mg 3× daily Enalapril 10–20 mg twice daily Lisinopril 20–40 mg daily Ramipril 10 mg daily *ARB* Candesartan 32 mg daily Losartan 150 mg daily Valsartan 160 mg twice daily	Symptomatic hypotension (ARNI>ACE-i/ARB) Worsening renal function Hyperkalemia Angioedema	Pregnancy Desire to become pregnant Bilateral renal artery stenosis

(continued)

TABLE 15.2 (continued)

Drug	Indications	Target doses	Monitor for	Avoid
β-blockers	LVEF is ≤40%	Bisoprolol 10 mg daily Carvedilol 25 mg twice daily for weight <85 kg, and 50 mg twice daily for weight ≥85 kg Metoprolol succinate 200 mg daily	Fluid retention Worsening HF symptoms Heart block	Low cardiac output state High-grade AV block Acute decompensated HF
MRAs	LVEF ≤35% and NYHA Class II to IV	Eplerenone 50 mg daily Spironolactone 25–50 mg daily	Worsening renal function Hyperkalemia	Serum creatinine >2.5 mg/dL or eGFR <30 mL/min/1.73m^2 Serum $K > 5.0$ mEq/L
SGLT2-i	LVEF is ≤40% and Class II–IV symptoms	Dapagliflozin 10 mg daily Empagliflozin 10 mg daily	Genito-urinary infections (typically manifests early during treatment) Rarely may cause necrotizing fasciitis of the perineum Diabetic ketoacidosis	Dapagliflozin and empagliflozin should be avoided in patients with eGFR <30 ml/min/1.73 m^2 and eGFR <20 ml/min/1.73 m^2, respectively

those with LVEF ≤35%, NYHA Class II–III symptoms, and >1 year survival. Importantly, ICDs should only be considered after a minimum of 3 months of appropriate GDMT [22]. This waiting period allows for optimization of medical therapy to improve ventricular remodelling and function, which may then render need for an ICD unnecessary.

Cardiac Resynchronization Therapy (CRT)

- CRT involves implantation of pacing leads in the right atrium and right ventricle and an epicardial lead overlying the left ventricle via the coronary sinus. The goal of CRT is to pace the ventricles in such a way as to maximize ventricular synchrony.
- CRT reduces all-cause mortality or heart failure hospitalization among select patients with HFrEF (MADIT-CRT, NEJM 2009) [23].
- CRT should be considered in patients with LVEF ≤35%, NYHA Class II–IV, in sinus rhythm with a left bundle branch block, and QRS duration ≥150 ms [22].
- CRT is also indicated in patients with an LVEF ≤50% who are undergoing placement of a permanent pacemaker and will require more than 40% pacing (2012 ACCF/AHA/HRS Focused Update Incorporated Into the ACCF/AHA/HRS 2008 Guidelines for Device-Based Therapy of Cardiac Rhythm Abnormalities: A Report of the American College of Cardiology Foundation/American Heart Association Task Force on Practice Guidelines and the Heart Rhythm Society Developed in Collaboration With the American Association for Thoracic Surgery and Society of Thoracic Surgeons).

Transcatheter Mitral Valve Repair

- Transcatheter mitral valve repair using the MitraClip (Abbott Laboratories, Lake Park, IL) has emerged as a potential treatment option in patients with HFrEF and severe secondary mitral regurgitation [24–26].

- In COAPT, the MitraClip reduced the primary end point of heart failure hospitalization and the secondary end point of all-cause mortality compared with placebo (COAPT, NEJM 2018) [26].
- It is possible that patients with severe secondary mitral regurgitation out of proportion to the degree of left ventricular remodeling stand to derive the most benefit from transcatheter mitral valve repair; however, this theory is controversial [27, 28].

Wireless Pulmonary Artery Pressure Monitors

- Implantation of a CardioMEMS Heart Sensor allows for wireless monitoring of pulmonary artery pressures.
- This device reduces HF hospitalizations among HF patients (HFrEF and HFpEF) with NYHA Class III symptoms (CHAMPION, JACC 2017) [29].
- The impact on mortality is unclear (GUIDE-HF).
- Contraindications to device placement include chest circumference > 165 cm, history of recurrent pulmonary embolism, mechanical tricuspid or pulmonic valve replacements, or any contraindication to right heart catheterization.

Cardiac Rehabilitation

- Supervised cardiac rehabilitation is both safe and effective among patients with chronic HFrEF.
- Supervised cardiac rehabilitation in this population reduces all-cause mortality, cardiovascular mortality, and HF hospitalizations (HF-ACTION, JAMA 2009) [30]. In addition exercise training improves functional capacity, exercise duration, and quality of life [31].
- For patients with infarct-mediated cardiomyopathy, cardiac rehabilitation should commence approximately 2 weeks after hospital discharge for an acute coronary

event and 6 weeks after coronary artery bypass surgery with no surgical complications [32].

Key Learning Points

- Patients with HFrEF should be on maximally tolerated or target doses of guideline-directed medical therapy.
- Quadruple therapy (ARNI, β-blocker, MRA, SGLT2-i) is the cornerstone of heart failure management.
- Device therapy including ICD, CRT, transcatheter mitral valve repair, and wireless pulmonary artery pressure monitors should be considered in the appropriate setting.
- Lifestyle and exercise interventions remain important features of heart failure management.

References

1. Mozaffarian D, Benjamin EJ, Go AS, et al. Executive summary: heart disease and stroke statistics – 2016 update: a report from the American heart association. Circulation. 2016;133:447–54.
2. Virani SS, Alonso A, Benjamin EJ, et al. Heart disease and stroke statistics-2020 update: a report from the American heart association. Circulation. 2020;141:e139–596.
3. Yancy CW, Jessup M, Bozkurt B, et al. 2017 ACC/AHA/HFSA Focused Update of the 2013 ACCF/AHA guideline for the management of heart failure: a report of the American college of cardiology/American heart association task force on clinical practice guidelines and the heart failure society of Ame. J Card Fail. 2017;23:628–51.
4. Greene SJ, Butler J, Albert NM, et al. Medical therapy for heart failure with reduced ejection fraction: the CHAMP-HF registry. J Am Coll Cardiol. 2018;72:351–66.

5. Santema BT, Ouwerkerk W, Tromp J, et al. Identifying optimal doses of heart failure medications in men compared with women: a prospective, observational, cohort study. Lancet (London, England). 2019;394:1254–63.
6. SOLVD Investigators, Yusuf S, Pitt B, Davis CE, Hood WB Jr, Cohn JN. Effect of enalapril on mortality and the development of heart failure in asymptomatic patients with reduced left ventricular ejection fractions. N Engl J Med. 1992;327:685–91.
7. CONSENSUS Trial Study Group. Effects of enalapril on mortality in severe congestive heart failure. N Engl J Med. 1987;316:1429–35.
8. Granger CB, McMurray JJV, Yusuf S, Held P, Michelson EL, Olofsson B, Ostergren J, Pfeffer MA, Swedberg K. Effects of candesartan in patients with chronic heart failure and reduced left-ventricular systolic function intolerant to angiotensin-converting-enzyme inhibitors: the CHARM-Alternative trial. Lancet (London, England). 2003;362:772–6.
9. McMurray JJV, Packer M, Desai AS, et al. Angiotensin–neprilysin inhibition versus enalapril in heart failure. N Engl J Med. 2014;371:993–1004.
10. Velazquez EJ, Morrow DA, DeVore AD, Duffy CI, Ambrosy AP, McCague K, Rocha R, Braunwald E. Angiotensin-neprilysin inhibition in acute decompensated heart failure. N Engl J Med. 2019;380:539–48.
11. Lee S, Oh J, Kim H, Ha J, Chun K-H, Lee CJ, Park S, Lee S-H, Kang S-M. Sacubitril/valsartan in patients with heart failure with reduced ejection fraction with end-stage of renal disease. ESC Hear Fail. 2020;7:1125–9.
12. The cardiac insufficiency bisoprolol study II (CIBIS-II): a randomised trial. Lancet (London, England). 1999;353:9–13.
13. Hjalmarson Å, Goldstein S, Fagerberg B, et al. Effects of controlled-release metoprolol on total mortality, hospitalizations, and well-being in patients with heart failure: the metoprolol CR/XL randomized intervention trial in congestive heart failure (MERIT-HF). JAMA. 2000;283:1295–302.
14. Packer M, Bristow MR, Cohn JN, Colucci WS, Fowler MB, Gilbert EM, Shusterman NH. The effect of carvedilol on morbidity and mortality in patients with chronic heart failure. N Engl J Med. 1996;334:1349–55.
15. Pitt B, Zannad F, Remme WJ, Cody R, Castaigne A, Perez A, Palensky J, Wittes J. The effect of spironolactone on morbidity

and mortality in patients with severe heart failure. N Engl J Med. 1999;341:709–17.
16. Zannad F, McMurray JJV, Krum H, van Veldhuisen DJ, Swedberg K, Shi H, Vincent J, Pocock SJ, Pitt B. Eplerenone in patients with systolic heart failure and mild symptoms. N Engl J Med. 2010;364:11–21.
17. McMurray JJV, Solomon SD, Inzucchi SE, et al. Dapagliflozin in patients with heart failure and reduced ejection fraction. N Engl J Med. 2019;381:1995–2008.
18. Packer M, Anker SD, Butler J, et al. Cardiovascular and renal outcomes with empagliflozin in heart failure. N Engl J Med. 2020;383:1413–24.
19. Maddox TM, Januzzi JLJ, Allen LA, et al. 2021 update to the 2017 ACC expert consensus decision pathway for optimization of heart failure treatment: answers to 10 pivotal issues about heart failure with reduced ejection fraction: a report of the American college of cardiology solution set oversi. J Am Coll Cardiol. 2021;77:772–810.
20. Swedberg K, Komajda M, Böhm M, Borer JS, Ford I, Dubost-Brama A, Lerebours G, Tavazzi L. Ivabradine and outcomes in chronic heart failure (SHIFT): a randomised placebo-controlled study. Lancet (London, England). 2010;376:875–85.
21. Taylor AL, Ziesche S, Yancy C, et al. Combination of isosorbide dinitrate and hydralazine in blacks with heart failure. N Engl J Med. 2004;351:2049–57.
22. Yancy CW, Jessup M, Bozkurt B, et al. 2017 ACC/AHA/HFSA focused update of the 2013 ACCF/AHA guideline for the management of heart failure: a report of the American college of cardiology/American heart association task force on clinical practice guidelines and the heart failure society of Ame. Circulation. 2017;136:e137–61.
23. Moss AJ, Hall WJ, Cannom DS, et al. Cardiac-resynchronization therapy for the prevention of heart-failure events. N Engl J Med. 2009;361:1329–38.
24. Obadia J-F, Messika-Zeitoun D, Leurent G, et al. Percutaneous repair or medical treatment for secondary mitral regurgitation. N Engl J Med. 2018;379:2297–306.
25. Feldman T, Foster E, Glower DD, et al. Percutaneous repair or surgery for mitral regurgitation. N Engl J Med. 2011;364:1395–406.
26. Stone GW, Lindenfeld J, Abraham WT, et al. Transcatheter mitral-valve repair in patients with heart failure. N Engl J Med. 2018;379:2307–18.

27. Grayburn PA, Sannino A, Packer M. Proportionate and disproportionate functional mitral regurgitation: a new conceptual framework that reconciles the results of the MITRA-FR and COAPT trials. JACC Cardiovasc Imaging. 2019;12:353–62.
28. Zimarino M, Ricci F, Capodanno D, et al. Left ventricular size predicts clinical benefit after percutaneous mitral valve repair for secondary mitral regurgitation: a systematic review and meta-regression analysis. Cardiovasc Revasc Med. 2020;21:857–64.
29. Givertz MM, Stevenson LW, Costanzo MR, Bourge RC, Bauman JG, Ginn G, Abraham WT. Pulmonary artery pressure-guided management of patients with heart failure and reduced ejection fraction. J Am Coll Cardiol. 2017;70:1875–86.
30. O'Connor CM, Whellan DJ, Lee KL, et al. Efficacy and safety of exercise training in patients with chronic heart failure: HF-ACTION randomized controlled trial. JAMA. 2009;301:1439–50.
31. Piepoli MF, Davos C, Francis DP, Coats AJ. ExTraMATCH collaborative. Exercise training metanalysis of trials in patients with chronic heart failure (ExTraMATCH). Br Med J. 2004;328:e95.
32. Leon AS, Franklin BA, Costa F, Balady GJ, Berra KA, Stewart KJ, Thompson PD, Williams MA, Lauer MS. Cardiac rehabilitation and secondary prevention of coronary heart disease: an American Heart Association scientific statement from the Council on Clinical Cardiology (Subcommittee on Exercise, Cardiac Rehabilitation, and Prevention) and the Council on Nut. Circulation. 2005;111:369–76.

Chapter 16
Heart Failure with Preserved Ejection Fraction

Nicolas Isaza and Pablo A. Quintero

Abbreviations

ACC	American College of Cardiology
AHA	American Heart Association
BNP	Serum brain natriuretic peptide
ECG	Electrocardiogram
FDA	Food and Drug Administration
HF	Heart failure
HFpEF	Heart failure with preserved ejection fraction
HFrEF	Heart failure with reduced ejection fraction
LV	Left ventricle
LVEDP	Left ventricular end-diastolic pressure
LVEF	Left ventricular ejection fraction

N. Isaza (✉)
Department of Medicine, Beth Israel Deaconess Medical Center, Harvard Medical School, Boston, MA, USA
e-mail: nisaza1@bidmc.harvard.edu

P. A. Quintero
Department of Medicine, Division of Cardiology, Beth Israel Deaconess Medical Center, Harvard Medical School, Boston, MA, USA

A. A. Bhargava et al. (eds.), *Handbook of Outpatient Cardiology*, https://doi.org/10.1007/978-3-030-88953-1_16

mPCWP	Mean pulmonary capillary wedge pressure
NT-proBNP	N-terminal pro-brain natriuretic peptide
PASP	Pulmonary artery systolic pressure

Introduction and Epidemiology [15]

- Population-based studies estimated that 51–63% of cases of heart failure are sub-classified as heart failure with preserved ejection fraction (HFpEF).
- HFpEF accounts for approximately 50% of the incidence of overall HF.
- The proportion of HF incidence attributed to HFpEF is higher in women and older and black populations.

Definition

- The main parameter to characterize left ventricular systolic function is the left ventricular ejection fraction (LVEF).
- A proportion of patients with heart failure do not have significant reductions in systolic function. This led to the understanding of the concept of diastolic dysfunction which later evolved to HFpEF.
- According to the professional societies' guidelines, the diagnosis of HFpEF requires signs and symptoms of heart failure and an LVEF ≥50%. Other sub-classifications include HF with mildly reduced EF (HFmrEF or HFpEF borderline) (LVEF 41–49%) and HF with recovered EF (HFrecEF or HFpEF improved) (patients who previously had and EF <40%) [18, 24].
- The conclusive diagnosis of HFpEF is complicated, and the H_2FPEF score and HFA-PEEF algorithm were developed to aid in its diagnosis (Figs. 16.1 and 16.2).

	Clinical Variable	Values	Points
H_2	Heavy	Body mass index > 30 kg/m^2	2
	Hypertensive	2 or more antihypertensive medicines	1
F	Atrial Fibrillation	Paroxysmal or Persistent	3
P	Pulmonary Hypertension	Doppler Echocardiographic estimated Pulmonary Artery Systolic Pressure > 35 mmHg	1
E	Elder	Age > 60 years	1
F	Filling Pressure	Doppler Echocardiographic E/e' > 9	1
	H_2FPEF score		Sum (0-9)

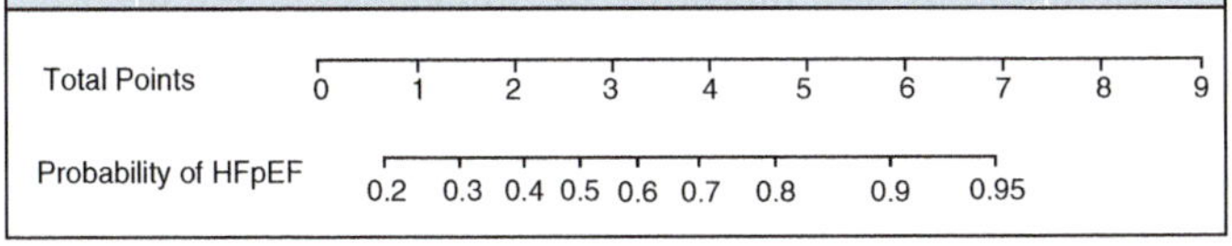

Figure 16.1 H_2FPEF score. (Adapted from Reddy et al. [19])

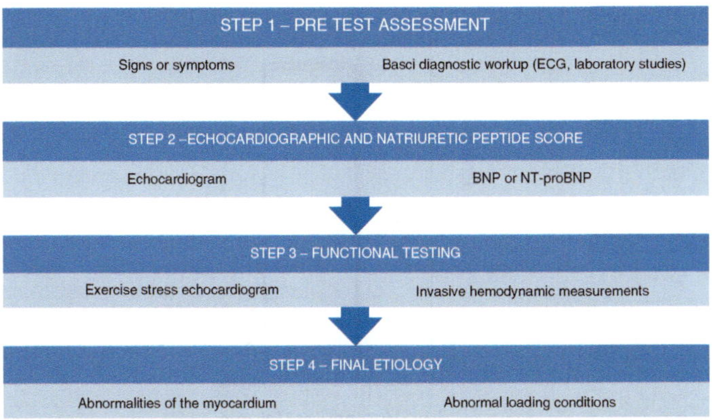

Figure 16.2 HFA-PEFF diagnostic algorithm. ECG electrocardiogram, BNP brain natriuretic peptide, NT-proBNP N-terminal pro-brain natriuretic peptide. (Adapted from Pieske et al. [16])

Pathophysiology [7]

- Most abnormalities in HFpEF are determined by an impaired LV relaxation and increased LV stiffness.
- The interaction between a reduced LV myocardial relaxation and an increased stiffness translates in a leftward shift in the ventricular pressure-volume loop that impairs left ventricular filling and therefore reduces cardiac output without compromising ejection fraction (Fig. 16.3).
- LV relaxation depends on cellular mechanisms to detach the actin-myosin cross-bridge, an active, energy-consuming process. In ischemia, the energy stores in cardiomyocytes are depleted, and therefore LV relaxation is impaired.
- LV stiffness is a passive process dependent on the myocardial compliance determined by the intracellular and extra-

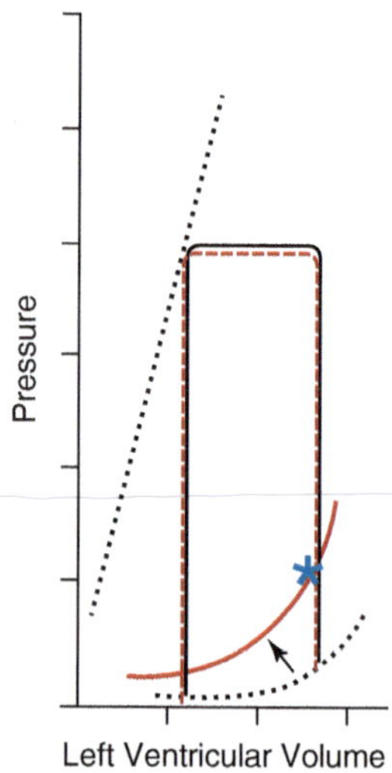

Figure 16.3 In diastolic dysfunction, the hallmark of heart failure with preserved ejection fraction (HFpEF), the diastolic normal pressure-volume line (black dotted line) is displaced upward and to the left (black arrow and red solid line); there is diminished capacity to fill at low left atrial pressures. In HFpEF, the ejection fraction is normal, and the end-diastolic pressure is elevated (blue asterisk)

cellular components. Extracellular fibrosis and collagen deposition (hypertensive heart disease), amyloid deposition, fibrosis caused by inflammatory mechanisms (cardiac sarcoidosis and eosinophilic endocarditis), and intracellular deposition of substances (Fabry, hemochromatosis) are causes of increased LV stiffness.

- The altered LV relaxation and stiffness lead to increased LV filling pressures and decreased organ perfusion resulting in the clinical syndrome of HF.

Clinical Presentation and Basic Diagnostic Testing

- Clinical syndrome is indistinguishable from other HF syndromes.
- Symptoms: exertional fatigue or dyspnea, orthopnea, paroxysmal nocturnal dyspnea, and peripheral edema. Abdominal fullness, anorexia, and early satiety might indicate advanced HFpEF with right-sided heart failure.
- Signs: elevated jugular venous pressure, hepatic congestion, ascites, lower extremity edema, and rales. An S4 on heart auscultation usually signifies left ventricular stiffness.
- Review history for comorbidities strongly linked to HFpEF, i.e., atrial fibrillation, obesity, diabetes, or metabolic syndrome.
- Electrocardiography (ECG) has low diagnostic value to identify HFpEF. ECG can help to detect conditions related to HFpEF such as hypertensive heart disease (LV hypertrophy) or cardiac amyloid (low voltages). It might suggest ischemic disease and detect atrial fibrillation which are predictive of underlying HFpEF [19].
- Initial laboratory testing: basic metabolic panel to assess electrolyte balance as well as estimated glomerular filtration rate.
- Other relevant labs: liver function tests, glycosylated hemoglobin, thyroid-stimulating hormone, complete blood count, and iron studies.

Echocardiography, Natriuretic Peptides, and Diagnostic Scores

Echocardiogram

- Useful to exclude patients with HFrEF or other causes of clinical heart failure with normal EF such as valvular disease or pericardial disease.
- A LVEF cut-off of >40% should be used when considering HFpEF (includes HFmrEF and HFrecEF).
- The most robust indicators that support the diagnosis of HFpEF include elevation in E/e' ratio (surrogate of LV filling pressures) and increase in estimated pulmonary artery systolic pressure (secondary to left atrial hypertension).
- There is no single diagnostic criterion for HFpEF. The echocardiographic evaluation should consider morphological and functional characteristics (Table 16.1) [16].

Natriuretic Peptides

- Serum brain natriuretic peptide (BNP) <35 ng/L or serum N-terminal pro-BNP (NT-proBNP) <125 ng/L has good negative predictive value to exclude heart failure [5].
- In HFpEF, where LV is not usually dilated and wall stress is compensated by hypertrophy, up to 20% of patients can have normal BNP/NT-proBNP [12].

Clinical Pearl

Elevated circulating natriuretic peptide levels are not necessary to diagnose HFpEF, but elevated concentrations increase the likelihood of HFpEF.

Table 16.1 Echocardiographic criteria for diagnosing heart failure with preserved ejection fraction

Echocardiographic parameter	**Suggestive of HFpEF**	**Observations**
Left ventricular ejection fraction – %	≥50%	
Left ventricular diastolic diameter – mm	≤5.9	
Septal mitral annular peak early diastolic velocity (e') – cm/s	<7	<5 in subjects aged ≥75 years
Lateral mitral annular peak early diastolic velocity (e') – cm/s	<10	<7 in subjects aged ≥75 years
Average septal-lateral E/e′ ratio	≥15	Values between 9 and 14 count as minor criterion in HFA-PEFF score
Tricuspid regurgitation peak velocity – m/s	>2.8	
Pulmonary arterial systolic pressure – mmHg	>35	
Left ventricular global longitudinal systolic strain – %	<−16	
Left atrial volume index – mL/m²	>34 in sinus rhythm >40 in atrial fibrillation	Values between 29 and 34 in sinus rhythm and between 34 and 40 in atrial fibrillation count as minor criterion in HFA-PEFF score

(continued)

Table 16.1 (continued)

Echocardiographic parameter	Suggestive of HFpEF	Observations
Left ventricular mass index – g/m^2	≥149 in men ≥122 in women	Values above 115 in men or 95 in women count as minor criterion in HFA-PEFF score
Relative wall thickness	>0.42	

Adapted from Pieske et al. [16]. *HFpEF* heart failure with preserved ejection fraction

HFA-PEFF Score [16]

- Three different domains: functional, morphological, and biomarkers (differentiated cut-offs depending of underlying rhythm, i.e., sinus rhythm vs. atrial fibrillation) (Table 16.2).
- Each domain can contribute 2 points if any major criterion is met or 1 point if no major but any minor criteria are positive. Several major criteria within a single domain still contribute *only* 2 points.
- A score ≥5 points is considered to be diagnostic for HFpEF, and a score ≤1 makes the diagnosis very unlikely. Scores between 2 and 4 need further functional testing.

H_2FPEF Score [19]

- The score is the sum of points assigned to the variables outlined in Figure 16.1.
- A score ≥6 points translates in a high likelihood of HFpEF, a score ≤1 makes the diagnosis very unlikely, and scores between 2 and 5 translate in an intermediate probability that should trigger the pursuit of functional testing.

TABLE 16.2 Echocardiographic and natriuretic peptide heart failure with preserved ejection fraction workup and scoring system

	Functional	Morphological	Biomarkers (sinus rhythm)	Biomarker (atrial fibrillation)
Major criteria	Septal e' <7 cm/s OR Lateral e' <10 cm/s OR Average E/e' ≥15 OR TR peak velocity ≥2.8 m/s OR PASP >35 mmHg	LA volume index >34 ml/m^2 OR LV mass index ≥149/122 (men/women) AND RWT >0.42	NT-proBNP >220 ng/L OR BNP >80 ng/L	NT-proBNP >660 ng/L OR BNP >240 ng/L
Minor criteria	Average E/e' 9–14 OR LV-GLS <16%	LA volume index 29–34 ml/m^2 OR LV mass index ≥115/95 (men/women) OR RWT ≥0.42 OR LV wall thickness ≥12 mm	NT-proBNP 125–220 ng/L OR BNP 23–80 ng/L	NT-proBNP 365–660 ng/L OR BNP 105–240 ng/L

TR tricuspid regurgitation, *PASP* pulmonary artery systolic pressure, *LV-GLS* left ventricular global longitudinal strain, *LA* left atrium, *LV* left ventricle, *RWT* relative wall thickness, *BNP* brain natriuretic peptide, *NT-proBNP* N-terminal pro-brain natriuretic peptide

Functional Testing [16]

Exercise Stress Echocardiography

- In HFpEF, impaired relaxation and increased stiffness prevent the physiologic increase in stroke volume and cardiac output seen during exertion. Instead, there are increased filling pressures and pulmonary artery systolic pressure (PASP).
- A ratio of the peak velocity of mitral inflow during early diastole (E) over the average of septal and lateral mitral annular early diastolic peak velocities (e′) ≥15 is highly suggestive of elevated filling pressures. This adds 2 points to the HFA-PEFF score.
- If, in addition to the E/e’ ≥15, the tricuspid regurgitation peak velocity increases to ≥3.4 m/s, an extra point is added to the HFA-PEFF score.

Invasive Hemodynamic Assessment

- The left ventricular end-diastolic pressure (LVEDP) is the goal standard for diagnosis. It can be obtained by direct measurement in a left heart catheterization or extrapolated from the mean pulmonary capillary wedge pressure (mPCWP) during a right heart catheterization.
- A LVEDP ≥16 mmHg or mPCWP ≥15 mmHg is diagnostic for HFpEF.
- Normal LVEDP or mPCWP during rest does not exclude HFpEF. Direct hemodynamic measurement cut-offs to diagnose HFpEF during exercise are LVEDP ≥25 mmHg or PCWP 20–23 mmHg.
- Normal filling pressures at rest with abnormal increase during exercise are associated with a twofold increase in mortality.

Specific Etiologies Investigation

Most cases of HFpEF are related to common risk factors and comorbidities, but the possibility of a specific underlying etiology should always be considered. A classification in phenotypes or phenogroups has been proposed, but there is no consensus yet [3, 20].

Abnormalities of the Myocardium

- Ischemia: Important to identify coronary artery disease if present and attempt revascularization if feasible. Cardiac magnetic resonance can also be helpful to identify areas of scar.
- Toxic: Recreational substances (alcohol and anabolic steroids), heavy metals (iron and copper), medications (chloroquine), and radiation.
- Immune/inflammatory: Infectious and non-infectious causes of myocarditis including autoimmune conditions such as systemic lupus erythematosus and other connective tissue disorders.
- Infiltrative: Cardiac amyloid, sarcoid, but other rarer causes include hemochromatosis and metabolic storage (Fabry and Pompe).
- Metabolic: Most common is thyroid disease but also seen in acromegaly and nutritional deficiency syndromes (thiamine and selenium).
- Genetic: Hypertrophic cardiomyopathy, restrictive cardiomyopathies, myocardial non-compaction, and other muscular dystrophies.

Clinical Pearl
Wild-type amyloid transthyretin cardiac amyloidosis (ATTRwt) may be present in 12–19% of people with HFpEF. Also, 3–4% of African Americans have an

ATTR mutation (V122I). It is important to recognize this condition as novel therapeutics such as tafamidis and patisiran have demonstrated efficacy in treating this disease. Tafamidis (transthyretin stabilizer) was approved by FDA in May 2019 for the treatment of ATTR cardiomyopathy.

Abnormal Loading Conditions

- Hypertension: Usually long-standing and causing LV hypertrophy
- Valvular and structural defects: Acquired and congenital
- Pericardial disease: Constrictive pericarditis
- High output states: Severe anemia, sepsis, pregnancy, and thyrotoxicosis
- Volume overload: Various causes including renal/liver failure
- Rhythm disorders: Atrial/ventricular arrhythmias and right ventricular pacing

Treatment

- The current ACC/AHA guideline recommendations for the treatment of HFpEF are summarized in Table 16.3 [24].

Lifestyle Interventions

- Improved cardiorespiratory fitness and quality of life from structured exercise training [13].
- The SECRET trial showed that structured exercise training and weight loss achieved through caloric restriction improved aerobic capacity and the effects of both interventions were additive [9].

TABLE 16.3 Guideline recommendations for the treatment of heart failure with preserved ejection fraction

Class of recommendations	**Recommendation**
Class I recommendations	
Blood pressure control	Systolic and diastolic blood pressure should be controlled in patients with HFpEF in accordance with published clinical practice guidelines to prevent morbidity
Diuretics	Diuretics should be used for relief of symptoms due to volume overload in patients with HFpEF
Class IIa recommendations	
Coronary revascularization	Coronary revascularization is reasonable in patients with CAD in whom symptoms (angina) or demonstrable myocardial ischemia is judged to be having an adverse effect on symptomatic HFpEF despite GDMT
Management of atrial fibrillation	Management of AF according to published clinical practice guidelines in patients with HFpEF is reasonable to improve symptomatic HF
Blood pressure medications	The use of beta-blocking agents, ACE inhibitors, and ARBs in patients with hypertension is reasonable to control blood pressure in patients with HFpEF
Class IIb recommendations	

(continued)

TABLE 16.3 (continued)

Class of recommendations	Recommendation
Aldosterone receptor antagonists	In appropriately selected patients with HFpEF (with EF ‡45%, elevated BNP levels or HF admission within 1 year, estimated glomerular filtration rate >30 mL/min, creatinine <2.5 mg/dL, potassium <5.0 mEq/L), aldosterone receptor antagonists might be considered to decrease hospitalizations
Angiotensin receptor blockers	The use of ARBs might be considered to decrease hospitalizations for patients with HFpEF
Class III recommendations (recommendation against)	
Nitrates or phosphodiesterase-5 inhibitors	Routine use of nitrates or phosphodiesterase-5 inhibitors to increase activity or QoL in patients with HFpEF is ineffective
Nutritional supplements	Routine use of nutritional supplements is not recommended for patients with HFpEF

Adapted from Yancy et al. [24]. *HFpEF* heart failure with preserved ejection fraction, *CAD* coronary artery disease, *GDMT* guideline-directed medical therapy, *AF* atrial fibrillation, *HF* heart failure, *ACE* angiotensin-converting enzyme, *ARB* angiotensin receptor blocker, *EF* ejection fraction, *BNP* brain natriuretic peptide, *QoL* quality of life

- The sodium-restricted dietary approaches to stop hypertension (DASH/SRD) diet showed improvement in diastolic function, but no clinical outcomes have been published [8].

Diuretics

- Diuretics should be used for symptomatic relief edema and pulmonary congestion.
- Loop diuretics including furosemide and torsemide are first line.
- In the case of diuretic resistance, thiazide or potassium-sparing diuretics can be used to augment diuresis.

Renin-Angiotensin-Aldosterone System Inhibitors

- No large randomized clinical trial studying renin-angiotensin-aldosterone system inhibitors has been able to show a mortality benefit in HFpEF.
- The CHARM-Preserved trial randomized patients to candesartan or placebo, and the composite primary endpoint of cardiovascular death or HF hospitalization was similar in both groups. Secondary analyses suggested a potential benefit in reducing heart failure hospitalizations [25].
- The I-PRESERVE trial randomized patients to irbesartan or placebo, and the composite primary endpoint of all-cause mortality or cardiovascular hospitalization was similar in both groups. The possible benefit in heart failure hospitalizations seen in CHARM-Preserved was not replicated [11].
- The PEP-CHF trial randomized patients to perindopril or placebo, and the composite primary endpoint of all-cause mortality or cardiovascular hospitalization was similar in both groups [2].
- The TOPCAT trial randomized patients to spironolactone or placebo, and the composite primary endpoint of cardiovascular death, HF hospitalization, or aborted cardiac arrest was similar in both groups. However, when analyzing patients recruited in the Americas, the primary endpoint was met and showed a 18% decrease in the primary outcome [17].

- The PARAGON-HF trial randomized patients to sacubitril-valsartan or placebo, and the composite primary endpoint of total hospitalizations for heart failure and death from cardiovascular causes was similar in both groups, but a signal toward benefit was seen (rate ratio, 0.87; 95% confidence interval, 0.75 to 1.01; $P = 0.06$). Based on this trial and secondary analyses, FDA approved the expanded indication of sacubitril-valsartan for the treatment of HFpEF [21].

Beta-blockers

- The Japanese Diastolic Heart Failure Study randomized patients to carvedilol or placebo. There was no significant difference in the composite of cardiovascular death and unplanned hospitalization for HF [23].
- The ELANDD trial result attempted to validate the theory that beta-blockers improved exercise capacity. Patients were randomized to nebivolol vs. placebo. There was no difference in the primary endpoint of change in six MWD from baseline or peak oxygen uptake [4].

Device Therapies

- An ancillary analysis of the CHAMPION trial showed that guided management using continuous hemodynamic monitoring with CardioMEMS reduced decompensation leading to hospitalization. Similar benefit in HFpEF was seen in HFrEF [1].

Other Treatment Targets [24]

- Hypertension should be controlled according to published guidelines to a goal systolic blood pressure of <130 mmHg.
- Coronary revascularization should be attempted if there are symptoms of ischemic heart disease and is judged to have a negative impact on symptomatic HFpEF.

- Atrial fibrillation management should be optimized to improve symptomatic HFpEF.

Ongoing Trials [14]

- The EMPEROR-Preserved trial enrolled patients with HFpEF and randomized them to empagliflozin, an SGLT-2 inhibitor, or placebo. In this study, empagliflozin was associated with a lower risk of HF hospitalization and cardiovascular death. The 21% reduction in the primary outcome was mainly driven by a reduction in HF hospitalizations [22].
- Studies of quality of life and exercise capacity outcomes are also ongoing with multiple molecules including inorganic nitrates, guanylate cyclase stimulators, endothelin receptor antagonists, calcium handling molecules, and molecules targeting mitochondrial dysfunction, among others.

Prognosis

- Higher mortality compared to individuals without heart failure.
- In comparison to HFrEF, some population studies have shown similar mortality in HFpEF. However, others suggest that HFpEF is associated to lower cardiovascular mortality while non-cardiovascular mortality is higher [6].
- Rates of hospitalization, hospitalization duration, and quality of life appear to be comparable between HFrEF and HFpEF [10].

Key Learning Points

- HFpEF is the clinical syndrome resulting from impaired left ventricular relaxation and increase LV stiffness with normal LVEF.
- The diagnosis of HFpEF is a multi-step process that includes clinical evaluation and basic laboratory

workup, echocardiographic evaluation, and investigation of etiologies.
- FDA expanded sacubitril/valsartan indication (Feb 2021) to reduce risk of cardiovascular death and hospitalization for adult patients with chronic heart failure, including HFpEF patients. Approval of empagliflozin in this population is expected.

References

1. Adamson PB, Abraham WT, Bourge RC, Costanzo MR, Hasan A, Yadav C, et al. Wireless pulmonary artery pressure monitoring guides management to reduce decompensation in heart failure with preserved ejection fraction. Circ Heart Fail. 2014;7(6):935–44. https://doi.org/10.1161/CIRCHEARTFAILURE.113.001229.
2. Cleland JG, Tendera M, Adamus J, Freemantle N, Polonski L, Taylor J, Investigators P-C. The perindopril in elderly people with chronic heart failure (PEP-CHF) study. Eur Heart J. 2006;27(19):2338–45. https://doi.org/10.1093/eurheartj/ehl250.
3. Cohen JB, Schrauben SJ, Zhao L, Basso MD, Cvijic ME, Li Z, et al. Clinical Phenogroups in Heart Failure With Preserved Ejection Fraction: Detailed Phenotypes, Prognosis, and Response to Spironolactone. JACC Heart Fail. 2020;8(3):172–84. https://doi.org/10.1016/j.jchf.2019.09.009.
4. Conraads VM, Metra M, Kamp O, De Keulenaer GW, Pieske B, Zamorano J, et al. Effects of the long-term administration of nebivolol on the clinical symptoms, exercise capacity, and left ventricular function of patients with diastolic dysfunction: results of the ELANDD study. Eur J Heart Fail. 2012;14(2):219–25. https://doi.org/10.1093/eurjhf/hfr161.
5. Doust JA, Glasziou PP, Pietrzak E, Dobson AJ. A systematic review of the diagnostic accuracy of natriuretic peptides for heart failure. Arch Intern Med. 2004;164(18):1978–84. https://doi.org/10.1001/archinte.164.18.1978.
6. Gerber Y, Weston SA, Redfield MM, Chamberlain AM, Manemann SM, Jiang R, et al. A contemporary appraisal of the heart failure epidemic in Olmsted County, Minnesota, 2000 to 2010. JAMA Intern Med. 2015;175(6):996–1004. https://doi.org/10.1001/jamainternmed.2015.0924.

7. Gevaert AB, Boen JRA, Segers VF, Van Craenenbroeck EM. Heart failure with preserved ejection fraction: a review of cardiac and noncardiac pathophysiology. Front Physiol. 2019;10:638. https://doi.org/10.3389/fphys.2019.00638.
8. Hummel SL, Seymour EM, Brook RD, Sheth SS, Ghosh E, Zhu S, et al. Low-sodium DASH diet improves diastolic function and ventricular-arterial coupling in hypertensive heart failure with preserved ejection fraction. Circ Heart Fail. 2013;6(6):1165–71. https://doi.org/10.1161/CIRCHEARTFAILURE.113.000481.
9. Kitzman DW, Brubaker P, Morgan T, Haykowsky M, Hundley G, Kraus WE, et al. Effect of caloric restriction or aerobic exercise training on peak oxygen consumption and quality of life in obese older patients with heart failure with preserved ejection fraction: a randomized clinical trial. JAMA. 2016;315(1):36–46. https://doi.org/10.1001/jama.2015.17346.
10. Loop MS, Van Dyke MK, Chen L, Brown TM, Durant RW, Safford MM, Levitan EB. Comparison of length of stay, 30-day mortality, and 30-day readmission rates in medicare patients with heart failure and with reduced versus preserved ejection fraction. Am J Cardiol. 2016;118(1):79–85. https://doi.org/10.1016/j.amjcard.2016.04.015.
11. Massie BM, Carson PE, McMurray JJ, Komajda M, McKelvie R, Zile MR, et al. Irbesartan in patients with heart failure and preserved ejection fraction. N Engl J Med. 2008;359(23):2456–67. https://doi.org/10.1056/NEJMoa0805450.
12. Meijers WC, Hoekstra T, Jaarsma T, van Veldhuisen DJ, de Boer RA. Patients with heart failure with preserved ejection fraction and low levels of natriuretic peptides. Neth Heart J. 2016;24(4):287–95. https://doi.org/10.1007/s12471-016-0816-8.
13. Pandey A, Parashar A, Kumbhani D, Agarwal S, Garg J, Kitzman D, et al. Exercise training in patients with heart failure and preserved ejection fraction: meta-analysis of randomized control trials. Circ Heart Fail. 2015;8(1):33–40. https://doi.org/10.1161/CIRCHEARTFAILURE.114.001615.
14. Parikh KS, Sharma K, Fiuzat M, Surks HK, George JT, Honarpour N, et al. Heart failure with preserved ejection fraction expert panel report: current controversies and implications for clinical trials. JACC Heart Fail. 2018;6(8):619–32. https://doi.org/10.1016/j.jchf.2018.06.008.
15. Pfeffer MA, Shah AM, Borlaug BA. Heart failure with preserved ejection fraction in perspective. Circ Res. 2019;124(11):1598–617. https://doi.org/10.1161/CIRCRESAHA.119.313572.

16. Pieske B, Tschope C, de Boer RA, Fraser AG, Anker SD, Donal E, et al. How to diagnose heart failure with preserved ejection fraction: the HFA-PEFF diagnostic algorithm: a consensus recommendation from the Heart Failure Association (HFA) of the European Society of Cardiology (ESC). Eur Heart J. 2019;40(40):3297–317. https://doi.org/10.1093/eurheartj/ehz641.
17. Pitt B, Pfeffer MA, Assmann SF, Boineau R, Anand IS, Claggett B, et al. Spironolactone for heart failure with preserved ejection fraction. N Engl J Med. 2014;370(15):1383–92. https://doi.org/10.1056/NEJMoa1313731.
18. Ponikowski P, Voors AA, Anker SD, Bueno H, Cleland JGF, Coats AJS, et al. 2016 ESC Guidelines for the diagnosis and treatment of acute and chronic heart failure: The Task Force for the diagnosis and treatment of acute and chronic heart failure of the European Society of Cardiology (ESC) Developed with the special contribution of the Heart Failure Association (HFA) of the ESC. Eur Heart J. 2016;37(27):2129–200. https://doi.org/10.1093/eurheartj/ehw128.
19. Reddy YNV, Carter RE, Obokata M, Redfield MM, Borlaug BA. A simple, evidence-based approach to help guide diagnosis of heart failure with preserved ejection fraction. Circulation. 2018;138(9):861–70. https://doi.org/10.1161/CIRCULATIONAHA.118.034646.
20. Samson R, Jaiswal A, Ennezat PV, Cassidy M, Le Jemtel TH. Clinical phenotypes in heart failure with preserved ejection fraction. J Am Heart Assoc. 2016;5(1) https://doi.org/10.1161/JAHA.115.002477.
21. Solomon SD, McMurray JJV, Anand IS, Ge J, Lam CSP, Maggioni AP, et al. Angiotensin-neprilysin inhibition in heart failure with preserved ejection fraction. N Engl J Med. 2019;381(17):1609–20. https://doi.org/10.1056/NEJMoa1908655.
22. Stefan D, Anker Javed, Butler Gerasimos, Filippatos João P, Ferreira Edimar, Bocchi Michael, Böhm Hans-Peter, Brunner–La Rocca Dong-Ju, Choi Vijay, Chopra Eduardo, Chuquiure-Valenzuela Nadia, Giannetti Juan Esteban, Gomez-Mesa Stefan, Janssens James L, Januzzi Jose R, Gonzalez-Juanatey Bela, Merkely Stephen J, Nicholls Sergio V, Perrone Ileana L, Piña Piotr, Ponikowski Michele, Senni David, Sim Jindrich, Spinar Iain, Squire Stefano, Taddei Hiroyuki, Tsutsui Subodh, Verma Dragos, Vinereanu Jian, Zhang Peter, Carson Carolyn Su Ping, Lam Nikolaus, Marx Cordula, Zeller Naveed, Sattar Waheed, Jamal Sven, Schnaidt Janet M, Schnee Martina, Brueckmann

Stuart J, Pocock Faiez, Zannad Milton, Packer. Empagliflozin in Heart Failure with a Preserved Ejection Fraction. N Engl J Med. 2021;385(16):1451–61. https://doi.org/10.1056/NEJMoa2107038.

23. Yamamoto K, Origasa H, Hori M, Investigators JD. Effects of carvedilol on heart failure with preserved ejection fraction: the Japanese Diastolic Heart Failure Study (J-DHF). Eur J Heart Fail. 2013;15(1):110–8. https://doi.org/10.1093/eurjhf/hfs141.
24. Yancy CW, Jessup M, Bozkurt B, Butler J, Casey DE Jr, Colvin MM, et al. 2017 ACC/AHA/HFSA Focused Update of the 2013 ACCF/AHA Guideline for the Management of Heart Failure: A Report of the American College of Cardiology/American Heart Association Task Force on Clinical Practice Guidelines and the Heart Failure Society of America. Circulation. 2017;136(6):e137–61. https://doi.org/10.1161/CIR.0000000000000509.
25. Yusuf S, Pfeffer MA, Swedberg K, Granger CB, Held P, McMurray JJ, et al. Effects of candesartan in patients with chronic heart failure and preserved left-ventricular ejection fraction: the CHARM-Preserved Trial. Lancet. 2003;362(9386):777–81. https://doi.org/10.1016/S0140-6736(03)14285-7.

Part VI
Valvular Heart Disease

Chapter 17
Aortic Valve Disease

Nikoloz Shekiladze and Joe X. Xie

Abbreviations

ACEI	Angiotensin-converting enzyme inhibitor
AR	Aortic regurgitation
ARB	Angiotensin II receptor blocker
AS	Aortic stenosis
AVA	Aortic valve area
AVR	Aortic valve replacement
AU	Agatston unit
BAV	Bicuspid aortic valve
CMRI	Cardiac magnetic resonance imaging
CT	Cardiac tomography
DSE	Dobutamine stress echo
EF	Ejection fraction
ESD	End-systolic diameter
GI	Gastrointestinal
IE	Infective endocarditis
LDL	Low-density lipoprotein
LGE	Late gadolinium enhancement
LVEDP	Left ventricular end-diastolic pressure

N. Shekiladze (✉) · J. X. Xie
Department of Medicine, Division of Cardiology, Emory University School of Medicine, Atlanta, GA, USA
e-mail: nshekil@emory.edu; joe.xie@emory.edu

A. A. Bhargava et al. (eds.), *Handbook of Outpatient Cardiology*, https://doi.org/10.1007/978-3-030-88953-1_17

LVEF	Left ventricular ejection fraction
LV	Left ventricle, left ventricular
LVESD	Left ventricular end-systolic diameter
MI	Myocardial infarction
MRI	Magnetic resonance imaging
SAVR	Surgical aortic valve replacement
SLE	Systemic lupus erythematosus
STS	Society of Thoracic Surgeons
TAVR	Transcatheter aortic valve replacement
TEE	Transesophageal echocardiogram
TTE	Transthoracic echocardiogram
VKA	Vitamin K antagonist

Aortic Stenosis (AS)

Epidemiology

- Aortic stenosis typically has an indolent course with a long latent period prior to onset of symptoms followed by a rapid decline in prognosis (Fig. 17.1).
- Prevalence of AS increases by age (in years): 0.3% in 18–44, 2–7% in 45–75, and 11.7% in individuals >75 [1, 2].
- Average survival after development of symptoms among patients with severe AS is 1–3 years.

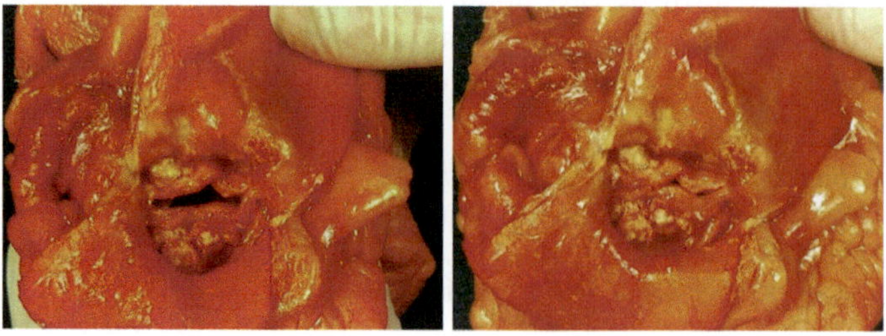

FIGURE 17.1 Intraoperative image of calcific bicuspid aortic valve in a patient with severe aortic stenosis

Anatomy and Pathology

- The aortic valve forms the bridge between the left ventricle and ascending aorta. The aortic valve annulus is a fibrous ring that is the transition point between the left ventricular outflow tract and the base of the aortic valve leaflets. The three cusps of the aortic valve are named the left, right, and non-coronary cusps and sit within the sinuses of Valsalva. The orifices of the coronary arteries also arise from the sinuses. Superiorly, the intersection of the sinuses and the ascending aorta is the sinotubular junction [3].
- Several forms of congenital aortic valve disease exist based on the number of aortic valve leaflets and include unicuspid (Fig. 17.2), bicuspid, and quadricuspid aortic valve disease [4].

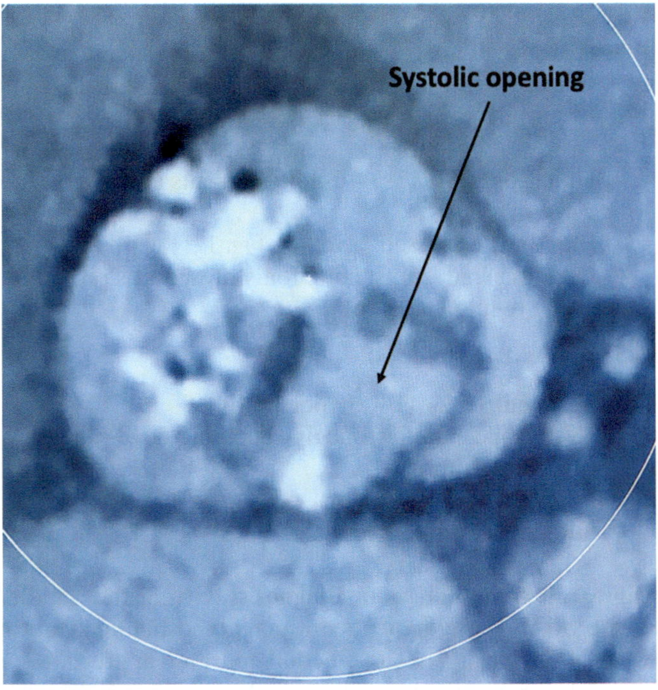

Figure 17.2 Multi-detector CT demonstrating severely calcified unicuspid valve

Common Causes of AS

- *Calcific AS* ("degenerative") is the most common cause of AS in adults.
  - Aortic sclerosis – initial stage; presence of calcified valve without hemodynamically significant stenosis.
  - Associations have been documented between calcific aortic valve disease and cardiovascular risk factors including hypertension, diabetes, dyslipidemia, and smoking [5].
- Rheumatic AS
  - Incidence is low in developed countries.
  - Similar to rheumatic mitral stenosis, the characteristic feature of rheumatic AS is fusion of the aortic valve commissures. The aortic valve orifice is subsequently reduced to a small triangular opening.
  - Aortic stenosis and regurgitation can present simultaneously.
- Congenital AS
  - Unicuspid (Fig. 17.2) – usually presents at a younger age with severe AS
  - Bicuspid (discussed later; see Fig. 17.1)
  - Quadricuspid – most commonly presents as progressive aortic regurgitation [6]
- Sequelae of Chronic AS
  - Left ventricular (LV) hypertrophy
  - LV systolic and diastolic dysfunction
  - Myocardial fibrosis
  - Pulmonary hypertension
  - Sub-endocardial ischemia

Clinical Presentation and Diagnosis: Given the indolent course of AS, many patients are diagnosed before symptom onset based on a systolic ejection murmur appreciated on physical examination followed by confirmation with echocardiography.

- Presenting Symptoms
  - Syncope (reduced cerebral perfusion from decreased cardiac output)
  - Angina (increased O2 demand due to decreased coronary flow reserve)
  - Heart failure: exertional dyspnea, paroxysmal nocturnal dyspnea, orthopnea, lower extremity edema, and fatigue
  - Heyde syndrome (GI bleeding from angiodysplasia) [7]

Physical Exam

- *Murmur* in severe aortic stenosis:
  - Systolic ejection murmur in the right upper sternal border.
  - Ejection click for bicuspid aortic valve (BAV).
  - Loudness of murmur is *not* necessarily associated with degree of stenosis.
  - Duration and timing of murmur *are* associated with stenosis severity. As aortic stenosis worsens, it takes longer for blood to be ejected through the valve. Thus, mild AS would have an early peaking murmur, while in severe AS, the murmur peaks later in systole.
  - Soft S2
- *Carotid pulse*: parvus et tardus (weak and delayed): slow-rising, late-peaking, low-amplitude carotid pulse
- *Heart failure*: lower extremity edema, elevated jugular venous pulsation, and crackles on lung auscultation

Diagnosis

Classification of AS (Fig. 17.3) [8]

- At risk (stage A, normal leaflet motion, no symptoms, aortic sclerosis, and no hemodynamic consequences).
- Progressive AS (stage B, leaflet calcification present, mild to moderate aortic stenosis by mean gradients and maxi-

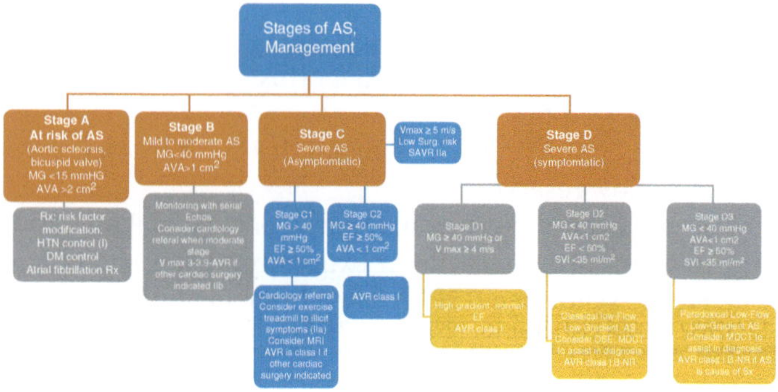

FIGURE 17.3 Recommendations and management based on AS staging

mum aortic velocity, no symptoms, LV ejection fraction (LVEF) preserved).

- Classic severe AS (stage C1 in asymptomatic patients and stage D1 in symptomatic patients).
- Severe low-flow, low-gradient aortic stenosis in patients with low LVEF (<50%) (stage C2 in asymptomatic and stage D2 in symptomatic patients). Dobutamine stress echo (DSE) can help distinguish pseudo-severe AS vs true severe AS (IIa).
- Severe low-flow, low-gradient aortic stenosis in patients with preserved LVEF (≥50%) ("paradoxical," stage D3). Evaluation of stroke volume index by echo and valve calcification by CT can be helpful in determining true severity of aortic stenosis.

Echocardiography: gold standard test for evaluation of AS

- Allows evaluation of valve anatomy and stenosis severity
- Evaluation of LV systolic/diastolic function
- Standard echo report delineating AS severity will include:
  - Doppler data of aortic valve jet velocity (Vmax), pressure gradient across the aortic valve, and aortic valve area (AVA), which have been well validated to predict clinical outcomes (Table 17.1)

TABLE 17.1 Echocardiographic grading of AS severity

AS grading and severity	Aortic sclerosis	Mild	Moderate	Severe
Peak velocity (m/s)	≤2.5 m/s	2.6–2.9	3.0–4.0	≥4.0
Mean gradient (mmHg)		<20	20–40	≥40
AVA (cm^2)		>1.5	1.0–1.5	<1.0

Baumgartner H et al. JASE (2017) 30(4):372–392

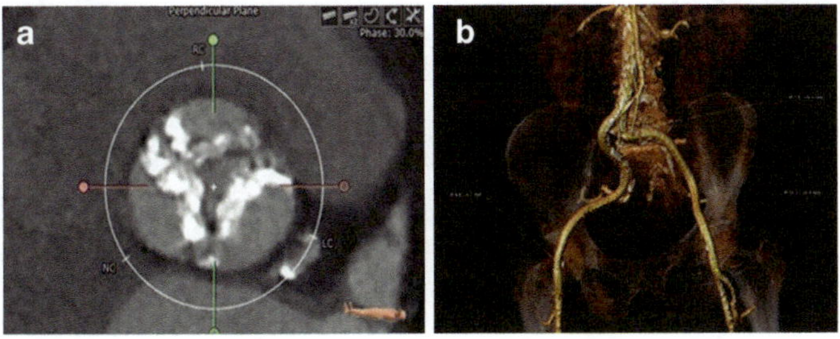

FIGURE 17.4 (**a**) Multi-detector CT (MDCT) demonstrating severely calcified leaflets of the patient with severe aortic stenosis drying systole. (**b**) CT angiogram run-off showing peripheral vasculature for sizing

Cardiac Computer Tomography (CT) (Fig. 17.4)

- Used for measurement of valve dimensions for transcatheter valve replacement planning.
- In stages D2 and D3, measurement of aortic valve calcium by CT imaging to confirm AS severity (IIa) [8].
- Current aortic valve calcium score thresholds for severe AS are female >1300 and male >2000 [9–12] (Fig. 17.5).
- Peripheral vascular anatomy for transcatheter intervention access.

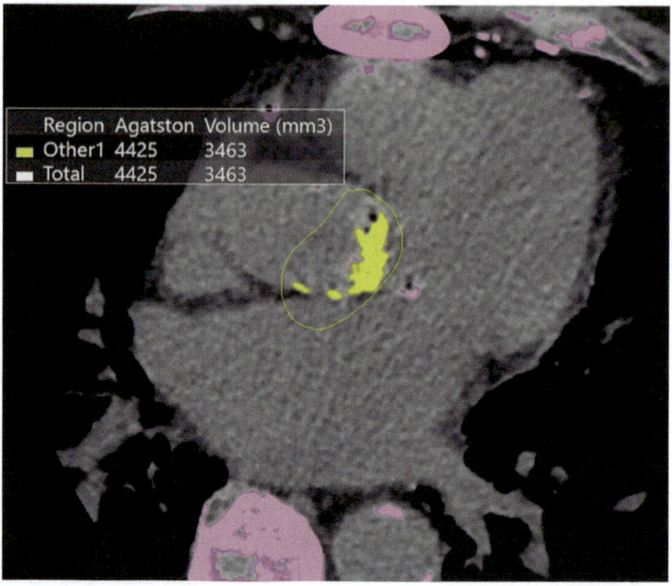

FIGURE 17.5 Aortic valve calcium score on MDCT indicating severe AS

Cardiac Catheterization

- Recommended when non-invasive tests are inconclusive
- Coronary evaluation before surgical evaluation [13]

Exercise Stress Testing

- Used to unmask symptoms in asymptomatic patients [14]
- Can be done in select patients under careful cardiology supervision

Cardiac Magnetic Resonance Imaging

- Late gadolinium enhancement suggesting myocardial fibrosis may be used to risk-stratify patients [15].

Treatment

- Surveillance with repeat imaging is important in asymptomatic patients: 3–5 years in mild AS, 1–2 years in moderate AS, and 6–12 months in severe AS [13].
- The role of early aortic valve replacement (AVR) in asymptomatic patients is unknown.
- AVR is superior to medical therapy in severe AS once symptoms develop [16].
- Medical therapy is always concurrently used to treat conventional cardiovascular risk factors:

  - Hypertension (no particular preference in class of medications, but diuretics should be used with caution to prevent sudden drops in preload).
  - Coronary artery disease, both primary and secondary prevention.
  - Statin therapy to treat aortic stenosis alone has not been shown to be beneficial (III) [8].
  - Tachyarrhythmias such as atrial fibrillation may result in further decline of cardiac output and unmask symptoms.

- AVR in symptomatic AS patients is recommended and can be performed with surgical (SAVR) or transcatheter (TAVR) approach [17].

  - Prohibitive or high surgical risk: STS>8%, ≥2 frailty measures, or ≤2 organ systems – TAVR (class I, if acceptable quality of life >1 year). Palliative care recommended if quality of life <1 year (class 1).
  - When surgical risk is NOT high or prohibitive: options are mechanical AVR (if VKA anticoagulation use is acceptable, and younger age, class IIa) or a bioprosthetic AVR (SAVR or TAVR) if VKA anticoagulation is contraindicated or not desired (class I).
  - Symptomatic severe AS (stages D1–D3) or severe AS with LVEF<50% with valve and vascular anatomy suitable for transcatheter aortic intervention:

TAVR (class I) is recommended in adult patients >80 y.
Both SAVR and TAVR are effective approaches in adults 65–80 years of age (class I).
SAVR is recommended in age group <65 y (class I) [8].

- Multidisciplinary heart valve team is recommended in decision for SAVR or TAVR candidacy [18].

> **Clinical Pearl**
> AVR (SAVR or TAVT) should be discussed at multidisciplinary team and patient age, and 1-year prognosis should be considered in decision-making according to recent guidelines.

Aortic Regurgitation (AR)

Epidemiology

- In the Framingham study, the prevalence of AR was estimated at 4.9%.
- Similar to AS, incidence and severity of AR increase with age [19, 20].

Causes [5]

- Primary (leaflet pathology):
  - Calcific, degenerative aortic valve disease affecting leaflet coaptation
  - Infective endocarditis (perforation and destruction of the leaflets)
  - Rheumatic fever (Fig. 17.6)
  - Congenital aortic valve disease
  - Autoimmune diseases involving aortic valve leaflets: lupus, Takayasu, ankylosing spondylitis, and Crohn's disease

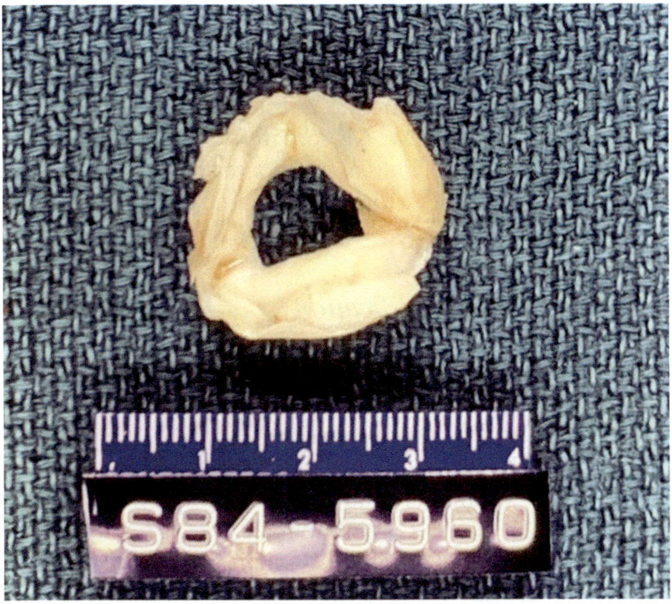

FIGURE 17.6 Gross anatomic image of excised rheumatic valve in patient with severe AI

- Secondary (aortic root disease):
  - Aortic dilation
  - Aortic dissection
  - Syphilitic aortitis
  - Reactive arthritis
  - Giant cell arteritis
  - Behcet's disease
  - Psoriatic arthritis
  - Relapsing polychondritis

Clinical Pearl
In chronic severe AR, there are eccentric LV hypertrophy and chamber dilation as a result of LV volume and pressure overload. As AR progresses over time, LV systolic function declines as compensatory LV hypertrophy fails to keep up with hemodynamic load.

Symptoms and Classification

Chronic AR Stages [8, 13]

- Stage A – At risk, asymptomatic.
- Stage B – Mild to moderate AR, normal LV function and normal LV volume or mild dilation, asymptomatic.
- Stage C – Severe AR, asymptomatic.
- C1: Normal EF (≥55%), LV dilation (LV end-systolic diameter LVESD ≤50 mm).
- C2: Depressed EF (<55%), LV dilation (LVESD >50 mm).
- Stage D – Severe AR, symptomatic; EF can be normal or reduced.

Chronic Severe AR

- Mostly asymptomatic until late stages when heart failure symptoms develop: dyspnea, orthopnea, and PND

Acute Severe AR

- Acute elevation in LV end-diastolic pressure from inability of LV to accommodate regurgitant volume leads to premature closure of mitral valve, decreased stroke volume, and decreased cardiac output.
- Patients become acutely sick and present with cardiovascular shock with profound hypotension, pulmonary congestion, and hypoxia [20].
- Most often occurs due to infectious endocarditis, aortic dissection, or trauma [21].

Physical Exam

- Wide pulse pressure.
- Laterally displaced apical impulse.
- Blowing diastolic decrescendo murmur immediately after A2 best heard at the level of upper sternal border. Longer duration of the murmur correlates with severity of AR.
- Austin Flint murmur (mid to late diastolic murmur) can also be heard due to regurgitant jet impinging opening of the anterior mitral leaflet.
- The first heart sound (S_1) may be diminished due to premature closure of mitral valve; S3 and S4 can also be present [22].
- *Characteristic Peripheral Signs of Chronic Severe AR*
  - *De Musset:* head bobbing with heartbeat
  - *Muller:* pulsation of the uvula with systole
  - *Quincke:* capillary pulsations when transmitting light through the patient's fingertips or exerting light pressure on the tip of the fingernail
  - *Traube:* "pistol shot" systolic and diastolic sounds over femoral arteries
  - *Corrigan:* abrupt distention and collapse of the pulses

Diagnosis

- *Echocardiography:* Transthoracic echo (TTE) is the preferred modality that incorporates use of color flow and Doppler echocardiography to estimate severity of the AR [5].
- Transesophageal echo (TEE) can be used when TTE images are suboptimal and to help identify etiology of the AR (IE, abscess, aortic dissection).
- *Cardiac Magnetic Resonance Imaging (CMRI*, Fig. 17.7): Useful in the evaluation of the severity of AR in patients with equivocal echocardiographic findings [23].

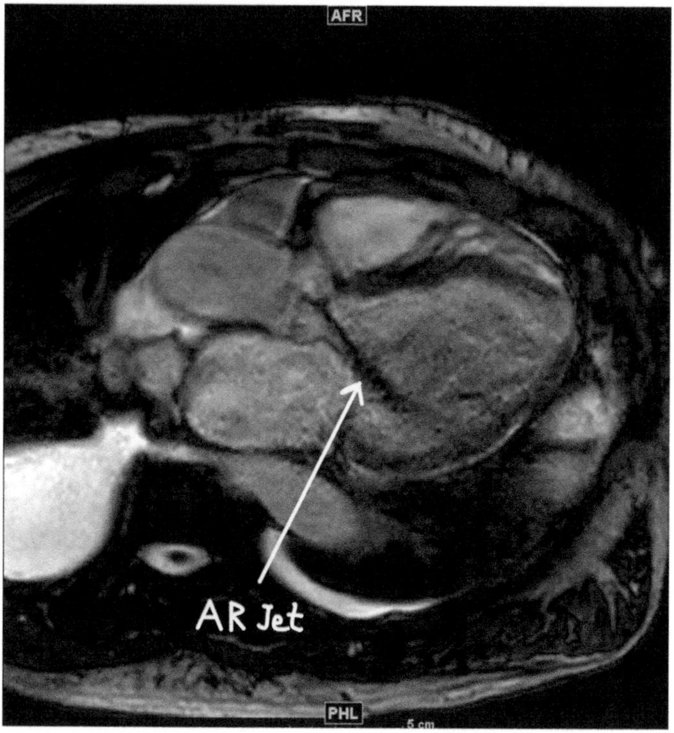

FIGURE 17.7 Cardiac magnetic resonance image of severe aortic regurgitation

Treatment

- *Acute Severe AR*
  - Urgent surgical intervention usually is required as this can lead to very rapid LV failure and circulatory collapse [13, 24].
  - Supportive care until surgical intervention includes medical therapy with inotropes and vasodilators to augment forward flow.
  - Surgery may be delayed for several days if the patient is stable, and antibiotic therapy is required for active IE [25].

- *Chronic Severe AR*
  - *Medical Management*

    In asymptomatic patients, TTE should be performed yearly to evaluate for the presence of systolic dysfunction and/or LV dilation [20].
    No dedicated medical therapy is recommended for severe AR [8].
    Treat uncontrolled hypertension: vasodilators such as dihydropyridine calcium channel blockers [26], angiotensin-converting enzyme inhibitors, or angiotensin II receptor blockers can be used. There are no definitive randomized clinical trials that show benefit of vasodilators in altering natural history of asymptomatic patients with chronic severe AR and normal LV systolic function [13, 20].
    In symptomatic inoperable patients, it is reasonable to treat them with aggressive HF regimen [13].

  - *Surgical Management* [8, 13]

    Symptomatic patients should undergo AVR regardless of LV systolic function.
    AVR is also indicated in asymptomatic patients with severe AR and LVEF ≤55% or end-systolic diameter (ESD) >50 mm (indexed LVESD >25 mm/m^2).
    AVR is indicated in severe AR and reasonable in moderate AR, if undergoing cardiac surgery for another indication.
    Transcatheter valve intervention in severe AR is not currently recommended, but there are reports on the use of transcatheter valves off-label, as well as ongoing research in the development of novel transcatheter valves specifically for AR [27].

Bicuspid Aortic Valve (BAV) Disease (Fig. 17.8)

- Congenital BAV presenting in 0.5–2% of the general population with 3:1 male-to-female predominance [28].

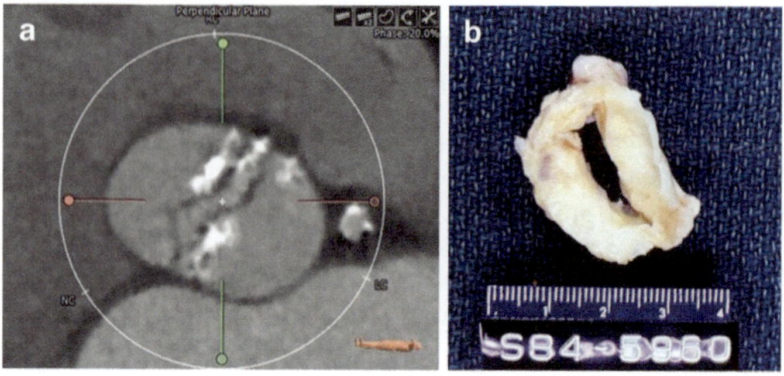

FIGURE 17.8 (**a**) Multi-detector CT demonstrating bicuspid Sievers type 0. (**b**) Gross anatomic picture of excised bicuspid aortic valve

- The most common type is fusion of left and right coronary cusps in 70% patients.
- Associated with aortopathy in about 20–40% of patients [28, 29].
- Diagnosis is with echocardiography and can be further confirmed by CT or MRI, which can also further delineate the size and morphology of the aortic root [8].
- Management of BAV differs based on hemodynamic consequences of valve dysfunction – AS or AR [5].

Key Points

- Important aspects of medical care in patients with AVD include accurate diagnosis of the etiology and severity.
- Monitoring of onset of symptoms and prompt recognition and treatment of associated cardiac conditions, i.e., hypertension, coronary artery disease, aortic dilation, and atrial fibrillation.
- Interval follow-up and surveillance by cardiac imaging.
- Indications and timing of surgical or transcatheter correction [17, 30].

References

1. Nkomo VT, Gardin JM, Skelton TN, Gottdiener JS, Scott CG, Enriquez-Sarano M. Burden of valvular heart diseases: a population-based study. Lancet. 2006;368(9540):1005–11.
2. Martinsson A, Li X, Andersson C, Nilsson J, Smith JG, Sundquist K. Temporal trends in the incidence and prognosis of aortic stenosis: a nationwide study of the Swedish population. Circulation. 2015;131(11):988–94.
3. Piazza N, de Jaegere P, Schultz C, Becker AE, Serruys PW, Anderson RH. Anatomy of the aortic valvar complex and its implications for transcatheter implantation of the aortic valve. Circ Cardiovasc Interv. 2008;1(1):74–81.
4. Singh GK. Congenital aortic valve stenosis. Children (Basel). 2019;6(5)
5. Zipes D. Braunwald's heart disease: a textbook of cardiovascular medicine, vol. 2. 11th ed; 2019. p. 3412–3.
6. Tutarel O. The quadricuspid aortic valve: a comprehensive review. J Heart Valve Dis. 2004;13(4):534–7.
7. Loscalzo J. From clinical observation to mechanism–Heyde's syndrome. N Engl J Med. 2012;367(20):1954–6.
8. Otto CM, Nishimura RA, Bonow RO, Carabello BA, Erwin JP 3rd, Gentile F, et al. ACC/AHA Guideline for the Management of Patients With Valvular Heart Disease: A Report of the American College of Cardiology/American Heart Association Joint Committee on Clinical Practice Guidelines. Circulation. 2020;2020:CIR0000000000000923.
9. Clavel MA, Pibarot P, Messika-Zeitoun D, Capoulade R, Malouf J, Aggarval S, et al. Impact of aortic valve calcification, as measured by MDCT, on survival in patients with aortic stenosis: results of an international registry study. J Am Coll Cardiol. 2014;64(12):1202–13.
10. Aggarwal SR, Clavel MA, Messika-Zeitoun D, Cueff C, Malouf J, Araoz PA, et al. Sex differences in aortic valve calcification measured by multidetector computed tomography in aortic stenosis. Circ Cardiovasc Imaging. 2013;6(1):40–7.
11. Messika-Zeitoun D, Aubry MC, Detaint D, Bielak LF, Peyser PA, Sheedy PF, et al. Evaluation and clinical implications of aortic valve calcification measured by electron-beam computed tomography. Circulation. 2004;110(3):356–62.

12. Pawade T, Clavel MA, Tribouilloy C, Dreyfus J, Mathieu T, Tastet L, et al. Computed tomography aortic valve calcium scoring in patients with aortic stenosis. Circ Cardiovasc Imaging. 2018;11(3):e007146.
13. Nishimura RA, Otto CM, Bonow RO, Carabello BA, Erwin JP 3rd, Guyton RA, et al. 2014 AHA/ACC Guideline for the Management of Patients With Valvular Heart Disease: a report of the American College of Cardiology/American Heart Association Task Force on Practice Guidelines. Circulation. 2014;129(23):e521–643.
14. Magne J, Lancellotti P, Pierard LA. Exercise testing in asymptomatic severe aortic stenosis. JACC Cardiovasc Imaging. 2014;7(2):188–99.
15. Dweck MR, Joshi S, Murigu T, Alpendurada F, Jabbour A, Melina G, et al. Midwall fibrosis is an independent predictor of mortality in patients with aortic stenosis. J Am Coll Cardiol. 2011;58(12):1271–9.
16. Leon MB, Smith CR, Mack M, Miller DC, Moses JW, Svensson LG, et al. Transcatheter aortic-valve implantation for aortic stenosis in patients who cannot undergo surgery. N Engl J Med. 2010;363(17):1597–607.
17. Nishimura RA, Otto CM, Bonow RO, Carabello BA, Erwin JP 3rd, Fleisher LA, et al. 2017 AHA/ACC Focused Update of the 2014 AHA/ACC Guideline for the Management of Patients With Valvular Heart Disease: A Report of the American College of Cardiology/American Heart Association Task Force on Clinical Practice Guidelines. J Am Coll Cardiol. 2017;70(2):252–89.
18. Holmes DR Jr, Mack MJ, Kaul S, Agnihotri A, Alexander KP, Bailey SR, et al. 2012 ACCF/AATS/SCAI/STS expert consensus document on transcatheter aortic valve replacement. J Am Coll Cardiol. 2012;59(13):1200–54.
19. Maurer G. Aortic regurgitation. Heart. 2006;92(7):994–1000.
20. Akinseye OA, Pathak A, Ibebuogu UN. Aortic valve regurgitation: a comprehensive review. Curr Probl Cardiol. 2018;43(8):315–34.
21. Stout KK, Verrier ED. Acute valvular regurgitation. Circulation. 2009;119(25):3232–41.
22. Griffin BP, Menon V, Wu WM, Cauthen CA, Dunn JM. Manual of cardiovascular medicine. 4th ed. Philadelphia, PA: Lippincott Williams & Wilkins; 2013.
23. Myerson SG, d'Arcy J, Mohiaddin R, Greenwood JP, Karamitsos TD, Francis JM, et al. Aortic regurgitation quantification using

cardiovascular magnetic resonance: association with clinical outcome. Circulation. 2012;126(12):1452–60.
24. Hamirani YS, Dietl CA, Voyles W, Peralta M, Begay D, Raizada V. Acute aortic regurgitation. Circulation. 2012;126(9):1121–6.
25. ROB CO. Valvular heart disease. In: Mann DL, Zipes DP, Libby P, Bonow RO, editors. Braunwald's heart disease. A textbook of cardiovascular medicine. 10th ed. Philadelphia: Elsevier Saunders; 2015.
26. Evangelista A, Tornos P, Sambola A, Permanyer-Miralda G, Soler-Soler J. Long-term vasodilator therapy in patients with severe aortic regurgitation. N Engl J Med. 2005;353(13):1342–9.
27. Franzone A, Piccolo R, Siontis GC, Lanz J, Stortecky S, Praz F, et al. Transcatheter aortic valve replacement for the treatment of pure native aortic valve regurgitation: a systematic review. JACC Cardiovasc Interv. 2016;9(22):2308–17.
28. Masri A, Svensson LG, Griffin BP, Desai MY. Contemporary natural history of bicuspid aortic valve disease: a systematic review. Heart. 2017;103(17):1323–30.
29. Verma S, Siu SC. Aortic dilatation in patients with bicuspid aortic valve. N Engl J Med. 2014;370(20):1920–9.
30. Baumgartner H, Falk V, Bax JJ, De Bonis M, Hamm C, Holm PJ, et al. ESC/EACTS Guidelines for the Management of Valvular Heart Disease. Rev Esp Cardiol (Engl Ed). 2017;71(2):110.

Chapter 18
Mitral, Tricuspid, and Pulmonic Valve Disease

John C. Lisko and Vasilis C. Babaliaros

Abbreviations

MR	Mitral regurgitation
MS	Mitral stenosis
PBMC	Percutaneous balloon mitral commissurotomy
RF	Regurgitant fraction
RHF	Rheumatic fever
TEE	Transesophageal echocardiography

Valvular heart disease remains a significant cause of morbidity and mortality related to heart failure. The mitral, tricuspid, and pulmonic valves are complex anatomic structures that may be primarily responsible for, or a consequence of, a patient's myocardial dysfunction and symptoms. Multimodality imaging and a heart team approach allows for thorough evaluation of a patient's valvular heart disease and appropriate medical, percutaneous, or surgical treatments.

J. C. Lisko (✉) · V. C. Babaliaros
Department of Medicine, Division of Cardiology, Emory University School of Medicine, Atlanta, GA, USA
e-mail: jlisko@emory.edu

A. A. Bhargava et al. (eds.), *Handbook of Outpatient Cardiology*, https://doi.org/10.1007/978-3-030-88953-1_18

Recent advances in percutaneous therapy may increase the number of patients eligible to undergo therapy.

Mitral Stenosis

- Background
  - MS is relatively uncommon in the United States.

    Often related to rheumatic valvular changes (Fig. 18.1) or severe mitral calcification (Fig. 18.2 and Table 18.1). History should include a detailed evaluation for prior rheumatic fever (RF), chest radiation, or significant renal disease.
  - Pathophysiology

    Narrowing of the mitral valve → left atrial pressure overload and enlargement → pulmonary hypertension

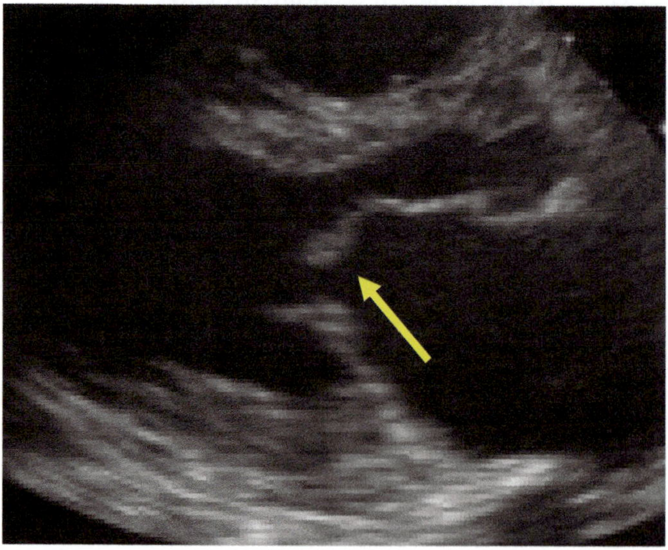

FIGURE 18.1 Rheumatic mitral valve disease. Parasternal long-axis view of a rheumatic mitral valve, note "hockey-stick" appearance (yellow arrow)

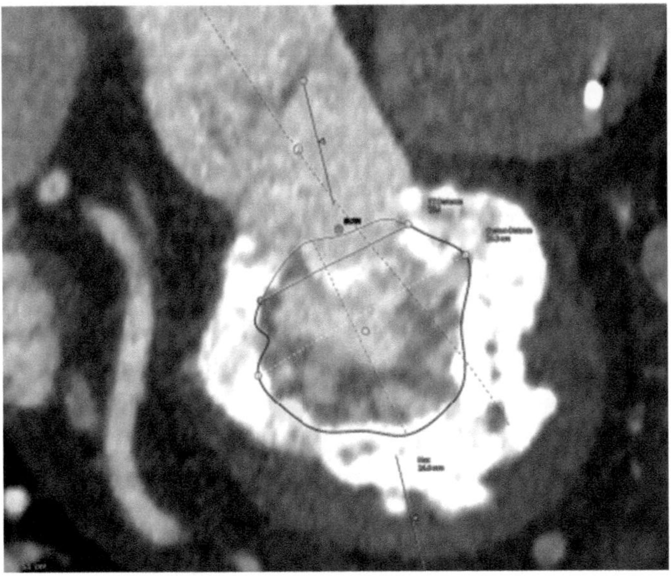

FIGURE 18.2 Mitral Annular Calcification. Above, computed tomography reconstruction of mitral annular calcification, note the circumferential calcium (white)

Clinical Pearl
The transthoracic echocardiogram is a simple, non-invasive, radiation-free modality for evaluating native valve disease.

- Diagnosis is primarily based on echocardiography [1].

  Planimetered mitral valve area $\leq$1.5 cm^2
  Diastolic pressure half-time $\geq$150 msec (narrowed orifice → delayed filling → increased time to pressurize)
  Gradient:

  - The gradient across the mitral valve is directly related to the patient's heart rate:

Table 18.1 Select criteria for diagnosing severe right-sided valvular heart disease

Valve	Severe stenosis criteria	Severe regurgitation criteria	Class I indications for surgery
Tricuspid	Mean gradient >5 mmHg Pressure 1/2 time ≥190 ms Valve area ≤1 cm^2	RA/RV: usually dilated IVC diameter: >2.5 cm Color flow: large central jet Systolic flow reversal in hepatic vein EROA (cm^2) ≥0.40	Stenosis Severe stenosis at the time of left-sided surgery Isolated, symptomatic severe stenosis Regurgitation Functional severe regurgitation at the time of left-sided valve surgery
Pulmonic	Peak velocity: >4 m/s Peak gradient: >64 mmHg	RV size: dilated Deceleration time <260 msec Pressure 1/2 time <100 msec Prominent diastolic flow reversal in PA RF >40%	Stenosis Moderate to severe stenosis and unexplained heart failure, cyanosis, or exercise intolerance→ balloon valvuloplasty, followed by surgical repair if failed valvuloplasty

A summary of select criteria, commonly found in echocardiogram, reports to denote severe right-sided valvular heart disease

- Mild MS: Mean gradient <5 mmHg
- Moderate MS: Mean gradient 5–10 mm Hg
- Severe MS: Mean gradient >10 mmHg

– Prognosis

Rheumatic MS is a progressive disease. The prognosis worsens once a patient becomes symptomatic. 44% 5-year survival in patients without correction [2].

- Presentation and Management
  - Presentation
    - Decreased exercise tolerance
    - Dyspnea on exertion/congestive heart failure
  - Physical Exam

    Classically an "opening snap" and "diastolic rumble," though these are often difficult to auscultate
    An earlier opening snap suggests severe MS.
    A late opening snap suggests mild MS.
  - Treatment [3]

    Surveillance

    - Echo every 3–5 years if mitral valve area > 1.5 cm^2
    - Echo every 1–2 years if mitral valve area 1.0 cm^2–1.5 cm^2
    - Echo every year if mitral valve area <1.0 cm^2

    - Medical therapy
      - Rate-controlling medications to reduce heart rate to the lowest tolerated rate in patients with:
        - Atrial fibrillation with a rapid ventricular response
        - Normal sinus rhythm and exercise induced symptoms
      - Anticoagulation in patients with concomitant atrial fibrillation

Clinical Pearl
Direct oral anticoagulants are not approved for patients with severe rheumatic mitral stenosis. A vitamin K antagonist such as warfarin is the drug of choice.

- Antibiotics for secondary prevention of rheumatic fever (RHF) [3]:
  - Penicillin G benzathine (1.2 million units IM every 4 weeks)
  - Penicillin V potassium (200 mg orally twice daily)
  - Sulfadiazine (1 g orally once daily)
  - Macrolide or azalide antibiotics for patients with allergies to penicillin and sulfadiazine (variable dose)
- Duration of secondary prophylaxis for RHF [3]:
  - RHF with carditis and residual heart disease (10 years or until age 40)
  - RHF with carditis but no residual heart disease (10 years or until age 21)
  - RHF without carditis (5 years or until patient is 21)

- Mechanical Correction [3]
  - Percutaneous balloon mitral commissurotomy (PBMC) in symptomatic patients with suitable anatomy.
  - PBMC can also be considered for asymptomatic patients with pulmonary artery systolic pressure >50 mmHg if performed at a comprehensive valve center.
  - Transesophageal echocardiography is necessary to determine a patient's anatomic suitability for valvuloplasty.

    Need to assess for left atrial thrombus.
    Patients cannot have > moderate MR.
    Favorability is determined by the Wilkins score [4]. Favorable characteristics include:

    - Highly mobile leaflets
    - Near normal leaflet thickness
    - Minimal leaflet calcification
    - Minimal thickening below the mitral leaflets
  - Mitral valve surgery is recommended for severely symptomatic patients who are not candidates for PBMC [3].

Mitral Regurgitation

- Background
  - Correctly defining the etiology of mitral regurgitation (MR) is essential to optimizing treatment [5].

    MR is classified as *primary* (degenerative) MR when the etiology of the MR is attributable to a problem with the mitral valve.
    MR is classified as *secondary* (functional) when the etiology of the MR is attributable to myocardial disease.

- Pathophysiology
  - MR leads to chronic LV volume overload → compensatory LV dilation → congestive heart failure.
- Diagnosis
  - Echocardiography is the main imaging modality for assessing the mitral valve [6].

    Severe MR is defined by the 4–5–6–7 rule:

    - Effective regurgitant orifice area (EROA) ≥0.40 cm
    - Regurgitant fraction ≥50%
    - Regurgitant volume ≥60 mL
    - Vena contracta width ≥0.7 cm

    TEE is often useful to better define the severity and etiology of MR.
    Cardiac MRI is useful to accurately quantify the degree of mitral regurgitation and for patients with suboptimal echocardiographic windows.

- Prognosis
  - Primary MR: 66% of asymptomatic patients require surgery within 5 years because of LV dysfunction, pulmonary HTN, or atrial fibrillation [7].
  - Secondary MR: 23.5% mortality rate at 24 months in the COAPT Trial [8].

Presentation and Management

- Presentation
  - The severity of a patient's symptoms is related to the severity of MR, associated pressure in the pulmonary artery, and associated arrhythmias (MR → atrial dilatation → atrial fibrillation).
  - Patients commonly present with symptoms of poor forward cardiac output (fatigue) and dyspnea on exertion.

> **Clinical Pearl**
> Changes in ventricular size or function should prompt cardiology consultation.

  - Acute MR may present as sudden onset dyspnea, flash pulmonary edema, and significant hemodynamic compromise → this raises the concern for a papillary muscle rupture, ruptured mitral chordae, or leaflet rupture from endocarditis.

> **Clinical Pearl**
> Consider exercise testing in patients with MR and unclear symptoms.

- Physical Exam: Holosystolic murmur best heard at the LV apex; in cases of mitral valve prolapse, there is often an audible mid-systolic click.
- Surveillance [3]
  - For asymptomatic patients with severe primary MR, repeat TTE is indicated every 6–12 months.
- Treatment
  - The complexity of the mitral valve and available therapies requires a heart team approach to patient care [3, 8–11].

- The mitral apparatus is a complex anatomic structure that often requires evaluation with multimodality cardiac imaging.
- Mechanical correction has shown survival benefit in patients with MR.

- Treatment of *primary* mitral regurgitation
  - Surgery remains the gold standard of treatment [3, 10, 11].
  - Mitral valve repair is preferred to replacement when:

    The MR is limited to the posterior leaflet
    The MR involves the anterior or both leaflets *and* durable repair can be accomplished

  - Class I recommendations for surgery in the following groups with chronic, severe, and primary MR:

    Symptomatic severe primary MR
    Asymptomatic patients with an EF < 60% or LVESD ≥40 mm → MV surgery

  - The MitraClip (Abbott Vascular) is a fully percutaneous edge-to-edge repair system that has shown efficacy in patients with severe primary MR at prohibitive surgical risk [12] (Fig. 18.3).

> **Clinical Pearl**
> Secondary MR is related to myocardial dysfunction.

- Treatment of *secondary* mitral regurgitation [5, 8–11]
  - The target of therapy for secondary mitral regurgitation is the underlying myocardial disease.
  - Prior to considering any mechanical correction to secondary MR, it is essential to:

    Evaluate for reversible ischemia and pursue revascularization if possible
    Optimize guideline-directed medical therapy (GDMT) for congestive heart failure

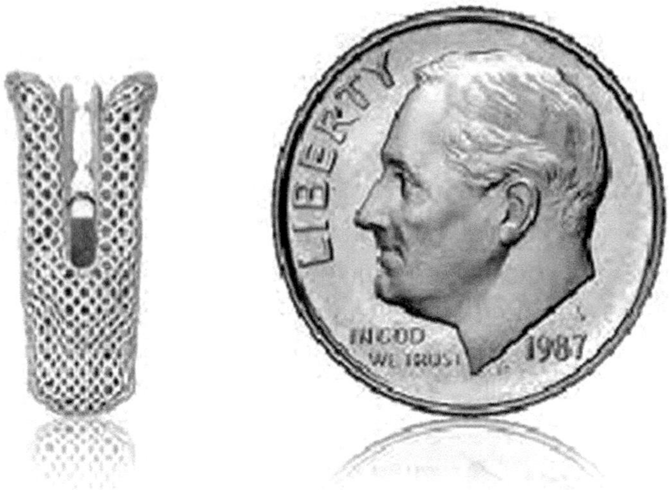

FIGURE 18.3 The MitraClip (Abbott) is a transcatheter edge-to-edge repair for patients with severe mitral regurgitation. Note the size compared to a US dime

Consider cardiac resynchronization therapy (typically reserved for patients with an underlying left bundle branch block and QRS duration >150 ms)

Consider consultation with advanced heart failure services

- Class IIA recommendation for transcatheter edge-to-edge repair for patients with secondary MR and NYHA class II–IV symptoms.
- The MitraClip has been studied in patients with secondary MR.
- Results from the two largest studies are conflicting.

The COAPT Trial demonstrated a significant reduction in HF hospitalization and all-cause death at 24 months in patients undergoing MitraClip + GMDT compared to GDMT alone [8]. There was a durable reduction in MR, mortality, and HF hospitalizations at 36 months.

The MITRA-FR Trial failed to show a significant in outcomes in patients undergoing MitraClip + GMDT compared to GDMT alone [9].
These differences may be attributable to:

- Patient selection
  - MITRA-FR patients included subjects with less severe MR and more severe LV dilation compared to COAPT.
- Operator experience
- Titration of medical therapy [13]

Patients should be evaluated by patients with expertise in heart failure management prior to undergoing MitraClip for secondary mitral regurgitation.

Right-Sided Valves

- Background
  - Right-sided valvular heart disease is much less common than left-sided disease.
  - Trace to mild disease is a common incidental echo finding [1, 3, 6, 10, 11, 14].
- Common Etiologies of Tricuspid Disease
  - Stenosis: Rheumatic heart disease, carcinoid syndrome, congenital abnormalities, pacemaker endocarditis, pacemaker-induced adhesions, lupus, and mechanical obstruction secondary to tumor.
  - Regurgitation: The most common cause is due to annular dilation. The most common primary cause is myxomatous degeneration.
- Common Etiologies of Pulmonic Disease
  - Stenosis: Congenital >>>acquired causes.
  - Regurgitation: Most likely to be from congenital disease or post-percutaneous valvuloplasty.
  - Acquired disease occurs in <1% of patients.

References

1. Baumgartner H, et al. Echocardiographic assessment of valve stenosis: EAE/ASE recommendations for clinical practice. J Am Soc Echocardiogr. 2009;22(1):1–23; quiz 101–2
2. Munoz S, et al. Influence of surgery on the natural history of rheumatic mitral and aortic valve disease. Am J Cardiol. 1975;35:234–42.
3. Otto CM, et al. 2020 ACC/AHA Guideline for the Management of Patients With Valvular Heart Disease: A Report of the American College of Cardiology/American Heart Association Joint Committee on Clinical Practice Guidelines. Circulation. 2021;143(5):e72–e227.
4. Wilkins GT, et al. Percutaneous balloon dilation of the mitral valve: an analysis of echocardiographic variables related to outcome and mechanism of dilatation. British Heart Journal. 1988;60:299–308.
5. Grayburn PA, Sannino A, Packer M. Proportionate and disproportionate functional mitral regurgitation: a new conceptual framework that reconciles the results of the MITRA-FR and COAPT trials. JACC Cardiovasc Imaging. 2019;12(2):353–62.
6. Zoghbi WA, et al. Recommendations for noninvasive evaluation of native valvular regurgitation: a report from the American Society of Echocardiography Developed in Collaboration with the Society for Cardiovascular Magnetic Resonance. J Am Soc Echocardiogr. 2017;30(4):303–71.
7. David TE, et al. Late outcomes of mitral valve repair for mitral regurgitation due to degenerative disease. Circulation. 2013;127(14):1485–92.
8. Stone GW, et al. Transcatheter mitral-valve repair in patients with heart failure. N Engl J Med. 2018;379(24):2307–18.
9. Obadia JF, et al. Percutaneous repair or medical treatment for secondary mitral regurgitation. N Engl J Med. 2018;379(24):2297–306.
10. Nishimura RA, et al. 2017 AHA/ACC Focused Update of the 2014 AHA/ACC Guideline for the Management of Patients With Valvular Heart Disease: A Report of the American College of Cardiology/American Heart Association Task Force on Clinical Practice Guidelines. Circulation. 2017;135(25):e1159–95.
11. Nishimura RA, et al. 2014 AHA/ACC Guideline for the Management of Patients With Valvular Heart Disease: execu-

tive summary: a report of the American College of Cardiology/American Heart Association Task Force on Practice Guidelines. Circulation. 2014;129(23):2440–92.

12. Feldman T, et al. Randomized comparison of prcutaneous repair and surgery for mitral regurgitation: 5-year results of EVEREST II. J Am Coll Cardiol. 2015;66(25):2844–54.
13. Mauricio R, Kumbhani DJ. MitraClip: how do we reconcile the inconsistent findings of MITRA-FR and COAPT? Curr Cardiol Rep. 2019;21(12):150.
14. Stout KK, et al. 2018 AHA/ACC Guideline for the Management of Adults With Congenital Heart Disease: A Report of the American College of Cardiology/American Heart Association Task Force on Clinical Practice Guidelines. Circulation. 2019;139(14):e698–800.

Chapter 19
Prosthetic Valve Disease

Ankit A. Bhargava and Allen Dollar

Abbreviations

ASA	Aspirin
AVR	Aortic valve replacement
CBC	Complete blood count
CMR	Cardiac magnetic resonance imaging
CT	Computed tomography
DOAC	Direct oral anticoagulant
ECG	Electrocardiogram
EGD	Esophagogastroduodenoscopy
FFP	Fresh frozen plasma
INR	International normalized ratio
LDH	Lactate dehydrogenase
LMWH	Low molecular weight heparin
MVR	Mitral valve replacement
PCC	Prothrombin complex concentrate
PPM	Patient prosthesis mismatch
PVL	Paravalvular leak
TAVR	Transcatheter aortic valve replacement

A. A. Bhargava (✉) · A. Dollar
Department of Medicine, Division of Cardiology, Emory University School of Medicine, Atlanta, GA, USA
e-mail: aabharg@emory.edu

A. A. Bhargava et al. (eds.), *Handbook of Outpatient Cardiology*, https://doi.org/10.1007/978-3-030-88953-1_19

TEE	Transesophageal echocardiogram
TTE	Transthoracic echocardiogram
UFH	Unfractionated heparin
VKA	Vitamin K antagonist
VTE	Venothromboembolism

Valve Types

There are two varieties of prosthetic heart valves: [1] mechanical and [2] bioprosthetic. Examples of surgically implanted heart valves are pictured in Fig. 19.1.

- **Mechanical valves** – Previous designs include the caged ball and single tilting disc. Essentially all contemporary mechanical valves utilize a bileaflet tilting disc design [1, 2].
  - Increased durability (they essentially never wear out)
  - Increased thrombogenicity (requiring lifelong anticoagulation)
- **Bioprosthetic valves** – These are typically xenografts (constructed from animal tissue such as bovine pericardium or porcine aortic valves). Autografts and homografts (derived from human valve tissue) [1] are uncommonly used in adults.
  - Decreased durability
  - Decreased thrombogenicity

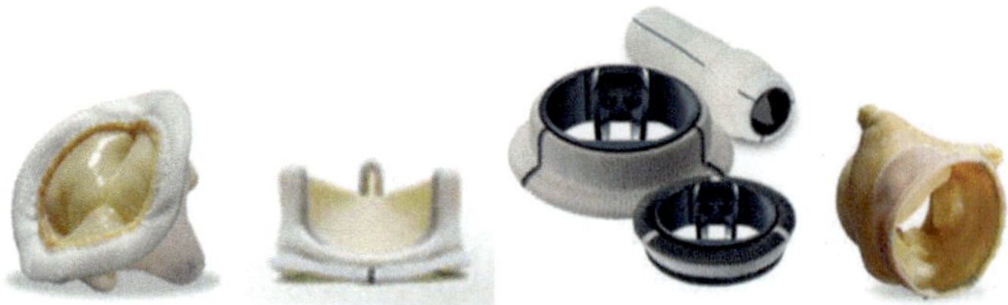

FIGURE 19.1 Examples of surgical prosthetic heart valves (from left to right): stented porcine aortic valve, stented bovine pericardial valve, bileaflet mechanical valves, and stentless porcine valve. (Source: Iaizzo et al. [2013] Heart Valves: From Design to Clinical Implantation, p 287, reprinted by permission from Springer)

- **Transcatheter valves** – All available forms are constructed from biological tissue. Examples of transcatheter valves are pictured in Fig. 19.2.

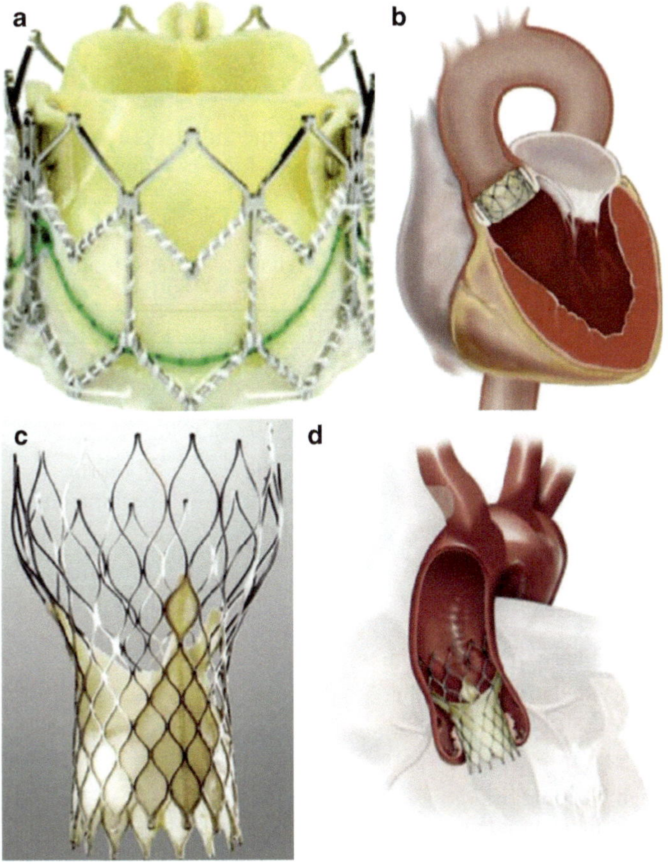

FIGURE 19.2 Examples of prosthetic heart valves deployed via transcatheter delivery systems. (**a**, **b**) The Edwards Sapien XT (Edwards Lifesciences, Irvine, CA, USA) valve and implantation in the aorta. (**c**, **d**) The third generation of the CoreValve prosthesis (Medtronic Inc., Minneapolis, MN, USA). (Source: Reimers et al. [2017] Percutaneous Interventions for Structural Heart Disease, p 47, reprinted by permission from Springer)

- To allow endovascular delivery, the valve is crimped and delivered via a stent frame that then expands once in the appropriate position. These stents can be either balloon-expandable or self-expanding [1].

Choice of Valve Prosthesis

The decision to implant either a mechanical or a bioprosthetic valve depends on several factors summarized in Table 19.1.

TABLE 19.1 Factors that favor mechanical versus bioprosthetic valves [3]

		Mechanical	**Bioprosthetic**
Age	*<50 years*[a]	✓ (aortic and mitral position)	
	50–65 years	✓ (aortic and mitral position)	✓ (aortic position only)
	>65 years		✓ (aortic and mitral position)
Shorter expected life span			✓
Anticoagulation for another reason (atrial fibrillation, VTE)		✓	
High bleeding risk/ contraindication to anticoagulation			✓
Higher morbidity/mortality with future re-intervention (e.g., porcelain aorta, prior radiation exposure)		✓	

[a]Uncommonly, in patients <50 years of age, a pulmonary autograft may be utilized instead of mechanical valve in the aortic valve position (Ross procedure) [3]

Other factors that influence the decision between mechanical and bioprosthetic valve:

- Patient frailty
- Cardiac and noncardiac comorbidities
- Valve anatomy
- Surgical risk
- Patient preference

Initial Follow-Up, Surveillance, and Clinical Assessment

The first postoperative visit should generally occur 3–4 weeks after valve replacement. In that first visit, the following should be obtained:

History:

- Progress of recovery, physical rehabilitation, and wound healing
- Medication reconciliation, particularly the antiplatelet/anticoagulation regimen
- Assessment of neurocognitive function
- Symptoms of heart failure
- Symptoms related to arrhythmia
- Identification of any bleeding issues
- Symptoms of infection
- Assessment for potential thromboembolism

Focused cardiovascular physical exam:

- Wound healing
- Prosthetic valve auscultation characteristics
- Signs of volume overload
- Detection of any arrhythmias
- Signs of infection

Baseline diagnostic tests:

- Chest X-ray.
- ECG.

- Baseline labs – INR (if on VKA), CBC, LDH, haptoglobin, and indirect bilirubin.
- Baseline TTE → ideally 1–3 months after valve implantation to establish baseline hemodynamics. The delay in performing this baseline allows anemia and other immediate postoperative abnormalities to resolve. Sometimes this TTE is completed on the index hospitalization for patient convenience [3].

Surveillance:

- Periodic surveillance generally performed by TTE.
- Interval of surveillance is based on type of valve prosthesis and length of time since implantation. General recommendations for timing of surveillance are summarized in Table 19.2.

Other factors that may necessitate more frequent or repeat imaging include changing signs/symptoms, monitoring for cardiac dysfunction, and during pregnancy.

Clinical Pearl #1
The following scenarios may indicate a potential valve complication and should prompt repeat imaging:

- Change in prosthetic valve auscultation characteristics (new or worsening murmur, softening or absence of a mechanical valve click with a mechanical valve)
- Change in clinical status (onset of heart failure symptoms, suspected embolic event, suspected bacteremia)

If TTE quality is poor (such as from shadowing from mechanical valves), alternative imaging modalities should be pursued → TEE, CT, CMR, or fluoroscopy.

TABLE 19.2 Surveillance frequency by valve intervention [3]

Valve intervention	Minimum imaging frequency
Mechanical valve (surgical)	Baseline, and then only if new problems arise or there is another cardiac dysfunction that requires monitoring
Bioprosthetic valve (surgical)	Baseline, 5 and 10 years after surgery, and then annually
Bioprosthetic valve (transcatheter)	Baseline, and then annually

Anticoagulation and Antiplatelet Management

Mechanical Valves

- Require lifelong anticoagulation in order to prevent valve thrombosis and thromboembolism [4, 5].
- Combination of thrombogenic valve material, abnormal flow conditions, and high shear stress leads to an environment of increased platelet activation → higher rates of thrombosis in the absence of anticoagulation [4, 5].
- The anticoagulant of choice remains VKAs such as warfarin, with heparin (unfractionated or low molecular weight) used as a bridging agent until the INR is at the designated therapeutic target [4, 5].
- *DOACs are contraindicated* and have been associated with both increased bleeding and thromboembolic events in patients with mechanical valves [6].

Bioprosthetic Valves

- Managed with aspirin therapy alone in the long term [4, 5]
- Reasonable to have a period of anticoagulation with a VKA in the first 3–6 months following valve replacement [5] to allow the cloth sewing ring to endothelialize

The INR goal for prosthetic valves is dependent on the *type of valve* (bioprosthetic vs. mechanical), *position of the valve* (aortic vs. mitral), and *presence of other risk factors for thromboembolism.*

Antiplatelet and anticoagulation therapies with INR goals are summarized in Table 19.3.

Clinical Pearl #2

Mechanical mitral valves have even higher thrombogenic potential than mechanical aortic valves due to a more sluggish blood flow across the valve. Anticoagulation goal for mechanical mitral valves is therefore an INR between 2.5 and 3.5, not 2.0 and 3.0 [5, 7].

TABLE 19.3 Antiplatelet and anticoagulation goals by valve type [3, 5]

Type	Position	Antiplatelet/anticoagulation goals	
Mechanical	Aortic	Without risk factors[a]	VKA (INR = 2.5) +/– ASA 75–100 mg QD
		With risk factors[a]	VKA (INR = 3.0) +/– ASA 75–100 mg QD
		On-X brand valve[b]	VKA (INR 1.5–2.0) ASA 75–100 mg QD
	Mitral	VKA (INR 3.0) ASA 75–100 mg QD	

Table 19.3 (continued)

Type	Position	Antiplatelet/anticoagulation goals
Bioprosthetic	Aortic	VKA (INR = 2.5) for the first 3–6 months is reasonable ASA 75–100mg QD
	Mitral	VKA (INR = 2.5) for the first 3–6 months is reasonable ASA 75–100mg QD
	TAVR	Clopidogrel 75 mg QD for the first 3–6 months ASA 75–100 mg QD lifelong *or* VKA for the first 3 months after implantation, followed by ASA 75–100 mg lifelong

[a]*Risk factors*: atrial fibrillation/flutter, prior thromboembolism, severe left ventricular dysfunction (ejection fraction <35%), older-generation valve, or hypercoagulable state
[b]In patients without risk factors who receive an *on -X brand mechanical aortic valve*, an even lower target INR of 1.5–2.0 may be reasonable starting 3 months after implantation

Bridging Therapy for Outpatient Procedures

Management strategy depends on type of valve and type of procedure, summarized in Table 19.4. [3].

Management of Anticoagulation During Pregnancy

Physiologic changes during pregnancy that can cause prosthetic valve problems:

- Increased plasma volume (nearly 50% above baseline) that can lead to heart failure if there is baseline ventricular or prosthetic valve dysfunction [8].

Table 19.4 Bridging strategy with respect to valve and procedure type

Bridging strategy	**Valve and procedure type**
Continue VKA with a therapeutic INR	Mechanical heart valve + minor procedure where bleeding is easily controlled (cataract surgery, dental extraction)
Temporary interruption of VKA without bridging	Bileaflet mechanical aortic valve replacement with no risk factors for thromboembolism and undergoing an invasive procedure
Bridging may be reasonable	Mechanical AVR and any thromboembolic risk factor Older-generation mechanical AVR Mechanical MVR Bioprosthetic heart valve on anticoagulation for atrial fibrillation → dependent on CHA_2DS_2-VASc

- Prothrombotic state of pregnancy increases risk of valve thrombosis [9].

Women with a prosthetic valve who are contemplating pregnancy should undergo pre-pregnancy assessment by a cardiologist with expertise in managing women with valvular heart disease in pregnancy.

- Pregnancy in women with **mechanical** heart valves = **very high risk**.
  - Maternal mortality rate >1% [10].
  - More than 1/3 women with mechanical heart valves will have a serious maternal or fetal complication during pregnancy [10].
  - No anticoagulation strategy has been shown to be consistently safe for both mother and baby.
  - Complications to mother and fetus are summarized in Table 19.5..

Clinical Pearl #3
VKA during pregnancy is associated with the lowest likelihood of maternal complications, but the highest likelihood of miscarriage, fetal death, and congenital abnormalities. This is of particular concern if taken during the first trimester and if the warfarin dose is >5 mg/day [3].

Considerations for anticoagulation in pregnant women with mechanical prosthetic heart valves [3]:

- Will need therapeutic anticoagulation with frequent monitoring throughout pregnancy.
- If able to maintain a therapeutic INR with warfarin ≤5 mg/day → can continue warfarin for all three trimesters.
- If only able to maintain a therapeutic INR with warfarin >5 mg/day → LMWH BID (or continuous IV unfractionated heparin if LMWH is unavailable) for the first trimester, followed by warfarin for the second and third trimesters. LMWH for all three trimesters is also acceptable if requiring >5 mg/day of warfarin.

Closer to delivery [3]:

- 1 week prior to delivery → stop VKA, and start IV UFH or LMWH.
- 36 hours prior to delivery → switch to IV UFH.
- 4–6 hours before planned delivery → stop IV heparin.

Table 19.5 Summary of maternal and fetal complications in pregnant patients with mechanical prosthetic valve [3]

Maternal complications	Fetal complications
Valve thrombosis	Spontaneous abortion
Thromboembolism	Teratogenicity related to VKAs
Hemorrhage	Fetal hemorrhage
Death	Fetal death

Antibiotic Prophylaxis in Patients with Prosthetic Heart Valves

Patients with prosthetic valves are a high-risk population for infective endocarditis. The risk of infective endocarditis is highest with dental procedures → antibiotic prophylaxis reasonable before dental procedures that involve [3]:

- Manipulation of gingival tissue
- Manipulation of periapical region of teeth
- Perforation of the oral mucosa

Clinical Pearl #4
In the absence of an active infection, antibiotic prophylaxis is not recommended for nondental procedures, including TEE, EGD, colonoscopy, or cystoscopy [3].

Antibiotic prophylaxis for dental procedures [11]:

- Dental procedures can result in transient viridans group streptococcal bacteremia and are therefore the target of prophylaxis.
- Antibiotics should be administered as a single dose prior to the procedure.
- Amoxicillin is the preferred choice for oral therapy (well-absorbed in the gastrointestinal tract, achieves high and sustained serum concentrations).
- For those who are allergic to penicillin/amoxicillin, alternative oral options include cephalexin, clindamycin, azithromycin, and clarithromycin.
- For those unable to take oral medications, intravenous or intramuscular preparations with ampicillin, ceftriaxone, or cefazolin may be used.

Prosthetic Valve Complications

The frequencies and types of complications depend on the type of prosthetic valve. Complications are summarized in Table 19.6.

TABLE 19.6 Summary of valve complications, diagnostic modalities, and management [5, 12–14]

Complication	Diagnostic orders	Management
Bleeding or supratherapeutic INR	CBC, INR	If INR 5–10 without bleed → hold VKA If INR>10 without bleed →hold VKA and give vitamin K PO 1 to 2.5 mg If needing urgent reversal of bleed → hold VKA and give PCC or FFP with vitamin K PO
Thromboembolism	TTE, TEE	Adjust anticoagulation regimen: Mechanical – increase INR goal by 0.5 Bioprosthetic – add VKA to ASA
Valve thrombosis/ pannus formation	TTE, TEE, fluoroscopy, CT	Mechanical – surgery (pannus/thrombus) vs. fibrinolysis (thrombus only) Bioprosthetic – UFH bridge to VKA
Patient prosthesis mismatch	TTE, TEE	Surgical consultation
Prosthetic valve stenosis	TTE, TEE, +/- blood cultures	Re-do surgery Valve-in-valve procedure if bioprosthetic valve

(continued)

Table 19.6 (continued)

Complication	Diagnostic orders	Management
Prosthetic valve regurgitation	TTE, TEE, +/- blood cultures, LDH if concerned for hemolysis	Re-do surgery Percutaneous paravalvular intervention
Hemolysis	TTE, TEE, LDH, haptoglobin, indirect bilirubin, reticulocyte count, peripheral smear	Usually occurs as a result of paravalvular regurgitation, would require re-do surgery or catheter closure of defect
Infective endocarditis	TTE, TEE, blood cultures	IV antibiotics tailored to organism +/- surgical intervention

These complications are typically evaluated and managed in the inpatient setting and are provided here as a reference.

Key Learning Points

1. Mechanical valves are more durable and more thrombogenic when compared to bioprosthetic valves. Mechanical valves therefore require lifelong VKA for anticoagulation, whereas bioprosthetic valves will typically only need aspirin lifelong.
2. The need for bridging anticoagulation for mechanical valves prior to a procedure is dependent on both the type of valve and the type of procedure.
3. Pregnant patients with mechanical heart valves are very high risk and require expert specialists for management. There has been no anticoagulation strategy that has been shown to be safe for both mother and fetus.
4. Antibiotic prophylaxis prior to dental procedures is recommended in all patients with a prosthetic valve.

References

1. Russo M, Taramasso M, Guidotti A, Pozzoli A, Nietilspach F, Segesser LK, et al. The evolution of surgical valves. Cardiovasc Med. 2017;20(12):285–92.
2. Dangas GD, Weitz JI, Giustino G, Makkar R, Mehran R. Prosthetic heart valve thrombosis. J Am Coll Cardiol. 2016;68(24):2670–89.
3. Otto CM, Nishimura RA, Bonow RO, Carabello BA, Erwin JP 3rd, Gentile F, et al. ACC/AHA Guideline for the Management of Patients With Valvular Heart Disease: A Report of the American College of Cardiology/American Heart Association Joint Committee on Clinical Practice Guidelines. Circulation. 2020;2020:Cir0000000000000923.
4. Nishimura RA, Otto CM, Bonow RO, Carabello BA, Erwin JP 3rd, Guyton RA, et al. 2014 AHA/ACC guideline for the management of patients with valvular heart disease: a report of the American College of Cardiology/American Heart Association Task Force on Practice Guidelines. J Am Coll Cardiol. 2014;63(22):e57–185.
5. Nishimura RA, Otto CM, Bonow RO, Carabello BA, Erwin JP 3rd, Fleisher LA, et al. 2017 AHA/ACC Focused Update of the 2014 AHA/ACC Guideline for the Management of Patients With Valvular Heart Disease: A Report of the American College of Cardiology/American Heart Association Task Force on Clinical Practice Guidelines. Circulation. 2017;135(25):e1159–e95.
6. Eikelboom JW, Connolly SJ, Brueckmann M, Granger CB, Kappetein AP, Mack MJ, et al. Dabigatran versus warfarin in patients with mechanical heart valves. N Engl J Med. 2013;369(13):1206–14.
7. Chikwe J, Chiang YP, Egorova NN, Itagaki S, Adams DH. Survival and outcomes following bioprosthetic vs mechanical mitral valve replacement in patients aged 50 to 69 years. JAMA. 2015;313(14):1435–42.
8. de Haas S, Ghossein-Doha C, van Kuijk SM, van Drongelen J, Spaanderman ME. Physiological adaptation of maternal plasma volume during pregnancy: a systematic review and meta-analysis. Ultrasound Obstet Gynecol. 2017;49(2):177–87.
9. Bremme KA. Haemostatic changes in pregnancy. Best Pract Res Clin Haematol. 2003;16(2):153–68.

10. van Hagen IM, Roos-Hesselink JW, Ruys TP, Merz WM, Goland S, Gabriel H, et al. Pregnancy in women with a mechanical heart valve: data of the European Society of Cardiology Registry of Pregnancy and Cardiac Disease (ROPAC). Circulation. 2015;132(2):132–42.
11. Wilson W, Taubert KA, Gewitz M, Lockhart PB, Baddour LM, Levison M, et al. Prevention of infective endocarditis: guidelines from the American Heart Association: a guideline from the American Heart Association Rheumatic Fever, Endocarditis, and Kawasaki Disease Committee, Council on Cardiovascular Disease in the Young, and the Council on Clinical Cardiology, Council on Cardiovascular Surgery and Anesthesia, and the Quality of Care and Outcomes Research Interdisciplinary Working Group. Circulation. 2007;116(15):1736–54.
12. Baumgartner H, Falk V, Bax JJ, De Bonis M, Hamm C, Holm PJ, et al. 2017 ESC/EACTS Guidelines for the management of valvular heart disease. Eur Heart J. 2017;38(36):2739–91.
13. Pernod G, Godier A, Gozalo C, Tremey B, Sie P. French clinical practice guidelines on the management of patients on vitamin K antagonists in at-risk situations (overdose, risk of bleeding, and active bleeding). Thromb Res. 2010;126(3):e167–74.
14. Baddour LM, Wilson WR, Bayer AS, Fowler VG Jr, Tleyjeh IM, Rybak MJ, et al. Infective endocarditis in adults: diagnosis, antimicrobial therapy, and management of complications: a Scientific Statement for Healthcare Professionals From the American Heart Association. Circulation. 2015;132(15):1435–86.

Part VII
Vascular Disease

Chapter 20
Peripheral Artery Disease

Dandan Chen and Bryan J. Wells

Abbreviations

ABI	Ankle-brachial index
ALI	Acute limb ischemia
CAS	Carotid artery stent
CEA	Carotid endarterectomy
CLI	Chronic limb ischemia
CTA	Computed tomography angiography
DM	Diabetes mellitus
DUS	Duplex ultrasound
FMD	Fibromuscular dysplasia
HLD	Hyperlipidemia
HTN	Hypertension
IC	Intermittent claudication
ICA	Internal carotid artery
MRA	Magnetic resonance angiography
PAD	Peripheral arterial disease
TBI	Toe-brachial index
TIA	Transient ischemic attack
TSPG	Translesional systolic pressure gradient

D. Chen (✉) · B. J. Wells
Department of Medicine, Division of Cardiology, Emory University School of Medicine, Atlanta, GA, USA
e-mail: dchen50@emory.edu; bjwells@emory.edu

A. A. Bhargava et al. (eds.), *Handbook of Outpatient Cardiology*, https://doi.org/10.1007/978-3-030-88953-1_20

Introduction and Risk Factors

- Peripheral arterial disease (PAD) is defined as narrowing and dynamic obstruction of blood flow of systemic arteries other than those of the cerebral and coronary circulation. The most common etiology is atherosclerosis; however, there are many causes of PAD including vasculitis (i.e., Takayasu and giant cell arteritis), degenerative conditions, fibromuscular dysplasia, thrombosis, and thromboembolism [2, 4, 7].
- Risk factors: Age >= 65 y, smoking, hypertension (HTN), hyperlipidemia (HLD), diabetes mellitus (DM), obesity, with known atherosclerotic disease in another vascular beds, family history of vascular disease, ionizing radiation, and repetitive injury (commonly associated with upper extremity PAD). *Smoking and DM are the strongest predictors of morbidity and mortality* [2, 9].

Clinical Manifestations of PAD (Table 20.1)

- Lower extremity PAD.
  - Asymptomatic PAD: Over 50% of patients.

TABLE 20.1 The Rutherford-Becker classifications for claudication

Rutherford-Becker stage	**Definition**
0	Asymptomatic
1	Mild claudication
2	Moderate claudication
3	Severe claudication
4	Rest pain
5	Ischemic ulcers of the digits of the foot (minor tissue loss)
6	Severe ischemic ulcers or gangrene (major tissue loss)

- Intermittent claudication (IC): Exertional aching pain typically in the calves and/or buttocks and relived by rest.
- Chronic limb ischemia (CLI): Resting pain, nonhealing wounds, or ulceration with or without tissue necrosis (gangrene). *Need early surgical consult and angiography.*
- Acute limb ischemia (ALI): "Six Ps": pain, pallor, paralysis, pulselessness, poikilothermia, and paranesthesia [11]. *This is a medical emergency and requires prompt revascularization.*

- Upper extremity PAD. Arm and hand claudication, digital ulceration, and neurologic symptoms caused by vertebral-subclavian steal.

Physical Examination

- Lower extremity PAD. Skin appearance (Burger test), temperature, palpation of all peripheral pulses (branchial, radial, femoral, popliteal, dorsalis, pedis, and posterior tibial arteries), auscultation for bruits (aortic, renal, femoral), and extremity neurologic examination.
- Upper extremity PAD. Besides the above physical findings, the simplest and appropriate screening test is to check blood pressure in both arms. A brachial blood pressure difference of >15–20 mm Hg is abnormal and suggestive of subclavian (or innominate) artery stenosis.

Diagnosis

- Ankle-brachial index (ABI). The initial diagnostic test for diagnosis and assessing the severity of PAD as well as monitoring the progress of existing disease and response to treatment. ABI <= 0.9 suggests PAD and ABI >1.4 indicates that arteries are not compressible, which may be due to end-stage renal disease and long-standing DM. *Toe-branchial index (TBI) is an alternative approach for these patients.* Exercise ABI testing is useful when the resting ABI is normal or borderline [2, 8, 9].

- Duplex ultrasound (DUS), computed tomography angiography (CTA), and magnetic resonance angiography (MRA) are useful noninvasive tests to evaluate anatomy and for surveillance after revascularization. *However, they should NOT be performed for the anatomic assessment in patients with asymptomatic PAD* [2, 8, 9].

Treatment

- Approaches to reduce CV events:
- Aggressive modification of risk factors: Lifestyle modification including smoking cessation, weight loss, and dietary intervention. Aggressive managements for HTN, DM, and HLD.
- Antiplatelet therapy: Aspirin alone (75–325 mg daily) or clopidogrel alone (75 mg daily). Dual antiplatelet therapy (aspirin and clopidogrel) may be reasonable to reduce the risk of limb-related events in patients with symptomatic PAD after revascularization [2, 8].
- Anticoagulation: The combination of low-dose rivaroxaban 2.5 mg twice a day and aspirin significantly lowers the incident of major adverse limb events, reduces composite CV events and the related complications, but increases the major bleeding risk (COMPASS trial) [15].

- Therapies for symptomatic relief:
  - Supervised exercise therapy (SET) has been shown to improve claudication symptom and walking distance and is the first-line therapy for claudication (CLEVER trial) [14].
  - Cilostazol (100 mg orally twice daily) is a phosphodiesterase-3 enzyme inhibitor, which can improve walking distance in patients with claudication. If symptoms remain unimproved after 3 months, it should be discontinued. *Cilostazol is contraindicated with congestive heart failure of any severity* [2, 8].
  - Revascularization. Patients with lifestyle-limiting claudication with an inadequate response to medical therapy and exercise should be considered for

revascularization. Percutaneous angioplasty with or without stenting is the first option. *Urgent or emergent vascular surgical consult and revascularization are required for ALI and CLI* [2, 6, 8].

Carotid Artery Disease

Introduction and Risk Factors

- Atherosclerotic carotid disease usually develops at branch points and bends especially at the bifurcation of the common carotid artery and origin of the internal carotid artery (ICA). The progression of carotid plaque results in carotid stenosis, obstruction, or plaque rupture, which can cause ischemic stroke or transient ischemic attack from embolization thrombosis or hemodynamic compromise. There is a linear increase in stroke risk as the stenosis increases to >70% [2, 3].
- Risk factors: Smoking, age, gender (men>>women if age <75 y; women>>men if age >75 y), HTN, HLD, DM, and other vascular diseases (e.g., CAD, PAD).

Clinical Manifestations

- Asymptomatic carotid atherosclerosis is a marker of increased risk for ischemic stroke, myocardial infarction, and vascular death.
  - Symptomatic carotid disease is defined as focal neurologic symptoms (e.g., amaurosis fugax, contralateral weakness or numbness, dysarthria or aphasia, spatial neglect, homonymous visual loss) in the distribution of a carotid artery with a significant stenosis. *All patients with a recent stroke or a transient ischemic attack (TIA) should be evaluated for the carotid artery disease* [2, 3].

Diagnosis: *NOT* recommended to screen asymptomatic individuals. However, it is reasonable to screen with DUS in asymptomatic individuals with a carotid bruit and in patients who have symptomatic atherosclerotic disease in another vascular bed (i.e., PAD, CAD, or aortic aneurysm) or have two or more risk factors for atherosclerotic disease.

- Noninvasive studies: *DUS*: The first-line screening test. *CTA:* High sensitivity, reproducibility, and the ability to visualize the entire carotid artery including extracranial and intracranial portions. It also provides information about adjacent bony and soft tissue structures. *Contrast-enhanced MRA:* High-quality images and less artifact when compared with CTA.
- Contrast angiography: The gold standard for the assessment of carotid atherosclerosis. Typically, only needed for diagnostic uncertainty or if intervention is considered.

Treatment

- Aggressive cardiovascular risk factor modifications as discussed in the PAD section.
- Antiplatelet therapy:
  - *Aspirin (75–325 mg daily)* in all patients with extracranial carotid or vertebral atherosclerosis to reduce ischemic cardiovascular events.
  - *Clopidogrel (75 mg daily)* may be used as an alternative to aspirin without increasing bleeding risk, when there is contraindication to aspirin therapy, aspirin allergy, or aspirin resistance (CAPRIE trial) [5].
  - *Low-dose aspirin (25 mg twice daily) plus dipyridamole (200 mg twice daily)* may be superior to aspirin alone or dipyridamole alone in the prevention of MI, stroke, or vascular death [14].
  - DAPT is *NOT* routinely used in patients with carotid atherosclerosis in the absence of an endovascular intervention alternate indication (e.g., coronary stenting).
- Anticoagulation: *NOT* recommended unless there is an alternate indication for anticoagulation (i.e., mechanical heart valve, atrial fibrillation).

- Invasive interventions: Carotid endarterectomy (CEA) and carotid artery stent (CAS) with embolic protection device (EPD) have similar safety and efficacy. ***Indications for invasive interventions***: Symptomatic, and low or average surgical risk, and ipsilateral ICA stenosis >50% as documented by noninvasive imaging, and the anticipated rate of perioperative stroke or mortality is <6%. Interventions should be performed within 2–4 weeks. It is reasonable to perform CEA in asymptomatic patients who have >70% of stenosis in the ICA if the risk of perioperative stroke, MI, and death is low. A full assessment of comorbid conditions and life expectancy and a thorough discussion of the risks and benefits of the procedure should be performed prior to the procedure. Prophylactic CAS might be considered in highly selected patients with asymptomatic carotid stenosis (minimum 60% of stenosis by catheter angiography and 70% by validated DUS). But its effectiveness may not be superior to medical therapy alone (Table 20.2) [3, 10, 11].

TABLE 20.2 Invasive interventions for carotid artery disease

Indications	CEA	CAS
Symptomatic carotid stenosis 50–69%	Consider: if older age (>75 yr) anatomic difficulty for stenting (Class IIa B indication)	Consider: if difficult surgical anatomy, prior neck irradiation, restenosis after CEA, or high surgical risks (Class IIb B indication)
Symptomatic carotid stenosis 70–99%	Prefer CEA (Class I A indication)	Consider if high risk for CEA (Class IIa B indication)
Asymptomatic carotid stenosis 60–99%	May consider CEA or CAS if life expectancy >5 yrs and favorable anatomy and higher stroke risk on medical management alone (Class II indication)	

Renal Arterial Disease

Introduction

- The most common causes of renal artery stenosis (RAS) are atherosclerosis and fibromuscular dysplasia (FMD). Atherosclerosis counting for 90% of RAS primarily affects over the age of 45 years and usually involves the ostium or the proximal main renal artery. This disorder is particularly common in patients with diffuse atherosclerosis. FMD accounts for <10% and most often affects women under the age of 50 years and typically involves the distal main renal artery or the segmental branches.

Clinical Manifestations and Physical Findings (Table 20.3)

- HTN: abrupt onset of HTN (age <30 y, often secondary to FMD; age >55 y, often due to atherosclerotic disease) or previously well-controlled chronic hypertension becoming resistant to medical therapy (three-drug regimen including a diuretic)

Table 20.3 Clinical situations (red flags) suspected for renal artery disease

Abrupt onset of HTN or rapid and persistent worsening of previously well-controlled HTN
New azotemia or worsening of renal function after administrations of ACEIs or ARBs
Acute hypertensive crisis (i.e., AKI, flash pulmonary edema with normal LV function, or hypertensive encephalopathy)
Unexplained atrophic kidney or discrepancy in kidney size or unexplained renal failure
Abdominal bruits, evidence of atherosclerosis in other vascular beds

- Azotemia: unexplained or an acute rise in serum creatinine following the administration of ACEIs or ARBs
- Recurrent flash pulmonary edema often with normal left ventricular function
- Epigastric bruits, evidence of atherosclerosis in other vascular beds (e.g., carotid or femoral bruits and diminished pedal pulses)
- Unilateral atrophic kidney or a size discrepancy between the two kidneys. If it is bilateral RAS, may see bilateral atrophic kidney and do not have size discrepancy between kidneys [16]

Diagnosis

- Laboratory study: Acute elevation of creatinine; rapid decline of estimated glomerular filtration rate (eGFR) and measured GFR.
  - Imaging studies: Duplex Doppler ultrasonography: It is highly useful for surveillance of renal arteries after stenting. MRA: Noninvasive and has ability to generate 3D reconstructions. CTA: Can be used to detect in-stent restenosis because of no significant imaging artifact with metal clips or stents [6].
  - Renal angiogram: The gold standard for the diagnosis of RAS [6].

Treatment

- Medical therapy: management for HTN: ACEIs and ARBs are preferred for unilateral RAS. *Notably, ACEIs and ARBs should not be used in patients with bilateral RAS or a solitary kidney with RAS* [1].
- Percutaneous revascularization: Early restoration of renal artery patency may improve hypertension management and minimize progressive renal dysfunction. *Cure of hypertension after revascularization is most likely in*

patients who have been hypertensive for less than 5 years. Indications: Severe RAS (>70% stenosis or 50%~70% stenosis with peak pressure gradient >20 mmHg or mean gradient >10 mmHg) *PLUS* progressive renal dysfunction, or poorly controlled HTN, or recurrent episodes of unstable angina, or recurrent unexplained flash pulmonary edema [13].

- Surgical revascularization: Including surgical bypass (aortorenal, celiac-renal, or mesenteric-renal) and endarterectomy. Indications: Patients with RAS and aortic diseases (either aneurysmal or occlusive); patients with significant atherosclerotic RAS and clinical indications for intervention with multiple renal arteries or early branching main renal artery; and patient with FMD associated with microaneurysms or complex disease involving segmental renal arteries [9, 12].

Clinical Pearls

- Peripheral artery disease is usually under-recognized at the early stage. Ankle-brachial index is the test of choice of initial diagnosis. Aggressive modification of risk factors and lifestyle modifications are the first-line therapies to prevent cardiovascular events.
- All patients with a recent stroke or a transient ischemic attack (TIA) should be evaluated for carotid artery disease.
- ACEIs and ARBs should not be used in patients with bilateral renal artery stenosis (RAS) or a solitary kidney with RAS. Cure of hypertension after revascularization is most likely in patients who have been hypertensive for less than five years.

Key Learning Points

- Diagnostic modalities for peripheral vascular diseases
- Guidelines-recommended medical management
- Indications for invasive interventions

References

1. ASTRAL Investigators, Wheatley K, Ives N, et al. Revascularization versus medical therapy for renal-artery stenosis. N Engl J Med. 2009;361:1953–62.
2. Griffin BP. Manual of cardiovascular medicine. 5th ed. Philadelphia: Wolters Kluwer; 2019. p. 407–19.
3. Brott TG, Halperin JL, Abbara S, Bacharach JM, Barr JD, Bush RL, Cates CU, Creager MA, Fowler SB, Friday G, Hertzberg VS, MI EB, Moore WS, Panagos PD, Riles TS, Rosenwasser RH, Taylor AJ. 2011 ASA/ACCF/AHA/AANN/AANS/ACR/ASNR/ CNS/SAIP/SCAI/SIR/SNIS/SVM/SVS guideline on the management of patients with extracranial carotid and vertebral artery disease: executive summary. A report of the American College of Cardiology Foundation/American Heart Association Task Force on Practice Guidelines, and the American Stroke Association, American Association of Neuroscience Nurses, American Association of Neurological Surgeons, American College of Radiology, American Society of Neuroradiology, Congress of Neurological Surgeons, Society of Atherosclerosis Imaging and Prevention, Society for Cardiovascular Angiography and Interventions, Society of Interventional Radiology, Society of NeuroInterventional Surgery, Society for Vascular Medicine, and Society for Vascular Surgery. Circulation. 2011;124(4):489–532.
4. Campia U, Gerhard-Herman M, Piazza G, Goldhaber SZ. Peripheral artery disease: past, present, and future. Am J Med. 2019;132(10):1133–41.
5. CAPRIES Steering Committee. A randomised, blinded, trial of clopidogrel versus aspirin in patients at risk of ischaemic events (CAPRIE). Lancet. 1996;348(9038):1329–39.
6. Chonchol M, Linas S. Diagnosis and management of ischemic nephropathy. Clin J Am Soc Nephrol. 2006;1(2):172–81.
7. Conte SM, Vale PR. Peripheral arterial disease. Heart Lung Circ. 2018;27(4):427–32.
8. Gerhard-Herman MD, Gornik HL, Barrett C, Barshes NR, Corriere MA, Drachman DE, Fleisher LA, Fowkes FGR, Hamburg NM, Kinlay S, Lookstein R, Misra S, Mureebe L, Olin JW, Patel RAG, Regensteiner JG, Schanzer A, Shishehbor MH, Stewart KJ, Treat-Jacobson D, Walsh ME. 2016 AHA/ACC guideline on the management of patients with lower extremity peripheral artery disease: executive summary: a report of the American College of Cardiology/American Heart Association

Task Force on Clinical Practice Guidelines. J Am Coll Cardiol. 2017;69(11):1465–508.

9. Levin SR, Arinze N, Siracuse JJ. Lower extremity critical limb ischemia: a review of clinical features and management. Trends Cardiovasc Med. 2019;30(3):125.
10. MRC European Carotid Surgery Trial: interim results for symptomatic patients with severe (70–99%) or with mild (0–29%) carotid stenosis. European Carotid Surgery Trialists' Collaborative Group. Lancet. 1991;337:1235–43.
11. Rutherford RB, Baker JD, Ernst C, et al. Recommended standards for reports dealing with lower extremity ischemia: revised version. J Vasc Surg. 1997;26:517–38.
12. Rundback JH, Sacks D, Kent KC, et al. AHA Councils on Cardiovascular Radiology, High Blood Pressure Research, Kidney in Cardiovascular Disease, Cardio-Thoracic and Vascular Surgery, and Clinical Cardiology, and the Society of Interventional Radiology FDA Device Forum Committee, et al. Guidelines for the reporting of renal artery revascularization in clinical trials. American Heart Association. Circulation. 2002;106(12):1572–85.
13. Textor SC, Misra S, Oderich GS. Percutaneous revascularization for ischemic nephropathy: the past, present, and future. Kidney Int. 2013;83:28–40.
14. Murphy TP, Cutlip DE, Regensteiner JG, et al. Supervised exercise versus primary stenting for claudication resulting from aortoiliac peripheral artery disease: six-month outcomes from the claudication: exercise versus endoluminal revascularization (CLEVER) study. Circulation. 2012;125:130–9.
15. Branch KR, Probstfield JL, Eikelboom JW, et al. Rivaroxaban with or without aspirin in patients with heart failure and chronic coronary or peripheral artery disease. Circulation. 2019;140:529–37.
16. Aboyans V, Ricco JB, ML ELB, et al. 2017 ESC Guidelines on the Diagnosis and Treatment of Peripheral Arterial Diseases, in collaboration with the European Society for Vascular Surgery (ESVS): Document covering atherosclerotic disease of extracranial carotid and vertebral, mesenteric, renal, upper and lower extremity arteries Endorsed by: the European Stroke Organization (ESO)The Task Force for the Diagnosis and Treatment of Peripheral Arterial Diseases of the European Society of Cardiology (ESC) and of the European Society for Vascular Surgery (ESVS). Eur Heart J. 2018;39:763–816.

Chapter 21
Aortic Aneurysms and Aortopathies

Dustin Staloch and Joe X. Xie

Abbreviations

AAA	Abdominal aortic aneurysm
AAS	Acute aortic syndrome
ACE-I	Angiotensin-converting enzyme inhibitor
ARB	Angiotensin receptor blocker
CTA	Computed tomography angiography
GCA	Giant cell arteritis
MRA	Magnetic resonance angiogram
MRI	Magnetic resonance imaging
TA	Takayasu arteritis
TAA	Thoracic aortic aneurysm
TEE	Transesophageal echocardiogram
TTE	Transthoracic echocardiogram

Overview

- Acute aortic syndromes are often a surgical emergency.

D. Staloch (✉) · J. X. Xie
Department of Medicine, Division of Cardiology, Emory University School of Medicine, Atlanta, GA, USA
e-mail: dustin.allen.staloch@emory.edu

A. A. Bhargava et al. (eds.), *Handbook of Outpatient Cardiology*, https://doi.org/10.1007/978-3-030-88953-1_21

- Feared complications of aortic disease include dissection/rupture, aortic regurgitation, or end-organ ischemia.
- Outpatient management of aneurysms and aortopathies center around surveillance to identify those at risk as well as medical therapies and risk factor modification to mitigate disease progression and complication.
- While more common risk factors such as hypertension or smoking are often implicated, aneurysms may present with or before recognition of genetic or systemic processes.

Definitions

- Aortic dissection: a tearing of the intimal layer of the aorta with longitudinal propagation and formation of a blood-filled false lumen, classified by location
- Aortic intramural hematoma: a collection of blood within the medial layer of the aorta without an intimal tear or false lumen
- Penetrating aortic ulcer: localized perforation at the site of an atherosclerotic plaque through the intima without creation of a false lumen
- Aortic aneurysm: abnormal focal dilatation of the aorta beyond 1.5 times normal caliber
  - True aneurysm: an aneurysm of normal wall histology (involving all three layers)
  - Pseudoaneurysm (false aneurysm): a contained rupture of the aortic wall where the segment is a collection of blood bounded not by the aortic wall but by a fibrous peel of periarterial connective tissue
  - Ectasia: modest (<150% normal caliber) and generalized enlargement of the aorta

Clinical Pearl
Aortic rupture is the most common cause of death from aortic disease and dissection, following by acute, severe aortic regurgitation [1].

Acute Aortic Syndromes

As aortic disease is identified incidentally on transthoracic echocardiogram (TTE), computed tomography (CT), or computed tomography angiogram (CTA) obtained for other reasons, it is important to exclude serendipitous recognition of acute processes at first identification to continue outpatient management.

Recognition

- Acute aortic syndrome (AAS) is a general term which includes acute aortic dissections, intramural hematomas, and penetrating ulcers.
- Chief risk factors for AAS include long-standing hypertension (up to 72% of patients) and prior aortic aneurysm. Other risk factors include smoking, drug use, and hyperlipidemia [2].
- Presentation is overwhelmingly (>90%) with chest or back pain, often sudden and severe [2].
- AAS should otherwise be suspected in the presence of the diastolic murmur of acute aortic regurgitation, syncope, a blood pressure or pulse differential (weak or absent owing to a compromised true lumen flow by external compression or an intimal flap), or evidence of end-organ ischemia (disproportionate abdominal pain, weakness/paraplegia, or worsened renal function) [1].

Clinical Pearl
Listen closely! The murmur of acute aortic regurgitation may be short due to rapid equalization of aortic and ventricular pressures.

Management

- Aortic dissections are classified based on the portion of the aorta involved (see Table 7.1).
- Emergent surgical intervention is warranted for dissections involving the ascending aorta (Stanford A or DeBakey I and II) or for high-risk features. If concerns for these exist, urgent surgical referral is indicated.
- In the absence of need for surgery, medical therapy aims to lower heart rate and blood pressure to minimize risk of propagation and complications. For these populations, surveillance imaging is warranted and future elective or urgent surgical intervention considered similar to chronic aneurysms [2].

Thoracic Aortic Aneurysms

Background

- Thoracic aortic aneurysm (TAA) is usually a degenerative disease of the media.
- Diagnosis is usually incidental as it is most often asymptomatic; less commonly, TAA may present with chest pain, an aortic regurgitation murmur, or compressive symptoms.
- The most common sites of involvement are the root (particularly in Marfan syndrome) and ascending aorta [2].

Table 7.1 Aortic dissection classification by dissection flap location

Stanford classification		**DeBakey classification**	
Type A:	Ascending ± descending aorta	Type I:	Ascending + descending aorta
		Type II:	Ascending aorta
Type B:	Descending aorta	Type III:	Descending aorta

- Lesser involved TAA sites include the transverse arch (10%), the descending thoracic aorta (distal to the left subclavian artery), and the thoracoabdominal aorta (involving both thoracic and abdominal components) [2].
- As with other degenerative disease, incidence increases with age with a mean age of 69 years at diagnosis and women being significantly older at presentation [3].

Associations and Risk Factors

- The largest modifiable risks for development of TAA include hypertension and smoking.
- Mycotic aneurysm risk is greatly increased by IV drug use or congenital abnormalities such as coarctation of the aorta.
- Though rare in the modern area, the late manifestations of syphilis, such as syphilitic aortitis and possible resultant aneurysm, should not be forgotten.
- Genetic disorders associated with medial degeneration include [1]:
  - Marfan syndrome
  - Bicuspid aortic valve
  - Turner syndrome
  - Ehlers-Danlos syndrome
  - Loeys-Dietz syndrome
  - Familial aortic aneurysm
- As discussed later, inflammatory disorders such as Takayasu arteritis, giant cell arteritis, and ankylosing spondylitis may present with aortic aneurysm.

Diagnosis

- Diagnosis requires focal enlargement >150% normal diameter, which varies based on gender, age, anatomic location, and imaging modality.

- With TTE, internal diameters are used by convention and judged against expected diameters based on age- and body size-adjusted nomograms.
- TTE has high specificity but low-moderate sensitivity for TAA. While it may be useful for diagnostic visualization of the aortic valve, root, and arch, TTE fails to consistently visualize and accurately measure the tubular portion of the ascending aorta [4].
- When diagnosis of TAA is made on TTE, full imaging of the aorta should be done with computed tomography angiography (CTA), magnetic resonance imaging (MRI), or magnetic resonance angiography (MRA) based on appropriateness of contrast agents.
- Unlike TTE, CT may struggle to define the aortic root unless properly protocolized. Also unlike TTE, there is no consensus on including or excluding the vessel wall when measuring aneurysm size with CTA or MRI/MRA [1].

Management

- Decision for surgical versus medical management is based around rate of rupture.
- Surgery, in general, should be considered urgently for patients with symptoms of expansion (chest or back pain) and electively for asymptomatic patients with rapidly growing (>0.5 cm/year) ascending TAA or any TAA ≥5.5 cm.
- Medical management aims at atherosclerotic risk reduction, including smoking cessation and statin therapy to target low-density lipid cholesterol <70 mg/dL.
- With anti-impulse benefits via reduced heart rate and shear wall stress, beta-blockers are the preferred antihypertensive agent, with blood pressure goals of lowest pressure tolerated or as dictated by comorbid conditions. Angiotensin-converting enzyme (ACE) inhibitors or angiotensin receptor blockers (ARBs) are also reasonable selections [5].

- Pregnant patients or those desiring pregnancy deserve specialist input as prophylactic surgery may be considered for progressive aortic dilatation or aortic valve regurgitation [1].

> **Clinical Pearl**
> Dimensional criteria for surgical intervention apply *only* to asymptomatic aneurysms. Symptomatic aneurysms at any level should undergo surgery – regardless of size.

Surveillance

- The goal of surveillance is to follow aneurysm enlargement, taking into account factors such as renal function, dissection location, and patient age.
- In general, serial imaging is best undertaken with the same modality and within the same institution to facilitate comparison.
- TTE's primary role is serial follow-up in patients with disease limited to the root. While CT may provide better anatomical detail, it comes at the expense of repeat radiation exposure – relevant in younger populations.
- The frequency of surveillance imaging is not entirely clear, due to lack of data to guide surveillance intervals. However, the mean rate of growth for all thoracic aortic aneurysms is approximately 1 mm/year [1, 6].
- It is prudent to obtain surveillance imaging on an annual basis provided the aneurysm size remains stable and every 2–3 years for stable, smaller aneurysms in older patients.

Abdominal Aortic Aneurysms

Background

- Like TAA, abdominal aortic aneurysm (AAA) is usually a degenerative disease of aging but may occur with inflammatory disorders, infectious processes, or congenital conditions.
- Like TAA, diagnosis of AAA requires full-thickness dilation of the abdominal aorta exceeding normal caliber (varying by age, sex, and body size) by >50% (usually ≥3 cm).
- Abdominal aortic aneurysms are considered small if less than 5.5 cm; above this cut-off, they are considered large AAA.
- In more than 90% of cases, the proximal edge remains infrarenal [7].
- A minority of patients will have symptoms warranting early detection. However, AAA without rupture may be a source of hematuria, gastrointestinal bleeding, or chronic abdominal or low back pain. With rupture, AAA may present with sudden-onset pain, syncope, or a pulsatile abdominal mass.

Associations and Risk Factors

- AAA is five times more common in smokers, in whom 89% of all aneurysm ruptures occur [1].
- Those most effected by AAA are men >65 years old. Other strong risk factors include family history of AAA, hypertension, and coronary artery disease.
- AAA is associated with most of the same congenital and inflammatory conditions TAA.

Diagnosis

- Abdominal ultrasound is the gold standard for diagnosis and monitoring in asymptomatic patients. For cost-effective screening of the general population, the US Preventive Services Task Force (USPSTF) recommends a one-time screening by ultrasound in men 65–75 years who have smoked. Due to low yield, it is recommended against screening women. There is no recommendation for or against men who have not smoked [8].
- CTA is typically performed for asymptomatic but large AAA or for symptomatic/ruptured AAA, as it is better suited for preoperative assessment and determination of repair method.

Clinical Pearl
Find the sweet spot! One-time ultrasound screening for AAA is recommended for men aged 65–75 who have ever smoked. Screening the remainder of the general population is not recommended.

Management and Surveillance

- Immediate surgical repair is indicated for aneurysms expanding >0.5 cm in 6 months or for any symptomatic aneurysms. Elective repair is usually considered for saccular aneurysms, AAA ≥5.5 cm for men, and ≥5.0 cm for women [9, 10].
- Smoking cessation is recommended for all patients to slow the growth of AAA.
- Evidence on medical management of AAA is mixed, as are society recommendations. While both statins and ACE inhibitors may be considered to reduce aortic complications in patients with small AAA, evidence is weak. These agents, along with ARBs and beta-blockers, are largely not

Table 7.2 Abdominal aortic aneurysm surveillance interval by aneurysm size

Aneurysm size	Surveillance interval
3.0–3.4 cm	Every 3 years
3.5–4.4 cm	Every 1 year
4.5–5.4 cm	Every 6 months

indicated for use solely to reduce risk of AAA expansion or rupture [9, 10].

- AAA without indication for operative intervention should be monitored with abdominal ultrasound at intervals based on aneurysm size (see Table 7.2) [11].

Inherited Aortopathies

Marfan Syndrome

- Characterized by long, thin extremities, ectopia lentis, and ligamentous redundancy, Marfan syndrome usually stems from an autosomal dominant FBN1 gene encoding fibrillin-1.
- Characteristic cardiovascular issues include fusiform enlargement of the aortic root involving enlargement of the aortic annulus (leading to aortic regurgitation) through the proximal ascending aorta. This lends a "flask-like" shape to the root characteristic of Marfan syndrome and other disorders of cystic medial necrosis.
- Abnormalities may involve the entire length of the aorta, though dissection is seen most commonly in the thoracic aorta. Nearly half of patients have mitral insufficiency [12].
- Beta-blockers and ARBs are indicated to slow aneurysm and aortic root dilation progression, but are not proven to impact clinical outcomes [2].
- Surgical repair of aortic aneurysms is recommended for aortic aneurysms ≥5 cm, severe aortic regurgitation, or

≥4.5 cm with family history of dissection or growth rate >0.3 cm/year.
- Women should be counseled against pregnancy; repair of aneurysms 4.1–4.5 cm is recommended for women anticipating pregnancy and may be considered if >4 cm for those desiring pregnancy [2, 10].

Ehlers-Danlos Syndrome

- Comprising a group of rare disorders of collagen synthesis, Ehlers-Danlos syndrome (EDS) occurs in 1 in 5000 persons worldwide with widely varying presentations from mild skin hyperextensibility to life-threatening cardiovascular complications.
- In the vascular EDS form, an autosomal dominant COL3A1 mutation leads to defective production of type III collagen and medial degeneration.
- Management strategies tend to parallel Marfan syndrome. Due to resultant challenges in healing, bleeding, and other complications, surgical intervention is avoided whenever possible.

Loeys-Dietz Syndrome

- With five subtypes, Loeys-Dietz syndrome (LDS) types 1 and 2 are classified as connective tissue diseases. While these patients were previously characterized as having Marfan syndrome of EDS, it is now recognized that LDS 1 and 2 are due to mutations of TGFBR1 and TGFBR2.
- With significant phenotypic overlap with the vascular EDS type, individuals are prone to pregnancy-related complications and rapidly enlarging aneurysms that are predisposed to rupture, with a mean age of death of 26 years.
- LDS 1 may be recognized by the triad of vascular aneurysms, cleft palate and/or bifid uvula, and hypertelorism; LDS 2 is notable for cutaneous manifestations akin to

vascular EDS such as easy bruising, atrophic scars, and velvety translucent skin [13].

Bicuspid Aortic Valve

- Structural abnormalities of the ascending aorta predispose those born with bicuspid aortic valves to aneurysm and dissection. In many, aneurysmal changes precede and are recognized prior to diagnosis of valvular dysfunction.
- These patients frequently undergo both aortic valve and aorta replacement owing to more rapid aneurysm growth compared to aneurysms of trileaflet patients, possibly due to excess matrix metalloproteinase activity [1].
- Repair or replacement of the ascending aorta or aortic root is recommended for:
  - Diameter ≥5.5 cm (class 1 indication)
  - Diameter >5 cm + family history of dissection or growth rate ≥0.5 cm/year (class 2a)
  - Diameter >5 cm + low surgical risk + experienced surgical team and center (class 2a)
  - Diameter >4.5 cm if aortic valve surgery is planned (class 2a) Aortic root repair/replacement or ascending aorta repair

Turner Syndrome

- In phenotypic females, Turner syndrome results from the absence of an X chromosome and resultant 45 XO genotype.
- Cardiovascular disease is common, including bicuspid aortic valve (up to 25%), coarctation of the aorta (up to 10%), and ascending aorta ectasia and aneurysm.
- Surveillance at routine intervals (typically annually) are recommended when abnormalities are identified or every 5–10 years in the absence of known cardiovascular complication [14].

Other Aortopathies

Takayasu Arteritis and Giant Cell Arteritis

- Takayasu arteritis (TA) and giant cell arteritis (GCA) are idiopathic vasculitides of the aorta and its branches with considerable phenotypic overlap.
- Both present predominately in women with indolent progression of systemic symptoms of fatigue, weight loss, fevers, and nonspecific elevations in inflammatory markers.
- A major distinction between the two is age, as TA diagnosed in younger patients (<40 years) and GCA in older patients (>50 years).
- Both may result in aneurysm of the aorta, but TA may also affect vascular beds from the coronary arteries through to arteries of the head, neck, and abdominal viscera.
- Treatment in general is with immunosuppression, and surgical intervention is avoided when possible (especially without disease quiescence) [15].

HLA-B27-Associated Spondyloarthropathies

- In patients with Reiter syndrome and ankylosing spondylitis, aortitis is common and is of highest prevalence in those with long-standing spondylitis, iritis, or peripheral arthritis.
- Driven by medial necrosis, aortic dissection has been reported as well as aortic regurgitation and cardiac conduction disease owing to local inflammation.

Infectious Aortopathies

- Primary infection of the aortic wall is uncommon but may be seen with *Staphylococcus*, *Salmonella*, and *Pseudomonas* species, giving rise to aortic aneurysms which are more often saccular. “Mycotic” or infectious aneurysms may be due otherwise to secondary infection of pre-existing aneurysms. Infection may lead to weakness of the aortic wall with high propensity for rupture.

- Though rare in the modern antibiotic era, syphilitic aortitis should not be forgotten. This form of tertiary syphilis occurs years after initial infection and may lead to aortic aneurysms.
- Tuberculous aneurysms may arise following infection extension from hilar lymph nodes leading to loss of aortic wall integrity from granulomatous medial destruction. Usually identified as saccular aneurysms arising from the posterior or posterolateral aortic wall, progression may give rise to perforation, aortoenteric fistulae, or pseudoaneurysm.

Key Learning Points

1. Outpatient management of aneurysms and aortopathies seek center on appropriate selection of imaging modality and intervals to identify surgical need.
2. While specific antihypertensive agents such as beta-blockers and ARBs are reasonable, evidence is not overwhelming. Blood pressure control, smoking cessation, and statin therapy are recommended for most.
3. Aortic aneurysms may not be a primary disorder, but instead a feature of congenital, systemic, or infectious conditions.

References

1. Elefteriades JA, Olin JW, Halperin JL. Diseases of the aorta. In: Fuster V, et al., editors. Hurst’s the heart. 14th ed. New York, NY: McGraw-Hill. p. 2261–89.
2. Hiratzka LF, Bakris GL, Becman JA, et al. 2010 ACCF/ AHA/ AATS/ ACR/ ASA/ SCA/ SCAI/ SIR/ STS/ SVM guidelines for

the diagnosis and management of patients with thoracic aortic disease. JACC. 2010;55(14):e27–129.

3. Ramanath VS, Oh JK, Sundt JM, et al. Acute aortic syndromes and thoracic aortic aneurysm. Mayo Clin Proc. 2009;84(5):465–81.
4. Cheitlin MD, Armstrong WF, Aurigemma GP, et al. ACC/AHA/ASE 2003 guideline update for the clinical application of echocardiography—summary article: a report of the American College of Cardiology/ American Heart Association Task Force on Practice Guidelines. JACC. 2003;42(5):954–70.
5. Whelton PK, Carey RM, Aronow WS, et al. 2017 ACC/ AHA/ AAPA/ ABC/ ACPM/ AGS/ APhA/ ASH/ ASPC/ NMA/ PCNA guidelines for the prevention, detection, evaluation, and management of high blood pressure in adults: a report of the American College of Cardiology/American Heart Association Task Force on Clinical Practice Guidelines. JACC. 2018;71(19):e127–248.
6. Davies RR, Goldstein LJ, Coady MA, et al. Yearly rupture or dissection rates for thoracic aortic aneurysms: a simple prediction based on size. Ann Thorac Surg. 2002;73:17–27.
7. Sakalihasan N, Michel JB, Katsargyris A, et al. Abdominal aortic aneurysms. Nat Rev Dis Primers. 2018;4(1):34.
8. Carnevale ML, Koleilat I, Lipsitz EC, et al. Extended screening guidelines for the diagnosis of abdominal aortic aneurysm. J Vasc Surg. 2020;72(6):1917–26.
9. Hirsch AT, Haskal ZJ, Hertzer NR, et al; ACC/AHA 2005 Practice Gui delines for the management of patients with peripheral arterial disease (lower extremity, renal, mesenteric, and abdominal aortic): a collaborative report from the American Association for Vascular Surgery/Society for Vascular Surgery, Society for Cardiovascular Angiography and Interventions, Society for Vascular Medicine and Biology, Society of Interventional Radiology, and the ACC/AHA Task Force on Practice Guidelines. Circulation. 2006;113(11):e463–654
10. Erbel R, Aboyans V, Boileau C, et al. ESC Committee for Practice Guidelines. 2014 ESC Guidelines on the diagnosis and treatment of aortic diseases: Document covering acute and chronic aortic diseases of the thoracic and abdominal aorta of the adult. The Task Force for the Diagnosis and Treatment of Aortic Diseases of the European Society of Cardiology (ESC). Eur Heart J. 2014;35(41):2873–926.
11. Chaikof EL, Dalman RL, Eskandari MK, et al. The Society for Vascular Surgery practice guidelines on the care of patients with an abdominal aortic aneurysm. J Vasc Surg. 2018;67(1):2–77.

12. Finkbohner R, Johnston D, Crawford ES, et al. Marfan syndrome: along-term survival and complications after aortic aneurysm repair. Circulation. 1995;91:728–33.
13. Loeys BL, Chen J, Neptune ER, et al. A syndrome of altered cardiovascular, craniofacial, neurocognitive and skeletal development caused by mutations in TGFBR1 or TGFBR2. Nat Genet. 2005;37:275–81.
14. Gravholt CH, Andersen NH, Conway GS, et al. Clinical practice guidelines for the care of girls and women with Turner syndrome: proceedings from the 2016 Cincinnati International Turner Syndrome Meeting. Eur J Endocrinol. 2017;177(3):g1–70.
15. Helmich B, Agueda, Monti S, et al. 2018 Update of the EULAR recommendations for the management of large vessel vasculitis. Ann Rheum Dis. 2020;79(1):19–30.

Chapter 22
Pulmonary Embolism and DVT

Stephanie Wang and Christine Kempton

Abbreviations

aPTT	Activated partial thromboplastin time
AHA	American Heart Association
BNP	Brain natriuretic peptide
CTPA	Computed tomography pulmonary angiogram
CTPH	Chronic thromboembolic pulmonary hypertension
DVT	Deep vein thrombosis
ESC	European Society of Cardiology
IFDVT	Iliofemoral DVT
LMWH	Low molecular weight heparin
DOAC	Direct oral anticoagulants
PE	Pulmonary embolism
PTP	Pretest probability
PTS	Post-thrombotic syndrome
VKA	Vitamin K antagonists

S. Wang (✉)
Department of Medicine, Division of Cardiology, Emory University School of Medicine, Atlanta, GA, USA
e-mail: szwang@emory.edu; stephanie.zi.wang@emory.edu

C. Kempton
Department of Hematology and Medical Oncology, Emory University School of Medicine, Atlanta, GA, USA

A. A. Bhargava et al. (eds.), *Handbook of Outpatient Cardiology*, https://doi.org/10.1007/978-3-030-88953-1_22

V/Q	Ventilation perfusion scan
VTE	Venous thromboembolism

Pulmonary Embolism

- Symptoms include pleuritic chest pain, dyspnea, tachypnea, and tachycardia.
- The main objectives in the outpatient setting are diagnosis, risk stratification, and treatment.
  - Treatment can be divided into three phases [1]:

    Initial management – time of diagnosis to 21 days
    Primary treatment – up to 3–6 months representing minimal duration of treatment for VTE
    Secondary treatment (aka extended anticoagulation) – post-primary treatment period and after determination of the risk of recurrent VTE

- *Diagnosis*
  - Initial Workup

    Pretest probability (PTP): Wells score, modified Wells score, Geneva score

    - Wells score: low <2, intermediate 2–6, high >6
      - Symptoms of DVT (3 points), less likely alternative diagnosis (3), heart rate >100 (1.5), immobilization for >3 days or surgery in the past 4 hours (1.5), prior DVT/PE (1.5), hemoptysis (1), malignancy (1)

    Diagnostic testing based on PTP [2–4]

    - High (>50%): empirically start anticoagulation and obtain computed tomography pulmonary angiogram (CTPA).
    - Intermediate (~20%): obtain D-dimer to exclude, followed by CTPA or ventilation perfusion scan

(V/Q) if needed. If patients are likely to have a nondiagnostic V/Q, they should undergo CT.
- Low (~5%): obtain D-dimer to exclude, and then obtain computed tomography pulmonary angiogram (CTPA) or V/Q if indicated based on D-dimer.
  - *Using age-adjusted cutoff for D-dimer (age × 10 in patients >50 years old) should be considered as alternative to fixed cutoff level (ESC 2019, ADJUST-PE)* [5]*(Clinical Pearl).*

- *Risk Stratification*
  - Vital signs
  - Clot burden and RV/LV dimensions on CTPA [6]
  - Cardiac echo

    Evidence of RV dysfunction may include RV hypokinesis, pulmonary hypertension, and McConnell's sign.
    Patent foramen ovale (seen on echo with bubble study) is an adverse predictor because paradoxical embolism is associated with increased risk of death, stroke, and other arterial embolisms; hence, more aggressive treatment of PE should be considered [7].

  - Biomarkers (troponin, BNP/proBNP, lactate)

- *Treatment Strategy* [8, 9, 10]
  - *Initial treatment strategy* is based on classification of severity of PE (see Table 22.1.).
  - In low-risk PE, patients can be considered for early discharge and outpatient treatment.

    In patients with low-risk PE, early discharge within 48 hours with rivaroxaban was not associated with increased risk of recurrent VTE or PE-related deaths within 3 months (HOT-PE, ESC 2020) [11].

Table 22.1 Summarization of PE findings and treatment

	Findings	Treatment
Massive	Shock – 15 minutes of sustained hypotension with SBP <90mmHg or 40mmHg lower than baseline or needing ionotrope	Systemic thrombolysis Catheter-directed therapies Surgical embolectomy Hemodynamic support Systemic anticoagulation in all
Submassive	RV dysfunction on echo or CT (RV/LV diameter >0.9) Positive biomarkers (troponin or BNP)	Half-dose thrombolytics Catheter-directed therapies Systemic anticoagulation in all
Low risk	Normotensive, normal biomarkers, no RV dysfunction	Systemic anticoagulation Single sub-segmental PE without proximal DVT can sometimes be managed with surveillance and no anticoagulation

– IVC filter considerations

Indicated for acute PE/proximal DVT with contraindications to anticoagulation including active bleeding; however, anticoagulation should be resumed as soon as contraindication is resolved (AHA Class I). *Does not reduce PE recurrence in patients with acute PE and compared with anticoagulation alone is associated with increased risk of DVT (PREPIC2, JAMA 2015)* [12] *(Clinical Pearl).*

– Anticoagulation for *initial and primary treatment* (see Table 22.2)

For outpatient treatment, options include low molecular weight heparin (LMWH), vitamin K antagonists (VKA) following LMWH, and direct oral anticoagulants (DOAC). DOAC use is associated with lower

TABLE 22.2 DOAC dosing for use in PE and DVT

DOAC	Initial and primary treatment	Secondary treatment (extended anticoagulation)
Apixaban	10 mg twice daily for 1 week and then 5mg twice daily Reduced dosing not studied for VTE	2.5 mg twice daily
Rivaroxaban	15 mg twice daily for 3 weeks and then 20 mg once daily	10 mg once daily
Dabigatran	150 mg twice daily following parenteral anticoagulation for 5–10 days initially	150 mg twice daily
Edoxaban	60 mg once daily following parenteral anticoagulation for 5–10 days initially	

risk of major bleeding and is preferred in the absence of contraindications [1, 9].

With exception of patients with gastrointestinal cancer, edoxaban, rivaroxaban, and apixaban can be considered as alternatives to LMWH in cancer patients [8].

Populations in which DOAC has not been studied extensively in or should be used with caution: triple positive antiphospholipid syndrome (only use VKA), liver disease, pregnancy (absolute contraindication), severe renal impairment (although apixaban has been used in end-stage renal patients), and severe morbid obesity. Potential drug-drug interactions should also be reviewed prior to initiation of DOAC therapy.

Primary treatment duration is usually 3 months.

– Decision to pursue *secondary treatment* [9, 24, 25]

Use of extended anticoagulation depends on risk of recurrence which is primarily based on presence or absence of reversible risk factors, which can be transient or chronic, and balanced against bleeding risk.

- Major transient risk factor: Surgery.
- Moderate transient risk factor: Immobility, hospitalization, pregnancy, estrogen/hormone use, long-haul air travel.
- Cancer and inflammatory bowel disease are also moderate risk factors that with adequate effective therapy are transient.

For provoked VTE with major transient risk factors, recommend only primary treatment.
For provoked VTE with moderate transient risk factors, primary treatment only is typically recommended, though it may be extended in some circumstances.
For provoked VTE with chronic risk factors (untreated cancer, hereditary disorders), recommend primary and secondary treatment with extended anticoagulation as long as risk factors are persistent.
For first unprovoked VTE, primary treatment is recommended for all patients. In those with low/moderate risk of bleeding, secondary treatment with extended anticoagulation is also recommended.

- The American College of Chest Physicians (ACCP) proposed a score to assess risk of bleeding based on factors such as age, previous bleeding, cancer, renal failure, etc. The score categorizes risk of major bleeding as low, moderate, and high based on the number of factors present [9].
- HAS-BLED score (used initially to assess risk of bleeding in anticoagulation for atrial fibrillation) has also been validated for use in VTE treatment [23].

- For recurrent unprovoked VTE with low to moderate risk of bleeding, recommend primary followed by secondary treatment; however, if there is high risk of bleeding that is not modifiable, recommend only 3 months for secondary anticoagulation.

- *Additional Treatment Care Considerations*
  - Testing for thrombophilias [13] (also applies to DVT)

    Perform testing if it will alter management, such as to extend anticoagulation duration or to aid in primary VTE prevention during periods of increased risk in relatives of hereditary disorders.

    - Testing includes lupus anticoagulants, factor V Leiden, prothrombin gene mutation, cardiolipin, beta-2 glycoprotein, and proteins C and S. Necessity and timing of these tests can differ based on clinical scenario.

    Thrombophilia testing is not recommended following episode of provoked VTE as a positive result is not sufficient to extend anticoagulation (Clinical Pearl).
    Testing is also not recommended following an episode of unprovoked VTE, as unprovoked episode would warrant extended anticoagulation (Clinical Pearl).
    Do not perform thrombophilia testing at the time of VTE diagnosis or during the initial 3-month course of treatment, unless there is a high suspicion of antiphospholipid antibody syndrome.

  - Evaluating for chronic thromboembolic pulmonary hypertension (CTPH)

    CTPH can be insidious in onset with continued dyspnea and functional limitation despite anticoagulation. With the first episode of PE, it can occur up to 4% at 2 years [14].

Diagnosed by evidence of pulmonary hypertension on echocardiogram and V/Q scan with mismatched perfusion defect.

Recommendation for referral to pulmonary hypertension center.

Deep Vein Thrombosis

- Symptoms include swelling, pain, and erythema.
- *Diagnosis* [3]
  - Pretest probability with Wells score as above

    Low probability: Use D-dimer to exclude.

    Intermediate probability: Lower extremity ultrasound. Can stop if whole leg US is negative, but if initial proximal ultrasound is negative, should be followed with repeat in 1 week if there is no alternative explanation.

    High probability: Proximal or whole leg ultrasound followed by repeat ultrasound in 1 week if initial one was negative.

    Isolated pelvic vein DVT may not be visualized on ultrasound, so venous CT or MRI should be considered.

- *Anatomy*
  - Distal lower extremity DVT: thrombosis in veins below the knee
  - Proximal lower extremity DVT: thrombosis in popliteal, femoral, and iliac veins and above and is associated with increased risk of embolization compared with distal DVT

    Iliofemoral DVT (IFDVT): thrombosis of any part of iliac or common femoral vein. It is associated with higher risk of recurrent DVT and post-thrombotic syndrome [15, 16].

Upper extremity DVT: thrombosis of ulnar, radial, interosseous, brachial, axillary, or subclavian veins

- *Treatment Approach* [8, 9, 17]
  - Most isolated DVT without PE can be treated in the outpatient setting unless there is massive obstructive DVT causing acrocyanosis, venous limb ischemia, or extension into inferior vena cava. Other reasons for inpatient treatment include patients with high-risk comorbidities or severe pain requiring inpatient pain management.
  - DVT with PE – refer to PE treatment above for anticoagulation guidelines.
  - Proximal DVT without PE

    Catheter-directed therapy (pharmacological/mechanical) should be considered in patients with phlegmasia cerulea dolens or with clot extension despite anticoagulation (AHA Class IIa) [19].
    Anticoagulation for at least 3 months.
    If the patient has contraindication to anticoagulation, then IVC filter should be placed. Anticoagulation should be resumed as soon as contraindication resolves (AHA Class I).
    Although some patients may experience pain reduction and edema with compression stockings, there is no consistent data to support the use of compression stockings in asymptomatic patients in order to reduce the risk of developing post-thrombotic syndrome (PTS) [1].

  - Isolated distal DVT

    Those at high risk of recurrence should be anticoagulated as above; otherwise, low-risk patients can be followed with ultrasound surveillance with serial imaging in 2 weeks. If there is extension of the clot, then anticoagulation should be initiated.
    High-risk conditions include prior VTE, age >50 years, cancer, presence of inflammatory diseases,

distal DVT involving popliteal trifurcation, and an unprovoked event.

- Upper extremity DVT

  Generally associated with catheters. If catheter can be removed, anticoagulate for 3 months. Otherwise anticoagulation is recommended for the duration of catheter placement. Do not remove the catheter as part of VTE management alone.

- *Recurrence* [9, 17, 18]
  - Aside from the previously noted high-risk factors for recurrence, anatomic abnormalities that result in venous compression such as May-Thurner and thoracic outlet syndromes may also cause recurrence.

    There are various scores/models for predicting risk of recurrence after the first unprovoked VTE: Vienna prediction model, DASH score, and HERDOO-2.

  - Definition/diagnosis

    DVT occurring after initial successful treatment based on symptoms and signs.
    Main diagnostic criterion on ultrasound is the presence of new, noncompressible venous segment.

    - If there was a previously abnormal segment, vein diameter increase by >4 mm indicates recurrence of ipsilateral DVT.

  - Surveillance

    Recommend baseline venous ultrasound and D-dimer at completion of anticoagulation to have baseline for future potential recurrences [20, 21] *(Clinical Pearl).*
    Elevation of D-dimer after it has normalized following anticoagulation treatment is associated with an increased risk of recurrence.

– Treatment

Please see discussion in the PE section about decision for prolonged anticoagulation (secondary treatment/extended anticoagulation) after unprovoked event.

If the patient had recurrent VTE on therapeutic VKA or DOAC, switch to LMWH can be made temporarily while investigating potential etiologies (cancer, compliance, true recurrence) [9, 22].

Key Learning Points

1. Massive and submassive PE require inpatient hospitalization for the evaluation of potential advanced therapies such as systemic thrombolysis, catheter-directed therapies, and catheter or surgical embolectomy.
2. Most low-risk PE and DVTs can be safely treated in the outpatient setting with anticoagulation.
3. DOACs are recommended over VKA and LMWH for anticoagulation for VTE in most patients.
4. Baseline imaging and D-dimer are recommended following the completion of initial treatment for DVT, to facilitate the potential future diagnosis of recurrent VTE.
5. Thrombophilia testing is indicated after VTE only if it will change management in terms of anticoagulation duration or support primary prevention at times of increased risk in relatives.

References

1. Ortel TL, Neumann I, Ageno W, et al. American Society of Hematology 2020 Guidelines for Management of Venous Thromboembolism: Treatment of Deep Vein Thrombosis and Pulmonary Embolism. Blood Adv. 2020;4(19):4693–738.

2. Kearon C, Ageno W, Cannegieter SC, Cosmi B, Geersing G-J, Kyrle PA. Categorization of patients as having provoked or unprovoked venous thromboembolism: guidance from the SSC of ISTH. J Thromb Haemost. 2016;14(7):1480–3.
3. Lim W, Le Gal G, Bates S, Righini M, Haramati L, Lang E, et al. American Society of Hematology 2018 guidelines for management of venous thromboembolism: diagnosis of venous thromboembolism. Blood Adv. 2018;2(22):3226–56.
4. Stein P, Fowler S, Goodman L, Gottschalk A, Hales C, Hull R, et al. Multidetector computed tomography for acute pulmonary embolism. N Engl J Med. 2006;354(22):2317–27.
5. Righini M, Van Es J, Den Exter PL, et al. Age-adjusted D-dimer cutoff levels to rule out pulmonary embolism: the ADJUST-PE study. JAMA. 2014;311(11):1117–24.
6. Furlan A, Aghayev A, Chang C, et al. Short-term mortality in acute pulmonary embolism: clot burden and signs of right heart dysfunction at CT pulmonary angiography. Radiology. 2012;265(1):283–93.
7. Konstantinides S, Geibel A, Kasper W, Olschewski M, Blümel L, Just H. Patent foramen ovale is an important predictor of adverse outcome in patients with major pulmonary embolism. Circulation. 1998;97(19):1946–51.
8. Stavros V Konstantinides, Guy Meyer, Cecilia Becattini, et al. ESC Scientific Document Group, 2019 ESC Guidelines for the diagnosis and management of acute pulmonary embolism developed in collaboration with the European Respiratory Society (ERS): The Task Force for the diagnosis and management of acute pulmonary embolism of the European Society of Cardiology (ESC). Eur Heart J. 2020;4(4):543–603.
9. Kearon C, Akl E, Ornelas J, Blaivas A, Jimenez D, Bounameaux H, et al. Antithrombotic therapy for VTE disease. Chest. 2016;149(2):315–52.
10. Jaff M, McMurtry M, Archer S, Cushman M, Goldenberg N, Goldhaber S, et al. Management of massive and submassive pulmonary embolism, iliofemoral deep vein thrombosis, and chronic thromboembolic pulmonary hypertension. Circulation. 2011;123(16):1788–830.
11. Barco S, Schmidtmann I, Ageno W, Bauersachs RM, Becattini C, Bernardi E, et al. Early discharge and home treatment of patients with low-risk pulmonary embolism with the oral factor Xa inhibitor rivaroxaban: an international multicentre single-arm clinical trial. Eur Heart J. 2019;

12. Mismetti P, Laporte S, Pellerin O, Ennezat P, Couturaud F, Elias A, et al. Effect of a retrievable inferior vena cava filter plus anticoagulation vs anticoagulation alone on risk of recurrent pulmonary embolism. JAMA. 2015;313(16):1627.
13. Stevens SM, Woller SC, Bauer KA, et al. Guidance for the evaluation and treatment of hereditary and acquired thrombophilia. J Thromb Thrombol. 2016;41(1):154–64.
14. Pengo V, Lensing A, Prins M, Marchiori A, Davidson B, Tiozzo F, et al. Incidence of chronic thromboembolic pulmonary hypertension after pulmonary embolism. N Engl J Med. 2004;350(22):2257–64.
15. Douketis J, Crowther M, Foster G, Ginsberg J. Does the location of thrombosis determine the risk of disease recurrence in patients with proximal deep vein thrombosis? Am J Med. 2001;110(7):515–9.
16. Kahn S. Determinants and time course of the postthrombotic syndrome after acute deep venous thrombosis. Ann Int Med. 2008;149(10):698.
17. Mazzolai L, Aboyans V, Ageno W, et al. Diagnosis and management of acute deep vein thrombosis: a joint consensus document from the European Society of Cardiology working groups of aorta and peripheral vascular diseases and pulmonary circulation and right ventricular function. Eur Heart J. 2018;39(47):4208–18.
18. Ageno W, Squizzato A, Wells PS, et al. The diagnosis of symptomatic recurrent pulmonary embolism and deep vein thrombosis: guidance from the SSC of the ISTH. J Thromb Haemost. 2013;11(8):1597–602.
19. Vedantham S, Goldhaber S, Julian J, Kahn S, Jaff M, Cohen D, et al. Pharmacomechanical catheter-directed thrombolysis for deep-vein thrombosis. N Engl J Med. 2017;377(23):2240–52.
20. Cosmi B, Legnani C, Tosetto A, et al. PROLONG Investigators (on behalf of Italian Federation of Anticoagulation Clinics). Usefulness of repeated D-dimer testing after stopping anticoagulation for a first episode of unprovoked venous thromboembolism: the PROLONG II prospective study. Blood. 2010;115(3):481–8.
21. Hamadah A, Alwasaidi T, LE Gal G, et al. Baseline imaging after therapy for unprovoked venous thromboembolism: a randomized controlled comparison of baseline imaging for diagnosis of suspected recurrence. J Thromb Haemost. 2011;9(12):2406–10.

22. Schulman S. How I treat recurrent venous thromboembolism in patients receiving anticoagulant therapy. Blood. 2017;129(25):3285–93.
23. Brown JD, Goodin AJ, Lip GYH, et al. Risk stratification for bleeding complications in patients with venous thromboembolism: application of the HAS-BLED bleeding score during the first 6 months of anticoagulant treatment. J Am Heart Assoc. 2018;7(6)
24. Heit JA, Mohr DN, Silverstein MD, et al. Predictors of recurrence after deep vein thrombosis and pulmonary embolism: a population-based cohort study. Arch Intern Med. 2000;160(6):761–8.
25. Baglin T, Luddington R, Brown K, Baglin C. Incidence of recurrent venous thromboembolism in relation to clinical and thrombophilic risk factors: prospective cohort study. Lancet. 2003;362(9383):523–6.

Part VIII
Arrhythmia

Chapter 23
Management of Atrial Fibrillation in the Outpatient Setting

Vladimir Kaplinskiy and Eli V. Gelfand

Abbreviations

AF	Atrial fibrillation
AV	Atrioventricular
CTI	Cavo-tricuspid isthmus
DAPT	Dual antiplatelet therapy
DCCV	Direct current cardioversion
DOAC	Direct oral anticoagulant
INR	International normalized ratio
LAA	Left atrial appendage
LV	Left ventricle
OAC	Oral anticoagulation
OSA	Obstructive sleep apnea
TEE	Transesophageal echocardiogram

V. Kaplinskiy (✉) · E. V. Gelfand
Department of Medicine, Division of Cardiology, Beth Israel Deaconess Medical Center, Harvard Medical School, Boston, MA, USA
e-mail: vkaplins@bidmc.harvard.edu

A. A. Bhargava et al. (eds.), *Handbook of Outpatient Cardiology*, https://doi.org/10.1007/978-3-030-88953-1_23

Terminology

- AF: Heart rhythm characterized by absence of discrete P-waves and with an R-R interval that follows no repetitive pattern (Fig. 23.1).
- Paroxysmal AF spontaneously terminates within 7 days of onset.
- Persistent AF lasts for >7 days and requires an intervention to restore sinus rhythm.
- Permanent or chronic AF is persistent AF which has been refractory to intervention or for which intervention to restore sinus has eventually been deemed futile, inappropriate, or otherwise undesired.
- Conversion pause: transient bradycardia caused by delayed sinus node recovery following termination of atrial fibrillation.
- Tachy-brady syndrome refers to co-existence of tachycardia during periods of atrial fibrillation and sinus pauses or sinus.

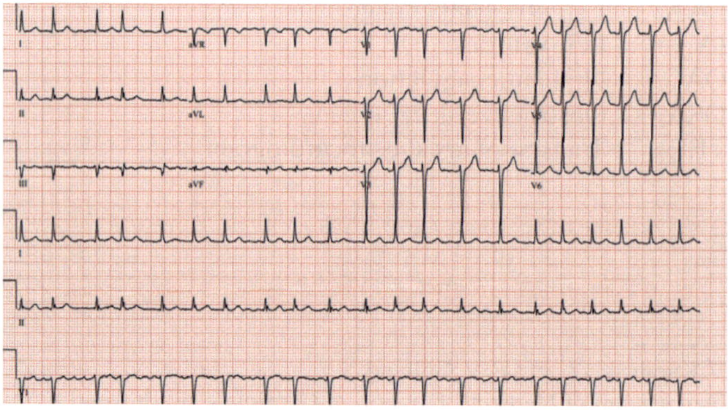

FIGURE 23.1 Atrial fibrillation

Epidemiology of Atrial Fibrillation

- Estimated prevalence ~34 million worldwide [1] and increases in frequency with age [2]. More frequent in men and North Americans. Whites have a higher risk of AF compared to Black, Hispanic, and Asian patients. Overall, 20–25% lifetime incidence.
- Risk factors for AF include age, hypertension, diabetes, obstructive sleep apnea, pulmonary disease, abnormal left ventricular systolic function, myo- and pericarditis, acute illness, alcohol intake, hyperthyroidism (including subclinical hyperthyroidism), and surgery (especially cardiac surgery) [3].
- AF is associated with multiple other conditions including coronary artery disease (though AF is rarely a manifestation of cardiac ischemia), sequelae of rheumatic fever, hypertrophic cardiomyopathy, obesity, chronic kidney disease, valvular heart disease, and alcohol overuse.
- Some literature suggests that a Mediterranean diet enriched with olive oil may decrease the risk of developing AF [4].
- Alcohol abstinence [5] and strict BP control [6] have been shown to reduce AF incidence.
- In patients on stable antiarrhythmic therapy, AF relapse is common, occurring in nearly 90% of subjects [7], and most of these recurrences are asymptomatic.

Clinical Pearl

There is no evidence to prove that excess caffeine consumption predisposes to the development of AF.

Consequences of Atrial Fibrillation

- Common symptoms of AF include palpitations, dyspnea, chest pain, and fatigue.
- Cardioembolic stroke.
- Patients whose ventricular filling is largely dependent on the atrial kick, such as those with severe LV diastolic dysfunction or restrictive cardiomyopathy, are more likely to develop symptoms due to loss of atrial contraction.
- Sustained rapid ventricular rates in AF beyond 7–10 days may lead to tachycardia-induced cardiomyopathy.
- Syncope may be a manifestation of a conversion pause.
- If a patient with atrial fibrillation is found to have a regular ventricular rhythm without clear organized atrial activity ("regularized" AF), third-degree (complete) heart block should be suspected and urgent evaluation undertaken.

Thromboembolic Risk

- Given the difficulty in establishing AF burden, paroxysmal and chronic AF should generally be approached similarly in terms of risk of thromboembolism.
  - Controversy exists regarding the threshold for anticoagulation in patients with brief (seconds to hours) episodes of AF detected with wearable or implanted cardiac devices such as smartwatches, pacemakers, and loop recorders. This should prompt a discussion with a cardiologist about the risks and benefits of anticoagulation on a patient-specific basis.
- CHA2DS2VASc score is a commonly used risk score to estimate the risk of thromboembolism (Table 23.1).
  - (C) Congestive heart failure (H) Hypertension (A) Age (D) Diabetes mellitus (S) History of stroke (VA) vascular disease, including history of coronary artery disease or peripheral vascular disease (Sc) Female gender.

Table 23.1 Risk of stroke in patients with atrial fibrillation [22]

CHA2DS2VASc score	Risk of stroke per 100 years at risk
0	0.2
1	0.6
2	2.2
3	3.2
4	4.8
5	7.2
6	9.7
7	11.2
8	10.8
9	12.2

- CHA2DS2VASc and other similar risk scores are not a perfect predictor of risk of stroke in an individual patient, and decisions for anticoagulation should take into account patient-specific factors, such as other comorbidities and risk of bleeding.

Evaluation of Patients with New Atrial Fibrillation

- Evaluate whether the patient requires acute inpatient treatment: symptoms and signs of hemodynamic compromise, significant debilitating symptoms, heart failure, or evidence of tachycardia-mediated cardiomyopathy.
- Assess for recent illness or surgery, alcohol use, presence of structural heart disease, hyperthyroidism, and risk factors for sleep apnea.
- Assess risk factors for thromboembolism.
- Perform transthoracic echocardiogram to assess ventricular and valvular function (to identify underlying structural

heart disease and/or systolic dysfunction consequent to AF).

- Laboratory evaluation: complete blood count, renal function, thyroid function, makers of coagulation, and glycosylated hemoglobin.
- Ambulatory cardiac monitoring should be considered in patients with new AF to assess burden and to correlate symptoms to paroxysms of AF.
- Patients with cryptogenic stroke or other arterial thromboembolic events without explanation should be considered for long-term cardiac monitoring to evaluate for occult AF.
  - In patients with cryptogenic stroke, occult AF was detected by an outpatient mobile monitor in up to 23% of subjects [8].
  - In patients with stroke risk factors but not known AF, implantable loop recorder resulted in the diagnosis of AF in 35% of subjects over an average of 40 months [9].
  - Short-term rhythm monitoring (24–48 hour Holter monitors) is generally less helpful in detecting AF.
- Routine screening for AF is not universally recommended. However, proof of concept data from the Apple Heart Study Investigators suggests that smartwatch applications may be a reliable method for incidental detection of AF in the future [10].

Anticoagulation for Atrial Fibrillation

- To reduce the risk of stroke, anticoagulation is recommended for any patient with CHA2DS2VASc score ≥2.
  - Anticoagulation should be strongly considered for any male patient with a score of 1 or female patient with a score of 2.
  - There is minimal data to guide decisions about anticoagulation in patients with a score of 0 (or 1 in females). Patient/physician discussion of risks and benefits is typically advised.

- Prior pulmonary vein isolation or MAZE procedure does not eliminate the risk of stroke, and anticoagulation should not be discontinued solely on the basis of having undergone the procedure or maintenance of sinus rhythm shortly thereafter.
- **Aspirin has no evidence of prevention of stroke and should not be used as monotherapy for stroke prevention.**
  - Aspirin plus clopidogrel has some benefit in stroke prevention but is inferior to the use of an anticoagulant [11] and should not be used as a substitute for oral anticoagulation in patients eligible for oral anticoagulation (OAC).
- Non-vitamin K anticoagulants (DOAC) (Table 23.2) are considered first line in the treatment of AF (except for patients with mechanical heart valves, moderate or severe rheumatic mitral stenosis) [12].
  - Rivaroxaban
  - Dabigatran
  - Apixaban
  - Edoxaban
- If warfarin is used for stroke prevention in atrial fibrillation, INR goal is generally 2.0–3.0.
  - For patients on warfarin, time in therapeutic range of >60% has been shown to achieve stroke risk reduction [13].
- In cases of severe bleeding:
  - Patients on warfarin can be treated with vitamin K, fresh frozen plasma, and prothrombin complex concentrates.
  - Novel reversal agents are available for direct oral anticoagulants.

    Andexanet alfa for rivaroxaban and apixaban
    Idarucizumab for dabigatran

Table 23.2 Common anticoagulants for atrial fibrillation

Anticoagulant	Mechanism	Common dosing	Bleeding risk (per year; vs. warfarin)	Reversal agent	Considerations
Dabigatran [23]	Direct thrombin inhibitor	150 mg PO BID[b]	Major: 3.1% vs. 3.4% Intracranial: 0.1% vs. 0.3%	Idarucizumab	Similar rates of stroke/ embolism to warfarin (1.7% vs. 1.5%) Lower rates of major hemorrhage
Apixaban [24]	Factor Xa inhibitor	5 mg PO BID[c]	Intracranial: 0.3% vs. 0.8% Major: 2.1% vs. 3.1%	Andexanet	Superior to warfarin in preventing strokes (1.3% vs. 1.6%) Shown to be safe in end-stage renal disease
Rivaroxaban [25]	Factor Xa inhibitor	20 mg PO daily (with evening meal)[d,e]	Intracranial: 0.5% vs. 0.7% Fatal: 0.2% vs. 0.5% Non-major clinically relevant: 11.8% vs. 11.4%	Andexanet	Similar rates of stroke/ embolism to warfarin (1.7% vs. 2.2%) No difference in overall bleeding but reduction in fatal and ICH bleeding Must be taken with a >500 kCal meal

Edoxaban [26]	Factor Xa inhibitor	60 mg PO daily	Major: 2.8% vs. 3.4% Intracranial: 0.4% vs. 0.9%	None	Similar rates of stroke/embolism (1.2% vs. 1.5%) Contraindicated if Cr clearance >95 mL/min

[a]Not intended for clinical care. Please refer to the most updated guidelines as per the manufacturer

[b]A dose of 110 mg BID can be considered (off-label) in patients with high bleeding risk. Lower doses (i.e., 75 mg BID) may be necessary in patients with reduced renal function

[c]A dose of 2.5 mg BID is indicated in patients with any two of the following: age ≥80 years, body weight ≤60 kg, or serum creatinine ≥1.5 mg/dL

[d]Post-percutaneous coronary intervention with stent placement and non-valvular AF, a dose of 15 mg daily in combination with an appropriate antithrombotic regimen (i.e., clopidogrel ∓ aspirin) is typically used

[e]A dose of 15 mg daily is typically used in patients with creatinine clearance of 15–50 mL/minute

[f]Dose should be reduced (i.e., 30 mg daily) for patients with creatinine clearance of 15–50 mL/minute. Some data (based on a Japanese geriatric population) suggests that 15 mg/day may be an acceptable dose in patients >80 years

- In cases when anticoagulation needs to be interrupted for a procedure:
  - Discussion with a cardiologist and the operator is often indicated to determine the balance of risks and the appropriate peri-procedural strategy.
  - Bridging anticoagulation (i.e., use of subcutaneous heparin products) should generally be pursued for patients on warfarin if CHADS2 score ≥5, if there is a history of prior stroke or recent venous thromboembolism, and for most patients with AF who also have mechanical heart valves. Bridging should be considered for patients with AF who have additional stroke risks, such as reduced LV ejection fraction.
  - Risks of interrupting anticoagulation may outweigh benefits in patients with highly elevated stroke risk (i.e., recent cardioversion, known atrial thrombus) undergoing a non-urgent procedure.
  - Patients on non-vitamin K-dependent anticoagulants generally do not require bridging anticoagulation, given the brief time necessary to interrupt the medicines prior to most procedures.
    - PAUSE trial [14] demonstrated that for most patients on DOAC, the medication can be held for 1 day prior to procedure with low bleeding risk and for 2 days prior to procedure with high bleeding risk.
    - Major bleeding risk was <2% and ischemic stroke risk was <0.5%.
- In patients with indication for dual antiplatelet therapy (DAPT) after percutaneous coronary interventions:
  - Rivaroxaban 15mg/day + clopidogrel showed equivalent level of cardiovascular mortality compared with warfarin + DAPT (PIONEER trial) [15].
  - A regimen that included apixaban and clopidogrel resulted in less bleeding and fewer hospitalizations without significant differences in stroke compared to

regimens that included warfarin, aspirin, or both (AUGUSTUS trial) [16].

- Surgical or percutaneous left atrial appendage (LAA) exclusion should be considered in patients for whom long-term anticoagulation is either not feasible or associated with unacceptable bleeding risk.
  - Watchman percutaneous LAA occlusion system is currently FDA-approved, but requires full anticoagulation for 45 days following implantation.
  - Surgical ligation can be done as a standalone procedure or as part of other cardiac surgery.

Heart Rate Control in Atrial Fibrillation

- Ventricular heart rate in AF is determined by multiple factors, such as balance between sympathetic and parasympathetic stimulation, medications that affect atrioventricular (AV) nodal conduction, and metabolic derangements.
  - Slow ventricular rate (i.e., less than 60 beats/minute) suggests slow AV conduction.
  - Very rapid ventricular rate (i.e., greater than 200 beats/minute) suggests the presence of an accessory pathway.
- Uncontrolled elevation in ventricular rate has been associated with the development of cardiomyopathy.
- Goal heart rate is generally <110 beats/minute.
  - RACE II trial randomized patients to lenient (<110 bpm) vs. strict (<80 bpm) rate control. There was no difference in 3-year incidence of cardiovascular death, HF hospitalization, stroke, systemic embolism, bleeding, and life-threatening arrhythmia.
  - Results may not be generalizable since the "lenient" group may have been treated more aggressively than expected (i.e., mean heart rate 86 bpm at 12 months) and the trial included only patients with permanent AF [17].

- Therapies for control of heart rate include:
  - Calcium channel blockade with non-dihydropyridine calcium channel blockers (i.e., verapamil or diltiazem)
  - Beta-blockers
  - Digoxin
- Caution must be exercised with the use of calcium channel blockers or beta-blockers in patients with significantly reduced ejection fraction and/or in whom there is concern for low cardiac output state, since they can exert negative inotropic effects and precipitate hypotension, bradycardia, and/or cardiogenic shock.
- Reversible causes of tachycardia (i.e., OSA, infection) should be identified.

Rhythm Control in Atrial Fibrillation

- Older randomized trials showed no significant difference in mortality or incidence of stroke between rate control and rhythm control strategies in AF (AFFIRM trial) [18].
  - Highly symptomatic patients may have been underrepresented.
  - Older patients were overrepresented.
  - Mortality may have been increased in the rhythm control group by discontinuation of anticoagulants.
- The more recent EAST-AFNET 4 trial [19] showed significant benefit to early rhythm control strategy.
  - Randomly assigned ~2800 patients with early AF (<12 months) at high risk for complications to early rhythm control with antiarrhythmic drugs and/or ablation vs. rate control.
  - High risk was defined as age >75 years, prior stroke or TIA, or two of the following: >65 years, female sex, heart failure, hypertension, diabetes, chronic kidney disease, and left ventricular hypertrophy.

 - Primary composite outcome (CV death, stroke, serious adverse events) occurred less often in rhythm control group.

- Spontaneous cardioversion will occur in ~70% of patients within the first 48 hours of AF, and early electrical cardioversion may not improve maintenance of sinus rhythm at 4 weeks compared with expectant management [20].
  - AV nodal-blocking agents do not promote restoration of sinus rhythm.
- Pharmacotherapy can restore sinus rhythm in up to 50% of cases.
- Electrical cardioversion (DCCV) is effective at restoring sinus rhythm in up to 90% of patients [21].
  - Risks of DCCV include burn at location of electrical pads, bradycardia, and post-cardioversion pulmonary edema.
  - **Consider reducing the dose of AV nodal-blocking medications prior to cardioversion.**
  - Ensure euvolemia in patients with volume overload prior to DCCV to reduce chance of AF recurrence.
  - Following restoration of sinus rhythm, there is a gradual recovery in mechanical atrial function over a period of 3 weeks.
  - Prior to cardioversion (pharmacologic or electrical), the risk of stroke should be assessed.

    In patients who are definitely known to have developed new atrial fibrillation within <48 hours, cardioversion may typically be performed without assessment for intracardiac thrombus provided that anticoagulation is achieved prior to cardioversion.

    A transesophageal echocardiogram (TEE) should be pursued to exclude a thrombus in the left atrial appendage in any patient who has been in AF >48 hours or in whom timing of AF onset is less certain, unless the patient has had documentation of full therapeutic anticoagulation for 4 weeks prior to cardioversion.

In stable asymptomatic patients with new atrial fibrillation, it is reasonable to pursue 4 weeks of therapeutic anticoagulation prior to cardioversion in order to forego a TEE.

- Anticoagulation should be maintained for at least 4 weeks after cardioversion in all patients. Thereafter, the need for chronic anticoagulation should be determined based on risk factors, as described earlier.
- Monitor for post-DCCV pulmonary edema and myocardial dysfunction due to transient stunning (typically lasting <48 hours).

• Pulmonary vein isolation should be considered early (often as first-line therapy), especially for patients with heart failure.
• AV node ablation (with pacemaker placement) should be considered for patients with AF refractory to other medical therapies above.

Antiarrhythmic Therapy

• Procainamide, ibutilide, and amiodarone are approved for pharmacologic cardioversion, but success rates are lower than with direct current cardioversion.
• Choice of antiarrhythmic medication (Table 23.3) is determined by the presence of structural heart disease, coronary artery disease, and renal disease.

- Type 1c agents (propafenone and flecainide) may be used in patients without structural heart disease.

  These should be used in combination with an AV nodal-blocking agent to avoid the organization of atrial flutter with 1:1 conduction.

- Sotalol, dofetilide, and amiodarone may be used in patients with coronary artery disease.

Table 23.3 Common antiarrhythmic medications for atrial fibrillation

Class	Medications	Mechanism	Appropriate for	Contraindications	Monitoring parameters	Common adverse reactions
1a	Procainamide Disopyramide	Na+ channel blockade K+ channel blockade Prolong action potential	Patients without structural heart disease Hypertrophic cardiomyopathy (disopyramide)	Coronary artery disease Structural heart disease	QTc interval CBC LFTs	Disopyramide: Anticholinergic effects and should be avoided in patients with prostate symptoms and glaucoma Agranulocytosis Quinidine Thrombocytopenia, granulomatous hepatitis, myasthenia gravis Procainamide: Agranulocytosis, lupus-like reaction

(continued)

TABLE 23.3 (continued)

Class	Medications	Mechanism	Appropriate for	Contraindications	Monitoring parameters	Common adverse reactions
1c	Flecainide Propafenone	Na+ channel blockade	Patients without structural heart disease	Coronary artery disease Structural heart disease		Flecainide: Associated with interstitial lung disease Propafenone: Agranulocytosis and lupus-like syndrome
III	Amiodarone Sotalol Dronedarone Dofetilide	K+ channel blockade Sotalol and amiodarone have beta-blocker effect Amiodarone also blocks Na+ and Ca2+ channels		Sotalol and dofetilide contraindicated with renal impairment Dronedarone contraindicated in patients with CHF	Amiodarone: Liver, thyroid, and pulmonary function should be checked every 6 months	Amiodarone: Interstitial lung disease Thyroid disease Transaminitis

- Amiodarone may be used in patients with structural heart disease.
- Dronedarone is contraindicated in patients with congestive heart failure.
- Due to risk of pharmacologic cardioversion, these agents should not be used in patients in whom duration in AF is not known and who had not been on therapeutic anticoagulation for at least 4 weeks (unless an LAA thrombus is excluded by TEE).

Clinical Pearl
Amiodarone and disopyramide may be particularly effective in hypertrophic cardiomyopathy.

Atrial Flutter (Fig. 23.2)

- Results from rapid regular atrial depolarizations at approximately 300 beats/minute and often leads to a pattern of regular intermittent conduction via the AV node.
- Lower incidence than atrial fibrillation.

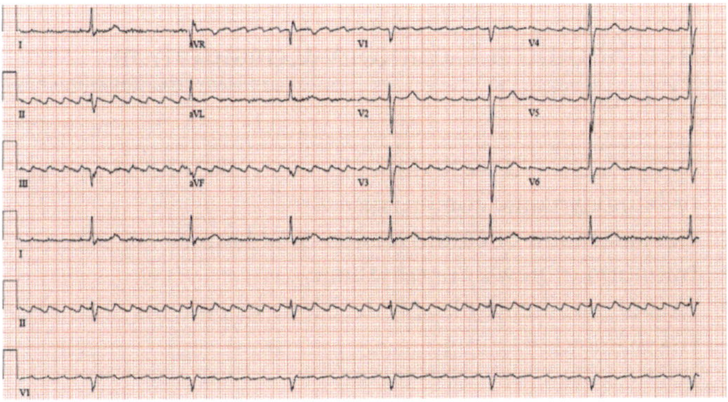

FIGURE 23.2 Atrial flutter

- Two general categories of atrial flutter:
  - Typical atrial flutter: Macro-reentrant circuit around the cavo-tricuspid isthmus (CTI) in the right atrium. Involves either a counterclockwise pattern of rotation ("sawtooth" appearance of the flutter waves, with inferior direction in the inferior ECG leads) or a "clockwise" circuit with positive flutter waves in the inferior ECG leads
  - Atypical atrial flutter: A reentrant circuit that can involve any region of the right or left atria (often around an area of a prior cardiotomy surgical scar). Can be difficult to distinguish from a focal atrial tachycardia

- Risk of thromboembolism extrapolated from atrial fibrillation and approach to anticoagulation should be guided by the same risk stratification scores (i.e., CHA2DS2VASc).
- Heart rate control is often more difficult to achieve, and patients may benefit from earlier consideration of electrical cardioversion, ablation, and/or initiation of anti-arrhythmic.
- Definitive treatment with ablation is preferred for most patients (particularly those with typical atrial flutter), as success rate is significantly higher than with AF.

When Should a Crdiology Consultation Be Considered

- Symptomatic AF with difficulty controlling heart rate and/or hemodynamic compromise
- Consideration of cardioversion or ablation
- Initiation of new antiarrhythmic
- Complex anticoagulation decisions in patients with high-risk AF and bleeding

Learning Points

1. Patients with a new diagnosis of atrial fibrillation should have an evaluation for reversible risk factors, including thyroid dysfunction, pericarditis, structural heart disease, and sleep apnea.
2. Early rhythm control strategy (including pulmonary vein isolation) is increasingly pursued as the treatment modality of choice and should be considered in all patients.
3. Assessment of stroke risk factors should be considered prior to initiation of an antiarrhythmic medication or cardioversion.
4. Patients who are taking antiarrhythmic medications and have undergone ablation procedures, MAZE surgery, or left atrial appendage occlusion may still be at risk for thromboembolism. Anticoagulation should be guided by general stroke risk factors and bleeding risk.

References

1. Chugh SS, Havmoeller R, Narayanan K, Singh D, Rienstra M, Benjamin EJ, et al. Worldwide epidemiology of atrial fibrillation: a Global Burden of Disease 2010 Study. Circulation. 2014;129(8):837–47.
2. Go AS, Hylek EM, Phillips KA, Chang Y, Henault LE, Selby JV, et al. Prevalence of diagnosed atrial fibrillation in adults: national implications for rhythm management and stroke prevention: the AnTicoagulation and Risk Factors in Atrial Fibrillation (ATRIA) Study. JAMA. 2001;285(18):2370–5.
3. Zimetbaum PJ, Buxton AE, Josephson ME. Practical clinical electrophysiology. Lippincott Williams & Wilkins; 2018. p. 67–89.

4. Martínez-González MÁ, Toledo E, Arós F, Fiol M, Corella D, Salas-Salvadó J, et al. Extravirgin olive oil consumption reduces risk of atrial fibrillation: the PREDIMED (Prevención con Dieta Mediterránea) trial. Circulation. 2014;130(1):18–26.
5. Voskoboinik A, Kalman JM, De Silva A, Nicholls T, Costello B, Nanayakkara S, et al. Alcohol abstinence in drinkers with atrial fibrillation. N Engl J Med. 2020;382(1):20–8.
6. Soliman EZ, Rahman AF, Zhang Z-M, Rodriguez CJ, Chang TI, Bates JT, et al. Effect of intensive blood pressure lowering on the risk of atrial fibrillation. Hypertension. 2020;75(6):1491–6.
7. Israel CW, Gronefeld G, Ehrlich JR, Li YG, Hohnloser SH. Long-term risk of recurrent atrial fibrillation as documented by an implantable monitoring device. Implications for optimal patient care [Internet]. ACC Curr J Rev. 2004;13:49–50. Available from: https://doi.org/10.1016/j.accreview.2004.03.016.
8. Tayal AH, Tian M, Kelly KM, Jones SC, Wright DG, Singh D, et al. Atrial fibrillation detected by mobile cardiac outpatient telemetry in cryptogenic TIA or stroke. Neurology. 2008;71(21):1696–701.
9. Diederichsen SZ, Haugan KJ, Kronborg C, Graff C, Højberg S, Køber L, et al. Comprehensive evaluation of rhythm monitoring strategies in screening for atrial fibrillation. [Internet]. Circulation. 2020;141:1510–22. Available from: https://doi.org/10.1161/circulationaha.119.044407.
10. Perez MV, Mahaffey KW, Hedlin H, Rumsfeld JS, Garcia A, Ferris T, et al. Large-scale assessment of a smartwatch to identify atrial fibrillation. N Engl J Med. 2019;381(20):1909–17.
11. Effect of clopidogrel added to aspirin in patients with atrial fibrillation. N Engl J Med. 2009;360(20):2066–78.
12. January CT, Wann LS, Calkins H, Chen LY, Cigarroa JE, Cleveland JC Jr, et al. 2019 AHA/ACC/HRS Focused Update of the 2014 AHA/ACC/HRS Guideline for the Management of Patients With Atrial Fibrillation: A Report of the American College of Cardiology/American Heart Association Task Force on Clinical Practice Guidelines and the Heart Rhythm Society in Collaboration With the Society of Thoracic Surgeons. Circulation. 2019;140(2):e125–51.
13. Connolly SJ, Pogue J, Eikelboom J, Flaker G, Commerford P, Franzosi MG, et al. Benefit of oral anticoagulant over antiplatelet therapy in atrial fibrillation depends on the quality of international normalized ratio control achieved by centers and

countries as measured by time in therapeutic range. Circulation. 2008;118(20):2029–37.

14. Douketis JD, Spyropoulos AC, Duncan J, Carrier M, Le Gal G, Tafur AJ, et al. Perioperative management of patients with atrial fibrillation receiving a direct oral anticoagulant. JAMA Intern Med [Internet]. 2019.; Available from: https://doi.org/10.1001/jamainternmed.2019.2431
15. Gibson CM, Mehran R, Bode C, Halperin J, Verheugt F, Wildgoose P, et al. An open-label, randomized, controlled, multicenter study exploring two treatment strategies of rivaroxaban and a dose-adjusted oral vitamin K antagonist treatment strategy in subjects with atrial fibrillation who undergo percutaneous coronary intervention (PIONEER AF-PCI). Am Heart J. 2015;169(4):472–8.
16. Lopes RD, Heizer G, Aronson R, Vora AN, Massaro T, Mehran R, et al. Antithrombotic therapy after acute coronary syndrome or PCI in atrial fibrillation. N Engl J Med. 2019;380(16):1509–24.
17. Van Gelder IC, Groenveld HF, Crijns HJGM, Tuininga YS, Tijssen JGP, Alings AM, et al. Lenient versus strict rate control in patients with atrial fibrillation. N Engl J Med. 2010;362(15):1363–73.
18. A comparison of rate control and rhythm control in patients with atrial fibrillation. N Engl J Med. 2002;347(23):1825–33.
19. Kirchhof P, Camm AJ, Goette A, Brandes A, Eckardt L, Elvan A, et al. Early rhythm-control therapy in patients with atrial fibrillation. N Engl J Med. 2020;383(14):1305–16.
20. Pluymaekers NAHA, Dudink EAMP, Luermans JGLM, Meeder JG, Lenderink T, Widdershoven J, et al. Early or delayed cardioversion in recent-onset atrial fibrillation. N Engl J Med. 2019;380(16):1499–508.
21. Abu-El-Haija B, Giudici MC. Predictors of long-term maintenance of normal sinus rhythm after successful electrical cardioversion. Clin Cardiol. 2014;37(6):381–5.
22. Friberg L, Rosenqvist M, Lip GYH. Evaluation of risk stratification schemes for ischaemic stroke and bleeding in 182 678 patients with atrial fibrillation: the Swedish Atrial Fibrillation cohort study. Eur Heart J. 2012;33(12):1500–10.
23. Connolly SJ, Ezekowitz MD, Yusuf S, Eikelboom J, Oldgren J, Parekh A, et al. Dabigatran versus warfarin in patients with atrial fibrillation. N Engl J Med. 2009;361(12):1139–51.

24. Granger CB, Alexander JH, McMurray JJV, Lopes RD, Hylek EM, Hanna M, et al. Apixaban versus warfarin in patients with atrial fibrillation. N Engl J Med. 2011;365(11):981–92.
25. Patel MR, Mahaffey KW, Garg J, Pan G, Singer DE, Hacke W, et al. Rivaroxaban versus warfarin in nonvalvular atrial fibrillation. N Engl J Med. 2011;365(10):883–91.
26. Giugliano RP, Ruff CT, Braunwald E, Murphy SA, Wiviott SD, Halperin JL, et al. Edoxaban versus warfarin in patients with atrial fibrillation. N Engl J Med. 2013;369(22):2093–104.

Chapter 24
Supraventricular Tachycardia

Sindhu Prabakaran, Rachel Slappy, and Faisal Merchant

Abbreviations

AT	Atrial tachycardia
AV	Atrioventricular
AVNRT	Atrioventricular nodal reentrant tachycardia
AVRT	Atrioventricular reentrant tachycardia
BB	Beta-blockers
BPM	Beats per minute
CCB	Calcium channel blockers
JT	Junctional tachycardia
MAT	Multifocal atrial tachycardia
PAC	Premature atrial contraction
PVC	Premature ventricular contraction

S. Prabakaran (✉)
Department of Medicine, Emory University School of Medicine, Atlanta, GA, USA
e-mail: sprabak@emory.edu

R. Slappy
Emory University School of Medicine, Atlanta, GA, USA

F. Merchant
Department of Medicine, Division of Cardiology, Emory University School of Medicine, Atlanta, GA, USA

A. A. Bhargava et al. (eds.), *Handbook of Outpatient Cardiology*, https://doi.org/10.1007/978-3-030-88953-1_24

SVT	Supraventricular tachycardia
VF	Ventricular fibrillation
VT	Ventricular tachycardia

Definition, Incidence, and Prevalence

- Supraventricular tachycardia (SVT) is a cardiac tachyarrhythmia that originates from the atrioventricular (AV) node or the atria. Generally, SVT causes a narrow complex tachycardia on ECG, but can cause wide complex tachycardia if conduction disease or other aberrant conduction is present.
- SVT is most often caused by a reentry circuit that occurs between the AV node and atrium or an atrioventricular accessory pathway. Other less common causes include triggered activity and enhanced automaticity of the atrium or AV node [1].
- The most common subtype of SVT is atrioventricular nodal reentrant tachycardia (AVNRT) followed by atrioventricular reentrant tachycardia (AVRT) and then atrial tachycardia (AT).
- The incidence of SVT is 36 per 100,000 person-years. SVT has a prevalence of 2.29 per 1000 persons [2].
- Atrial fibrillation and atrial flutter are excluded from this chapter and presented in a separate chapter.

Clinical Pearl
In the patient with suspected SVT, obtaining a 12-lead ECG is an essential first step.

AV Nodal Reentrant Tachycardia

- AVNRT is caused by the presence of two conduction pathways within the AV node with differing speeds of impulse conduction and repolarization. The fast pathway conducts impulses quickly and has a longer refractory period.

Conversely, the slow pathway conducts impulses slowly and has a shorter refractory period.

- AVNRT is more frequent in women than in men. The typical ventricular rate is between 180 and 200 beats per minute (BPM). However, ventricular rates as low as 110 BPM and as high as >250 BPM have been observed [3].

Typical AVNRT

- Typical AVNRT refers to a reentrant circuit that is initiated by antegrade conduction through the slow pathway followed by retrograde conduction via the fast pathway (Fig. 24.1).
- AVNRT can also be initiated through the retrograde conduction of a premature ventricular conduction (PVC) via the fast pathway.
- Since the retrograde P wave will appear close to the QRS complex, the RP interval will be short. P waves can also manifest in the anterior precordial leads as a pseudo-r'

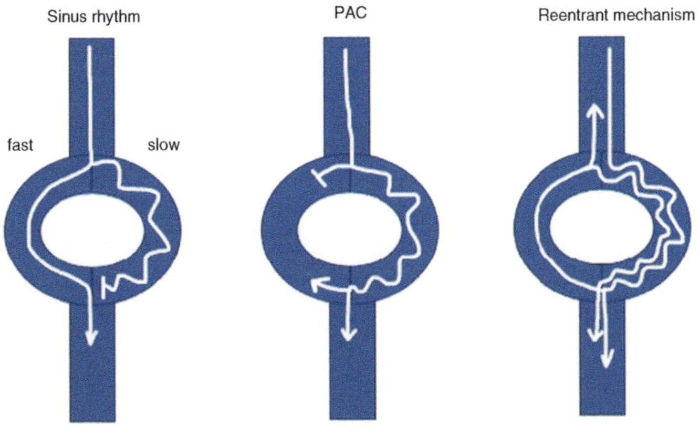

Figure 24.1 After a premature atrial contraction (PAC), unidirectional block occurs in the fast pathway. Conduction proceeds antegrade down the slow pathway as a result. As the impulse travels down the slow pathway, the fast pathway may repolarize and permit retrograde conduction of the impulse completing the reentrant circuit

pattern. In the inferior leads, retrograde P waves can cause pseudo-S waves. If the retrograde P wave axis is inferiorly directed, AVNRT is excluded (Fig. 24.2.). Frequently, the RP may be so short that the retrograde P wave is buried in the QRS complex and no P wave is visible during AVNRT.

- For symptomatic patients, first-line treatment of AVNRT is catheter ablation of the slow pathway. Beta-blockers (BB), diltiazem, or verapamil is recommended for patients who are not candidates for ablation. Flecainide, propafenone, amiodarone, digoxin, dofetilide, and sotalol can also be useful for the treatment of AVNRT.
- Minimally symptomatic patients with infrequent tachycardic episodes may choose long-term outpatient follow-up without any interventions. It may be useful to offer medications such as BB, diltiazem, or verapamil to be self-administered during any episodes. Additionally, these patients should be taught how to perform vagal maneuvers as well as when to pursue emergency care.

Atypical AVNRT

- In atypical AVNRT, the arrhythmia begins with antegrade conduction of the impulse down the fast pathway followed by retrograde conduction up the slow pathway.
- Since the retrograde P wave is conducted up the slow pathway, the P wave will occur later, which will increase the RP interval (Fig. 24.3).
- Treatment of atypical AVNRT follows the same recommendations as typical AVNRT.

Clinical Pearl

Minimally symptomatic AVNRT patients with infrequent episodes may choose long-term outpatient follow-up without any interventions. It may be useful to offer medications to be self-administered during any episodes, and patients should be taught how to perform vagal maneuvers as well as when to pursue emergency care.

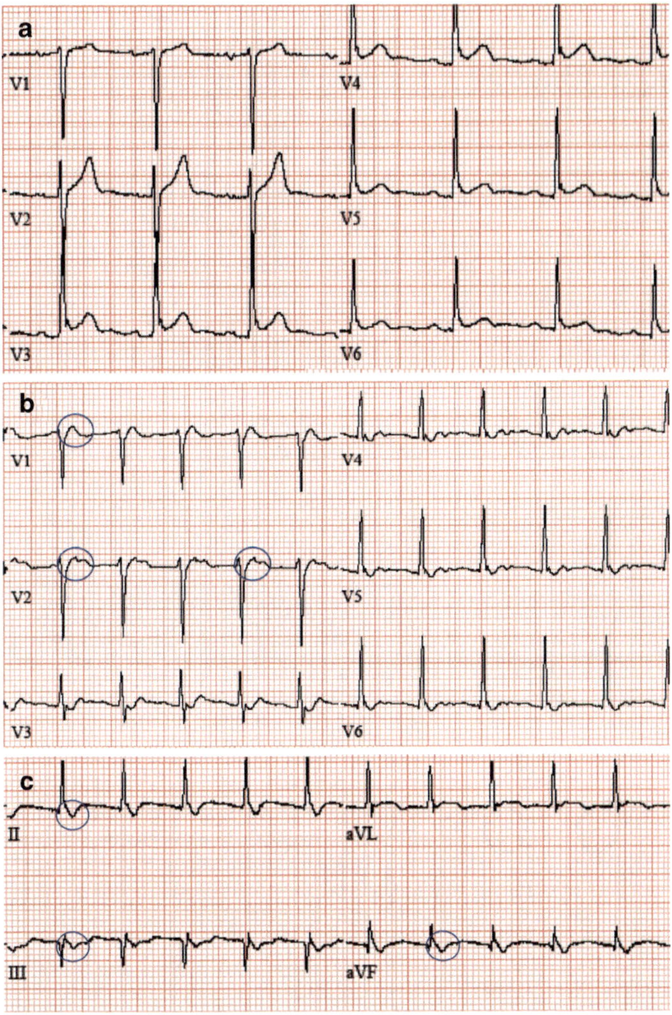

FIGURE 24.2 (**a**) This is an ECG from the precordial leads of a 32-year-old male who was diagnosed with typical AVRT. (**b**) During a tachycardic episode in the same patient, retrograde P waves contributed to a pseudo-r' pattern. This resulted in a shortened RP interval. (**c**) Pseudo-S waves were also observed in the inferior leads during a tachycardic episode in the same patient due to the superior axis of the retrograde P waves

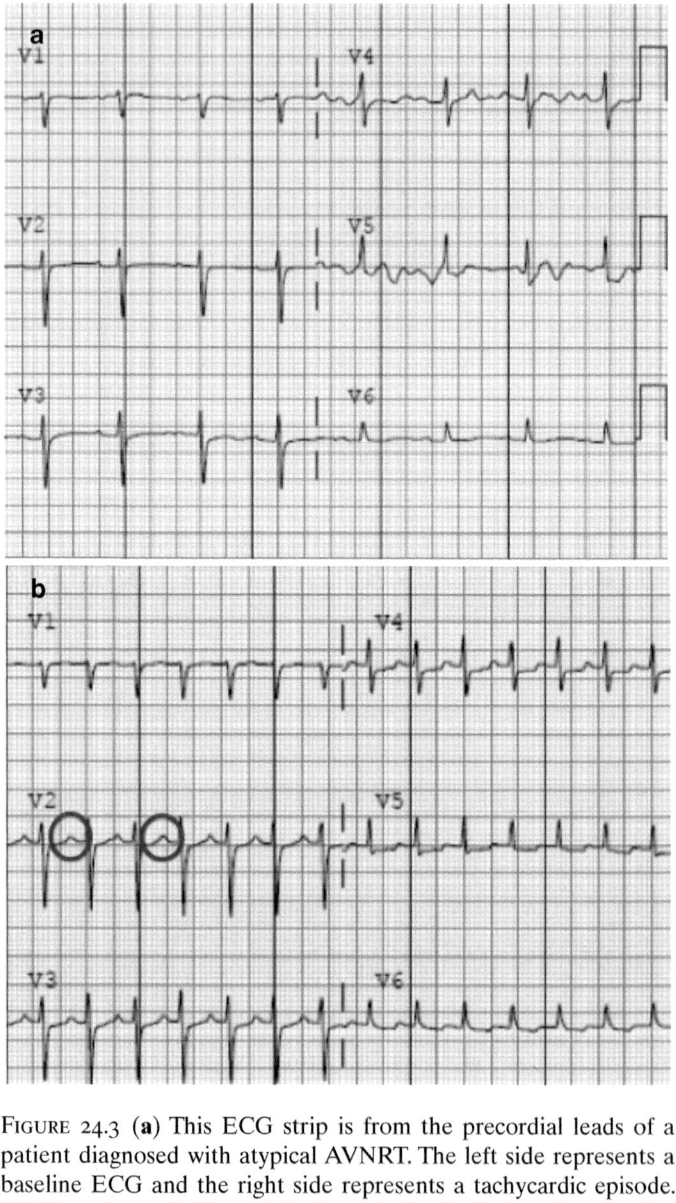

FIGURE 24.3 (**a**) This ECG strip is from the precordial leads of a patient diagnosed with atypical AVNRT. The left side represents a baseline ECG and the right side represents a tachycardic episode. (**b**) The retrograde P waves in the anterior leads show lengthening of the RP interval as compared to the PR interval

AVRT

- AVRT consists of a reentrant circuit that is completed via an accessory pathway located external to the AV node. These accessory pathways can result in antegrade or retrograde conduction.
- Depending on conduction direction, accessory pathways may result in changes on ECG and are thus described as manifest. If manifest pathways conduct antegrade, they will cause pre-excitation in the ventricles during sinus rhythm resulting in a delta wave on ECG, described as Wolff-Parkinson-White (WPW) pattern. Retrograde conduction through the accessory pathway will lead to a concealed pathway and not produce delta waves (Fig. 24.4).

Pre-excited Atrial Fibrillation

- Patients with manifest pathways are at an increased risk of ventricular fibrillation (VF) if AF occurs due to quick impulse conduction from the atria to the ventricles (Fig. 24.5).

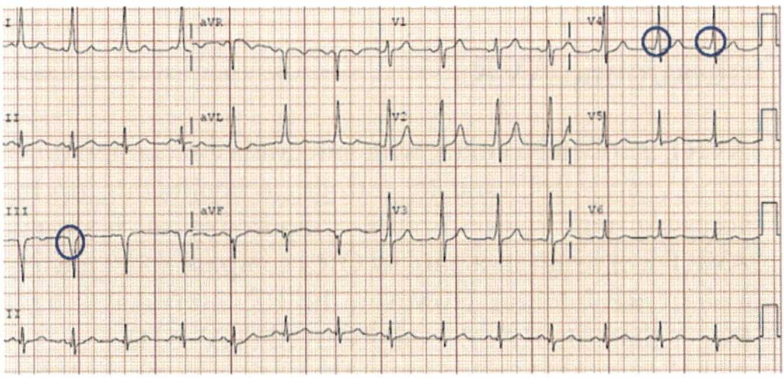

FIGURE 24.4 This 12-lead ECG demonstrates ventricular pre-excitation with a shortened PR interval and a delta wave in both the precordial and inferior limb leads

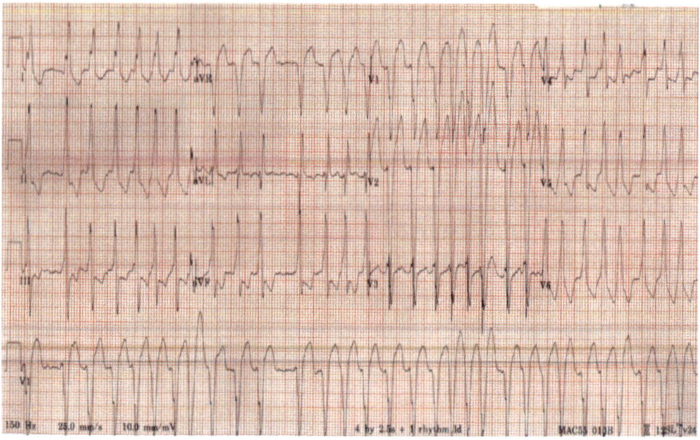

FIGURE 24.5 This is a 12-lead ECG from a 32-year-old male patient diagnosed with pre-excited atrial fibrillation

- In patients with pre-excited AF, catheter ablation of the accessory pathway is recommended. Second-line treatment options such as flecainide or propafenone may be useful. Dofetilide, sotalol, or amiodarone may also be considered in these patients.
- Drugs that are contraindicated in the treatment of pre-excited AF include nodal agents such as BB, diltiazem, verapamil, and digoxin.

Orthodromic AVRT

- AVRT involving a circuit with antegrade conduction down the AV node followed by retrograde conduction up the accessory pathway is termed orthodromic. Orthodromic AVRT will result in a narrow QRS complex and, typically, a short RP interval. However, the RP interval is usually longer than the RP interval observed in AVNRT.
- Ablation of the accessory pathway is recommended in patients with orthodromic AVRT both with and without pre-excitation on ECG. BB, diltiazem, or verapamil may be used as first-line treatment instead of ablation in patients without pre-excitation.

- In patients with and without pre-excitation on ECG, flecainide or propafenone may be considered as second-line options. In patients without pre-excitation, amiodarone, digoxin, dofetilide, or sotalol may be reasonable to consider.

Antidromic AVRT

- AVRT involving a circuit with antegrade conduction down the accessory pathway followed by retrograde conduction up the AV node is termed antidromic and occurs in 5–10% of patients with accessory pathways [3]. On ECG, antidromic AVRT appears as a wide complex tachycardia because antegrade impulses do not conduct through the His-Purkinje system. It may appear very similar to ventricular tachycardia (VT).
- Antidromic AVRT should be treated with the same interventions as orthodromic AVRT.

Atrial Tachycardia

- AT is a regular atrial rhythm originating outside of the sinus node. AT, when used, typically refers to focal atrial tachycardia, which arises from a single focus or small (<2 cm) micro-reentrant circuit. It can produce rates between 100 and 250 BPM [3].
- AT often occurs in healthy individuals without structural heart disease. Other potential etiologies include hypoxia, pulmonary disease, ischemic heart disease, stimulants, alcohol, and heightened sympathetic tone [4].
- Patients may complain of palpitations, lightheadedness, chest pain, or pressure. Symptoms can be paroxysmal or persistent in nature.
- AT can be gradual or abrupt in onset. It may conduct 1:1 to the ventricle, although this varies. On 12-lead ECG, focal AT generally appears as a long RP tachycardia (Fig. 24.6). It is important to note, however, that the RP

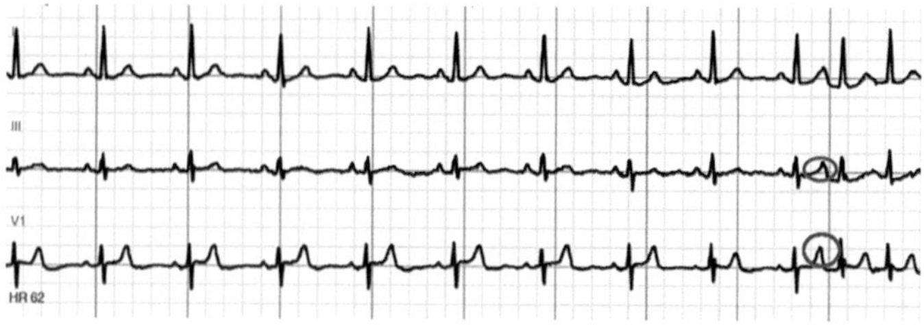

FIGURE 24.6 This 3-lead telemetry strip captures the onset of atrial tachycardia in a patient with palpitations. Note the increased rate as well as change in T wave morphology with a superimposed P wave, resulting in a long RP interval

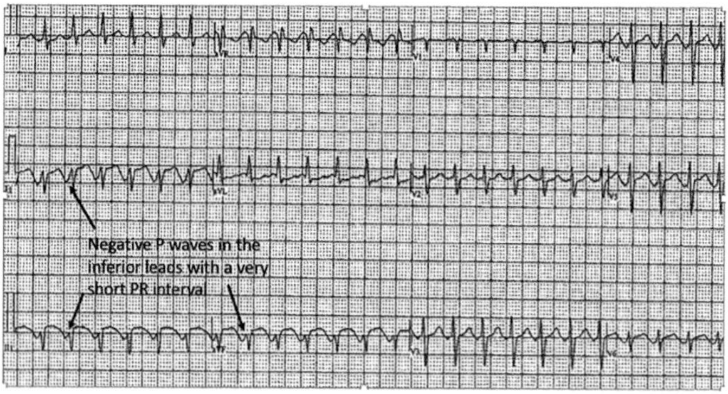

FIGURE 24.7 This is the 12-lead ECG for a patient with recurrent atrial tachycardia. Note the consistent negative P waves with long RP interval

interval will be short if concomitant first-degree AV block is present [3].

- The P wave axis should have subtle differences when compared to sinus rhythm. P waves should be unifocal and similar in morphology to each other; they can potentially be inverted. A consistent PP interval despite variable PR and RP intervals on ECG suggests AT (Fig. 24.7).
- Initial management of AT should focus on addressing underlying causes. Ventricular rate can be controlled with

the use of BB or calcium channel blockers (CCB). Class IA, IC, or III antiarrhythmics can be considered if BB or CCB fail to control the rate. Catheter ablation may be appropriate in patients failing medical therapy [4]. Electrical cardioversion will likely result in recurrence given that many focal AT are driven by enhanced automaticity.

Multifocal Atrial Tachycardia

- Multifocal atrial tachycardia (MAT) is a rapid, irregular atrial rhythm caused by multiple ectopic foci within the atria. It manifests as three distinct P wave morphologies in the same lead and a heart rate >100 BPM. There should be irregular PP intervals [5].
- MAT is typically seen in elderly patients with underlying severe pulmonary disease, cardiac disease, electrolyte abnormalities, and renal failure. Most patients with MAT are asymptomatic and retain hemodynamic stability. It is often incidentally found [5].
- The treatment of MAT should focus on the management of underlying medical conditions. Specific treatment is indicated if there is persistent symptomatic arrhythmia despite adequate treatment of underlying conditions [5]. Treatment options include non-dihydropyridine calcium channel blockers, beta-blockers, and AV nodal ablation with pacemaker implantation.

Junctional Tachycardia

- Junctional tachycardia (JT) arises from the AV junction, specifically from perinodal tissue and the His bundle. The AV junction's intrinsic rate is 40–60 BPM, and an accelerated junctional rhythm is slightly faster at 60–100 BPM. This becomes junctional tachycardia at rates >100 BPM.

- In addition to a ventricular rate >100 BPM, JT can have a short or long RP interval, with P waves before, after, or within the QRS complex.
- JT rarely occurs in adults and is more common in infants and children. It can be seen transiently after valve surgery [3].
- Treatment options for JT include BB, diltiazem, verapamil, or procainamide [3].

Interventions for SVT

- Vagal maneuvers should be considered as first-line treatment for patients with hemodynamically stable SVT. These typically include the Valsalva maneuver and the modified Valsalva maneuver.
- To perform the Valsalva maneuver, patients should be counseled to inhale followed by exhaling against a closed glottis for 10–15 seconds while in a supine or semi-recumbent position.
- The modified Valsalva is significantly more effective at converting patients out of SVT and involves supine positioning with a passive leg raise at the end of strain [3].
- Adenosine can be considered if a patient fails vagal maneuvers. At the time that this is being considered, the patient should be in an inpatient setting. Adenosine functions by decreasing the heart rate and slowing conduction through the AV node.
- If patients in an SVT are hemodynamically unstable, they should undergo immediate synchronized electrical cardioversion.

Approach to the Patient with SVT

- In the patient with suspected SVT, obtaining a 12-lead ECG is an essential first step.

- The RP interval, in particular, can aid in diagnosis. It is defined as the interval between the onset of the R wave and the onset of the next P wave.
  - Short RP tachycardias include typical AVNRT, most AVRTs, and rarely AT with concomitant first-degree AV block.
  - Long RP tachycardias include atrial tachycardia, atypical AVNRT, and, rarely, AVRT.
- Response to adenosine can help delineate the type of SVT. At the time that adenosine is being considered, patients should ideally be in an inpatient setting.
  - Adenosine-responsive SVTs include AVNRT, AVRT, JT, and some focal AT.
  - If adenosine fails to terminate the rhythm, it may still aid in diagnosis by revealing discrete atrial activity.
- Adenosine can be considered if a patient fails vagal maneuvers. At the time that this is being considered, the patient should be in an inpatient setting.

Clinical Pearl

Adenosine can be considered if a patient fails vagal maneuvers. At the time that this is being considered, the patient should be in an inpatient setting.

Key Learning Points

- SVT is a tachyarrhythmia that originates from the AV node or atria and most commonly manifests as a narrow complex tachycardia on ECG though in some cases it may appear as a wide complex tachycardia.
- The most common subtype of SVT is atrioventricular nodal reentrant tachycardia (AVNRT) followed by atrioventricular reentrant tachycardia (AVRT) and

then atrial tachycardia (AT), although prevalence varies with age at presentation.
- Vagal maneuvers should be considered as first-line treatment for patients with hemodynamically stable SVT. These typically include the Valsalva maneuver and the modified Valsalva maneuver.
- Response to adenosine can help delineate type of SVT. Adenosine-responsive SVTs include AVNRT, AVRT, JT, and some focal AT.

References

1. Lilly LS. Pathophysiology of heart disease: a collaborative project of medical students and faculty. 6th, North American ed. Wolters Kluwer; 2015.
2. Page RL, Joglar JA, Caldwell MA, Calkins H, Conti JB, Deal BJ, Estes NAM, Field ME, Goldberger ZD, Hammill SC, Indik JH, Lindsay BD, Olshansky B, Russo AM, Shen W-K, Tracy CM, Al-Khatib SM. 2015 ACC/AHA/HRS guideline for the management of adult patients with supraventricular tachycardia. J Am Coll Cardiol. 2016;67(13):e27–e115. https://doi.org/10.1016/j.jacc.2015.08.856.
3. Wells BJ, Quintero PA, Southmayd G. Handbook of inpatient cardiology. 1st ed. Springer; 2020.
4. Liwanag M, Willoughby C. Atrial Tachycardia. [Updated 2020 Nov 20]. In: StatPearls [Internet]. Treasure Island (FL): StatPearls Publishing; 2021.
5. Custer AM, Yelamanchili VS, Lappin SL. Multifocal Atrial Tachycardia. [Updated 2020 Jul 19]. In: StatPearls [Internet]. Treasure Island (FL): StatPearls Publishing; 2021.

Chapter 25
Bradyarrhythmia

Thomas E. Bigham and Michael S. Lloyd

Abbreviations

AV	Atrioventricular
BPM	Beats per minute
CSH	Carotid sinus hypersensitivity
EKG	Electrocardiogram
OSA	Obstructive sleep apnea
PPM	Permanent pacemaker
SA	Sinoatrial
SND	Sinus node dysfunction

T. E. Bigham (✉)
Department of Medicine, Emory University School of Medicine, Atlanta, GA, USA
e-mail: Thomas.bigham@emory.edu

M. S. Lloyd
Department of Medicine, Division of Cardiology, Emory University School of Medicine, Atlanta, GA, USA

A. A. Bhargava et al. (eds.), *Handbook of Outpatient Cardiology*, https://doi.org/10.1007/978-3-030-88953-1_25

Sinus Bradycardia

- *Sinus bradycardia* is defined as a heart rate less than 50 beats per minute (BPM) with a normal sinus P wave morphology (positive P wave deflection in I, II, and aVL and negative P wave in aV) on electrocardiogram (EKG) [1].
- It is commonly a benign, asymptomatic arrhythmia seen in young adults, well-trained athletes with low resting heart rates, and sleeping elderly adults.
- Resting bradycardia (heart rate less than 40 BPM) is considered abnormal and associated with underlying pathology.

Sinus Node Dysfunction

- *Sinus node dysfunction (SND)*, or sick sinus syndrome, is a broad term for several underlying conduction abnormalities.
- SND manifests with arrhythmias including sinus bradycardia, SA exit block, sinus pause, sinus arrest, and chronotropic incompetence.
- SND most often occurs in patients older than 50 years and is generally asymptomatic.
- Sinus node dysfunction commonly coincides with atrial tachycardias (estimated in 40–70% of cases). In settings of sole sinus node dysfunction, development of atrial tachycardias is common over time. This is commonly seen with *tachy-brady syndrome* which refers to the coexistence of SND and paroxysmal atrial fibrillation [2].
- Tachy-brady syndrome, a common disorder of the elderly, includes symptoms of palpitations followed by lightheadedness or syncope during the conversion to sinus rhythm and is associated with a long post-conversion sinus pause.

Etiology

- Sinus node dysfunction may be categorized into two major groups, intrinsic (most commonly caused by idiopathic degenerative sinus node disorder) or extrinsic (most commonly caused by medications) (Table 25.1).

TABLE 25.1 Intrinsic and extrinsic causes of sinus node dysfunction

Intrinsic causes	
Idiopathic degeneration	Mild inherited or spontaneous mutations in sodium or potassium channels
Myocardial ischemia	Acute or chronic myocardial ischemia, especially in the right coronary artery distribution
Cardiomyopathy	Dilated cardiomyopathy, hypertensive heart disease, congenital heart disease
Infiltrative disease	Amyloidosis, hemochromatosis, sarcoidosis
Infectious/inflammatory disorders	Lyme disease, viral myocarditis, rheumatic fever
Extrinsic causes	
Medications	AV nodal blockers (beta-blockers, calcium channel blockers, digoxin), antiarrhythmics, sympatholytic medications (clonidine), anticholinergics, lithium, phenytoin, opioids, sedatives
Systemic illness	Hypothyroidism, hypothermia, sepsis
Metabolic derangements	Hypoxia, hypokalemia or hyperkalemia, hypocalcemia
Autonomic dysfunction	Carotid sinus hypersensitivity, vasovagal syncope
Increased vagal tone	Obstructive sleep apnea, carotid sinus massage, increased intracranial pressure

Classification of Sinus Node Dysfunction

Sinus Pauses and Sinus Arrest

- Sinus pauses and sinus arrest are abnormalities in SA node depolarization.
- On EKG, sinus pause and arrest have a prolonged period of P wave absence followed by return of either sinus rhythm or an escape beat (Fig. 25.1).
- The pause or arrest is not a multiple of the baseline PP interval.
- Benign sinus pauses up to 3 seconds are common; however, pauses greater than 3 seconds, while commonly asymptomatic, should be considered abnormal [3].

Sinoatrial Exit Block

- Sinoatrial (SA) exit block is a pathologic condition of impaired conduction between the sinus node and the surrounding atrial tissues, with three main categories, characterized as follows:
- First-degree SA exit block is delayed or slowed conduction of an SA nodal impulse to the surrounding atria. EKG appears normal. Typically, there is little or no clinical significance.
- Second-degree SA exit block is defined as intermittent blocked conduction from SA node to atrial tissue.

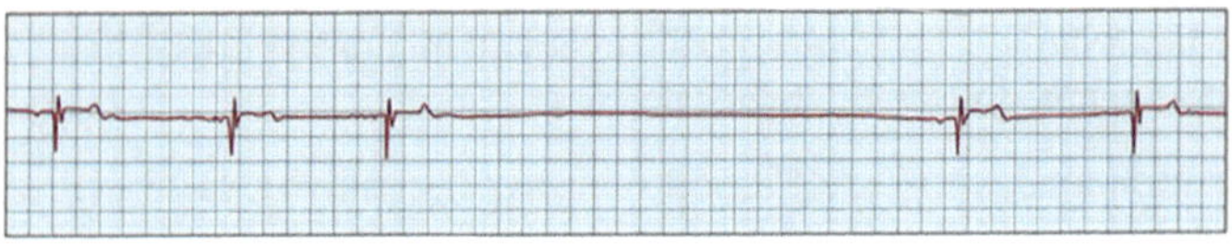

FIGURE 25.1 Telemetry strip demonstrating progressive worsening sinus bradycardia with associated sinus pause. (Imaged reproduced with permission from Vijayaraman et al., McGraw-Hill Education) [3]

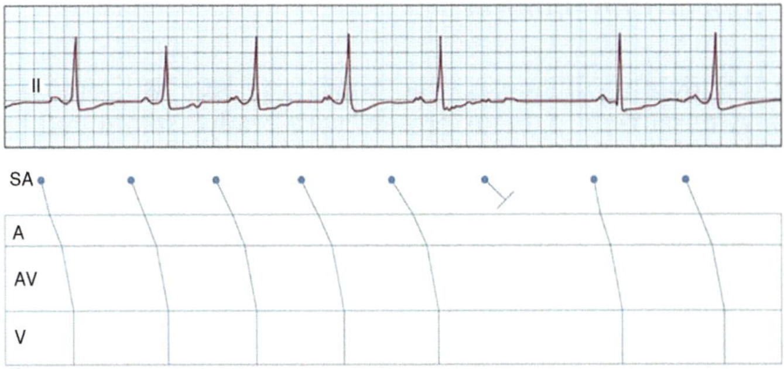

FIGURE 25.2 Telemetry strip and correlating ladder diagram demonstrating second-degree Mobitz type 1 sinoatrial exit block. Note the constant PP interval with progressively prolonged SA intervals, as detailed on the ladder diagram, leading to progressive shortening of the RR intervals. (Imaged reproduced with permission from Vijayaraman et al., Ellenbogen, McGraw-Hill Education) [3]

- In second-degree type 1 (Wenckebach), progressive prolongation of the SA conduction time is followed by a non-conducting sinus impulse. EKG shows shortening of the PP interval prior to sinus pause (Fig. 25.2).
- Second-degree type 2 SA block has a constant sinus node conduction interval followed by a subsequent sinus pause. EKG shows a constant PP interval with subsequent sinus pause. In type 1 and type 2 SA exit block, grouped beating is characteristic.
- Third-degree SA block presents as sinus arrest on EKG.

Chronotropic Incompetence

- Chronotropic incompetence is the inability of the sinus node to respond to activity or demand to achieve a targeted heart rate. There is no formal definition of this target heart rate; however, it is typically defined by 85% of (220- age) or failure to achieve a heart rate greater than 100 BPM [1].
- Development of chronotropic incompetence increases the risk of cardiovascular disease and mortality [4, 5].

Clinical Presentation

- Incidental diagnosis via routine EKG is common. Alternatively, patients present with bradycardia found by smartwatches, home pulse oximetry, or EKG devices.
- Syncope and presyncope are common symptoms associated with SND. However, patients may present with vague symptoms including exercise intolerance, fatigue, angina, dyspnea, or palpitations.
- The hallmark symptom of chronotropic incompetence is exertional intolerance, which is evaluated with exercise treadmill test.

Evaluation of Sinus Node Dysfunction

- A 12-lead EKG while symptomatic is the gold standard for diagnostic evaluation.
- Ambulatory monitoring should be considered for diagnostic evaluation of SND.
  - Ambulatory monitoring identifies infrequent episodes of SND in the setting of non-diagnostic EKGs.
  - Ambulatory monitoring assists in correlating symptoms with rhythm changes in the setting of sinus node dysfunction.
- Carotid sinus massage with prolonged sinus pause may demonstrate underlying carotid sinus hypersensitivity (CSH).
- Exercise treadmill test can identify chronotropic incompetence or patients with exertional intolerance.
- In patients with concern for underlying structural heart disease, consider echocardiogram; however, in asymptomatic patients with SND and no suspicion for structural heart disease, routine cardiac imaging with TTE is not indicated [1].
- An electrophysiology (EP) study may diagnose SND when a thorough workup has been otherwise unrevealing.

Clinical Pearls
There is no minimum heart rate capable of inducing symptoms among all patients. Likelihood of symptomatology inversely correlates to an individual's cardiac output, which is a product of heart rate and stroke volume. With sufficiently increased stroke volume, cardiac output is maintained, accounting for asymptomatic cases (as similar to athletes). Therefore, there is no minimum heart rate necessitating permanent pacing for sinus node dysfunction.

Treatment of SND

- Management of SND depends on the ability to **correlate** symptoms with documented bradycardia.
- There is no established heart rate cut-off for asymptomatic bradycardia necessitating PPM placement.
- In symptomatic bradycardia due to reversible causes, management should focus on the underlying etiology [1].
- In patients on guideline-directed medical therapy (GDMT) who are unable to discontinue or reduce dosing, PPM placement may be indicated in order to continue GDMT [1].
- Patients with symptomatic bradycardia due to SND may benefit from PPM to improve heart rate and symptoms [1].

Clinical Pearls
In patients with history of vasovagal syncope, physical exam should include carotid sinus massage following carotid bruit auscultation. Diagnosis of CSH is made in the presence of symptoms and carotid auscultation demonstrating sinus pause greater than 3 seconds and symptoms.

Atrioventricular Conduction Disease

- Atrioventricular (AV) conduction disease may potentiate clinically significant bradycardia. AV conduction disease is classified by the extent of the effect on AV conduction, ranging from delayed conduction to intermittent atrioventricular conduction to complete AV dyssynchrony.
- AV conduction disease occurs at different levels (AV node and the His-Purkinje system) determining the effect of sympathetic and vagal input, as well as risk of disease progression.
- In contrast to sinus node disease, most patients with second-degree AV block or higher require inpatient evaluation and treatment.

Etiology

- AV conduction disease can be characterized as intrinsic or extrinsic (Table 25.2).
- The most common etiology of intrinsic AV block is idiopathic degeneration of the conduction system.

Classification

First-Degree AV Block

- First-degree AV block is a misnomer, as there is only a conduction delay with prolonged atria-ventricular conduction time. This is defined as EKG PR interval greater than 200 msec.
- First-degree AV block may be a normal variant in younger patients.
- In older patients, the most common etiology is idiopathic degeneration of the conduction system.

TABLE 25.2 Intrinsic and extrinsic causes of atrioventricular block

Intrinsic causes	
Idiopathic/ degenerative	Inherited or acquired age-related mutations causing channelopathies (sodium or potassium channels)
Myocardial ischemia	Acute or chronic myocardial ischemia, especially inferior wall
Infiltrative/ inflammatory	Cardiomyopathies, amyloidosis, hemochromatosis, sarcoidosis, rheumatologic (including lupus, systemic scleroderma, rheumatic arthritis)
Infectious	Lyme carditis, endocarditis, viral myocarditis, rheumatic fever
Neuromuscular	Myotonic dystrophy, Kearns-Sayre syndrome
Congenital	Congenital heart disease, maternal lupus erythematosus
Iatrogenic	History of valve repair/replacement, including transcatheter, alcoholic septal ablation, surgical myectomy, catheter ablation
Extrinsic causes	
Medications	AV nodal blockers (beta-blockers, calcium channel blockers, digoxin), antiarrhythmics, lithium
Metabolic	Hyperkalemia, hypermagnesemia, hypo-/ hyperthyroidism
Autonomic dysfunction	Carotid sinus hypersensitivity, vasovagal syncope
Increased vagal tone	Highly conditioned, athletes, obstructive sleep apnea, carotid sinus hypersensitivity, increased intracranial pressure

Second-Degree AV Block

- Blocked premature atrial contractions are most commonly mistaken for second-degree AV block, but can be distinguished from true second-degree AV block by assessing for prematurity of the blocked P wave.
- **Second-degree AV block** is an intermittent, non-conducting atrial impulse, commonly grouped.
- The Mobitz type 1 (or Wenckebach) pattern is progressive PR interval prolongation prior to a non-conducting P wave. The PR interval before the non-conducted P wave is longer than the PR interval following the non-conducting P wave (Fig. 25.3).
- Wenckebach commonly occurs at the AV node, with a subsequently narrow QRS [6, 7].
- Mobitz type 2 is a constant PR interval followed by a non-conducting P wave. The PR interval to non-conducting P wave is the same as the PR interval after the non-conducting P wave.
- Mobitz type 2 commonly occurs at or below the level of the His bundle; thus, it has a wide QRS (70% of cases) [6].
- 2:1 AV block is a constant PP interval in which every other P wave fails to conduct (Fig. 25.5). This type of block includes Mobitz type 1 or type 2.

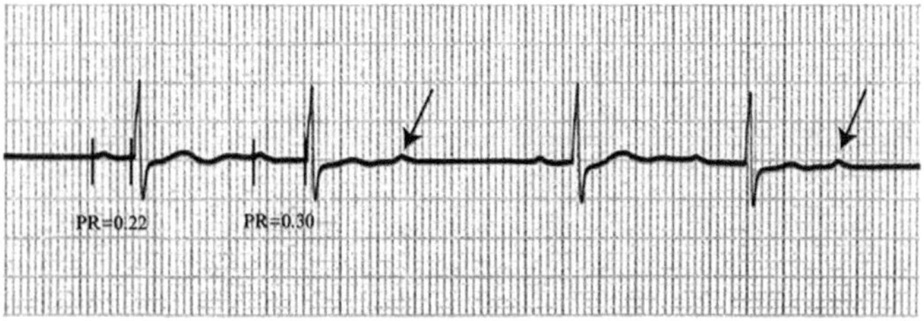

FIGURE 25.3 Telemetry strip demonstrating a 3:2 second-degree Mobitz type 1 AV block. Note the PR interval progressively lengthens until the non-conducting P wave. The PR interval after the non-conducting P wave is shorter than the prior PR interval. (Imaged reproduced with permission from Petty, Springer New York) [7]

- High-degree AV block is described as two or more consecutive non-conducting P waves at a constant PP rate. It is most commonly seen during vagotonic pauses (such as those during apneic phase of sleep apnea) (Fig. 25.4). High-grade AV block while awake may portend severe infranodal conduction disease [3].

Third-Degree AV Block

- Complete atrioventricular dyssynchrony defines third-degree AV block.
- EKG shows a constant but unrelated PP interval and RR interval. The ventricular rate is determined by either a junctional or ventricular escape rhythm (Fig. 25.6) [7].

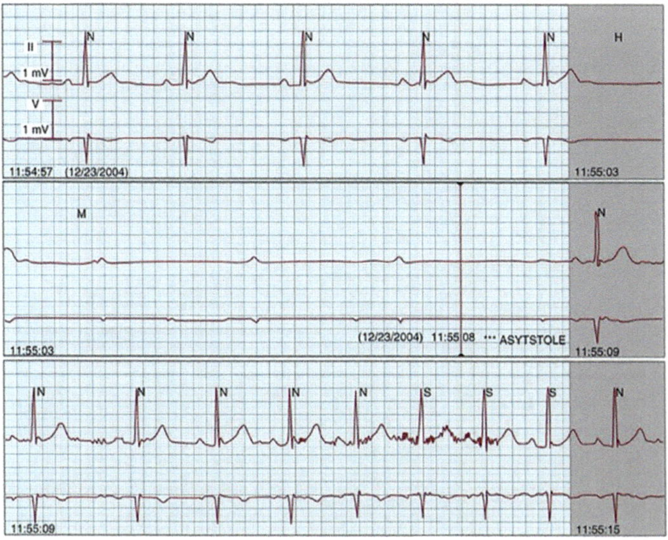

FIGURE 25.4 Telemetry strip of a sleeping patient with an episode of high-grade AV block with underlying sinus bradycardia, suggesting increased vagal tone while asleep. (Reproduced with permission from Vijayaraman et al., Ellenbogen, McGraw-Hill Education) [3]

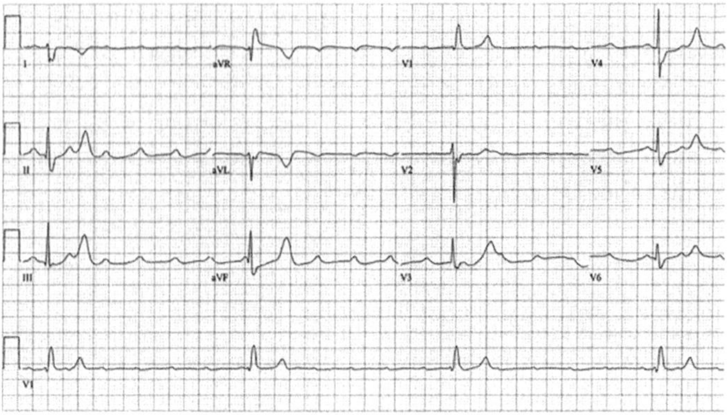

Figure 25.5 12-lead EKG with sinus tachycardia and third-degree AV block with slow ventricular escape rhythm. (Reproduced with permission from Petty, Springer New York) [7]

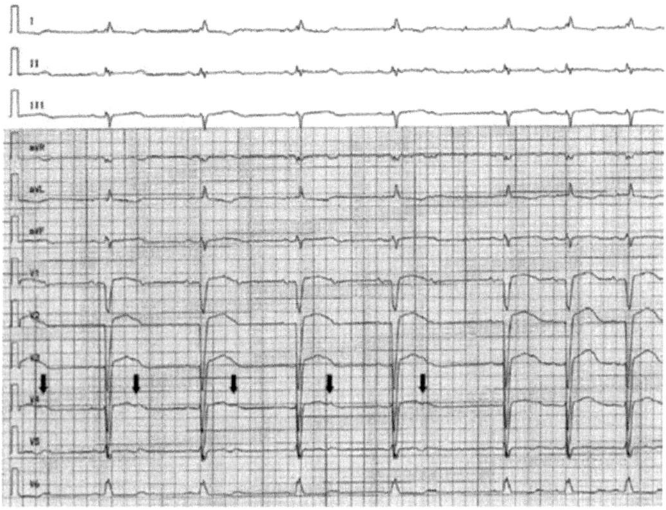

Figure 25.6 12-lead rhythm strip demonstrating 2:1 AV block which improves to 1:1 conduction which carotid sinus suggesting second-degree Mobitz type 2 AV block. (Reproduced with permission from Ojo and Buxton, Springer International Publishing) [9]

Presentation

- AV conduction disorders may be asymptomatic or produce symptoms of lightheadedness, syncope, palpitations, or dyspnea with exertion.
- First-degree AV block and Wenckebach are generally asymptomatic, whereas Mobitz type 2 and third-degree AV block may be symptomatic or asymptomatic.
- An elderly patient with history of symptomatic heart failure, with or without syncope, constitutes the most common presentation of complete AV block.
- Counterintuitively, systolic *hypertension* is the rule, due to long diastolic intervals with bradycardia; however, this should not lessen consideration of temporary pacing.

Diagnosis and Evaluation

- Diagnosis relies on 12-lead EKG; however, ambulatory EKG monitoring may be useful as it is often difficult to determine the relationship between symptoms and arrhythmias.
- Routine labs including electrolytes and thyroid studies should be obtained. The decision for further specific laboratory tests depends on history and physical.
- Cardiac imaging with TTE is indicated in patients Mobitz type 2, high-degree AV block, and complete heart block. Routine TTE is not indicated in asymptomatic first-degree AV block [1].
- In patients with 2:1 AV block or in unspecified second-degree AV block, location of the block may be determined by the length of the QRS or response to exercise, atropine, or carotid massage (Fig. 25.5 and Table 25.3) [8].
- Location of the block, often diagnosed on EP study, dictates treatment necessity. Intra-Hisian and infra-Hisian diseases are more likely to progress to complete heart block and require pacemaker even in asymptomatic cases [9].

TABLE 25.3 Characteristics and maneuvers that may aid in differentiation of 2:1 AV block or otherwise unspecified AV block

	QRS width	Exercise	Atropine	Carotid sinus massage
Mobitz type 1	Narrow	Improves	Improves	Worsens
Mobitz type 2	Wide	Worsens	Worsens	Improves

Clinical Pearls
In patients with Mobitz type 2, high-degree, or third-degree AV block, hemodynamically stable patients should be monitored continuously with plan for urgent coordination of PPM placement.

Therapy

- In acquired AV conduction disease, an initial focus to determine underlying etiology is essential to potentially identify treatments to reverse the effects on the conduction system.
- In patients with symptomatic first-degree AV or Mobitz type 1, PPM implantation is reasonable and indicated. Pacemaker is not indicated for asymptomatic cases.
- In acquired, irreversible second-degree Mobitz type 2, high-grade AV block, or complete heart block, PPM is indicated regardless of symptoms. Patients require urgent cardiology evaluation for pacemaker implantation upon initial presentation.
- Patients with symptomatic AV conduction disturbances will benefit from urgent cardiology referral for PPM evaluation.

Bradycardia in Special Circumstances

Bradycardia in the Sleeping (Including Obtunded, Intubated, or Sedated) Patient

- Bradycardia in such a clinical context is common and can lead to a variety of arrhythmias, including sinus arrest, high-grade AV block, or combinations of the two, with or without substantial pauses greater than 3 seconds. Vagal tone is the most common cause, and such bradycardias are atropine responsive. Despite rare use of pacing, electrophysiologic consultation is often required for refractory cases.
- Patients should be screened for sleep apnea, as appropriate treatment often reverses nocturnal bradyarrhythmias.
- Progressive prolongation of the PP intervals (indicating rising sinus nodal vagal tone) just prior to the bradyarrhythmia of concern suggests vagotonic etiology.

Clinical Pearls
Patients with nocturnal bradyarrhythmias require nighttime polysomnography, as OSA is associated with increased vagal tone, inducing bradyarrhythmias (1).

Carotid Sinus Hypersensitivity (CSH)

- CSH is a special type of reflexogenic (vagal related) bradycardia, manifesting as sinus arrest or AV block during head-turning or carotid sinus pressure, and often requires pacing.
- Following carotid bruit auscultation, gentle carotid massage is an essential part of any physical exam for bradycardia evaluation.

- CSH is characterized by greater than 3 second pause **with symptoms** during carotid sinus massage.
- PPM may alleviate, but not necessarily eliminate, symptoms.

Key Learning Points
1. PPM insertion is indicated in patients with symptomatic SND.
2. In patients on guideline-directed medical therapy leading to symptomatic SND or AV block, PPM may be indicated if the medication cannot be withdrawn or dose reduced.
3. PPM implantation is not indicated in patients with asymptomatic first-degree AV block or Wenckebach.
4. Type 2 second-degree AV block and high-grade AV block are indications for urgent evaluation as they are at high risk for becoming symptomatic or progressing to complete heart block. In these patients and those with third-degree heart block, PPM is indicated.

References

1. Kusumoto FM, Schoenfeld MH, Barrett C, Edgerton JR, Ellenbogen KA, Gold MR, et al. ACC/AHA/HRS Guideline on the Evaluation and Management of Patients With Bradycardia and Cardiac Conduction Delay: A Report of the American College of Cardiology/American Heart Association Task Force on Clinical Practice Guidelines and the Heart Rhythm. Circulation. 2018;2019:140(8).
2. John RM, Kumar S. Sinus node and atrial arrhythmias. Circulation. 2016;133(19):1892–900.
3. Vijayaraman P, Ellenbogen KA. Bradyarrhythmias. In: Fuster V, Harrington RA, Narula J, Eapen ZJ, editors. Hurst's the heart, 14e. New York, NY: McGraw-Hill Education; 2017.

4. Engeseth K, Hodnesdal C, Grundvold I, Liestøl K, Gjesdal K, Kjeldsen SE, et al. Temporal reduction in chronotropic index predicts risk of cardiovascular death among healthy middle-aged men: a 28-year follow-up study. J Am Heart Assoc. 2016;5(12):e004555.
5. Lauer MS. Impaired chronotropic response to exercise stress testing as a predictor of mortality. JAMA. 1999;281(6):524.
6. Katritsis DG, Josephson ME. Electrophysiological testing for the investigation of bradycardias. Arrhythm Electrophysiol Rev. 2017;6(1):24.
7. Petty BG. Atrioventricular (AV) Block. Basic electrocardiography. New York, NY: Springer New York; 2016. p. 65–77.
8. Mangiardi LM, Bonamini R, Conte M, Gaita F, Orzan F, Presbitero P, et al. Bedside evaluation of atrioventricular block with narrow QRS complexes: usefulness of carotid sinus massage and atropine administration. Am J Cardiol. 1982;49(5):1136–45.
9. Ojo AO, Buxton AE. Bradyarrhythmias and AV block. In: Wells BJ, Quintero PA, Southmayd G, editors. Handbook of inpatient cardiology. Cham: Springer; 2020. p. 87–102.

Chapter 26
Device Management

Marvin Louis Roy Lu and Hakeem Ayinde

Abbreviations

ATP	Anti-tachycardia pacing
CIED	Cardiac implantable electronic devices
CRT	Cardiac resynchronization therapy
ECG	Electrocardiogram
EF	Ejection fraction
EOL	End of life
ERI	Effective replacement indication
ICD	Implantable cardioverter-defibrillator
PPM	Permanent pacemaker
SCD	Sudden cardiac death
VF	Ventricular fibrillation
VT	Ventricular tachycardia

M. L. R. Lu (✉)
Department of Medicine, Division of Cardiology, Emory University School of Medicine, Atlanta, GA, USA
e-mail: mylu2@emory.edu

H. Ayinde
Departments of Heart & Vascular Institute, Novant Health Presbyterian Medical Center, Charlotte, NC, USA

A. A. Bhargava et al. (eds.), *Handbook of Outpatient Cardiology*, https://doi.org/10.1007/978-3-030-88953-1_26

Introduction

Pacemakers

- Permanent pacemakers (PPM) are devices capable of pacing the heart and are used mainly to treat symptomatic bradyarrhythmias by providing adequate heart rate to sustain cardiac output and hemodynamics. It consist of mainly two components:
  - A pulse generator (Fig. 26.1a) provides the electrical impulse and contains the battery, circuitry, and capacitors. It is implanted via a small incision in the deltopectoral groove into the prepectoral or subpectoral position.
  - One to three leads that have electrodes able to sense or deliver (pace) the electrical impulse to stimulate the myocardium. Leads are placed transvenously via the axillary/subclavian or cephalic vein into the cardiac chambers (Figs. 26.1b, c and 26.2a).
- A single-chamber pacemaker will have a lead inserted in either the right atrium or right ventricle. A dual-chamber pacemaker has leads inserted in both the right atrium and right ventricle (Fig. 26.2b). A biventricular pacemaker that is used for cardiac resynchronization therapy (CRT) will have a third lead inserted into the coronary sinus and its branches (Fig. 26.2a).
- Leadless cardiac pacing systems such as the Micra Medtronic system are fully implanted into the right ventricle (Fig. 26.1d).

Defibrillators

- Implantable cardioverter-defibrillators (ICD) are devices that are capable of delivering an electrical shock to the myocardium.

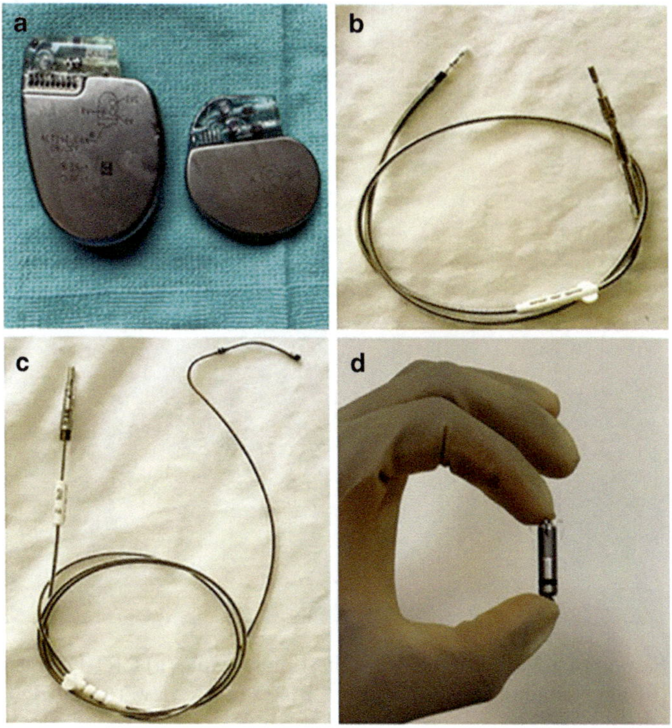

FIGURE 26.1 (**a**) Side-by-side comparison of a single-chamber ICD and a dual-chamber pacemaker. (**b**) An active fixation pacemaker lead with proximal pin and distal electrodes shown. (**c**) A left ventricular pacemaker lead. (**d**) A leadless pacemaker showing the tines used for attachment to the right ventricle [1]

- The high voltage lead of an ICD has one or two coils to maximize the density of current flow to the myocardium during the shock (Fig. 26.2a). Just like PPM, these leads are also capable of sensing and pacing the myocardium. ICD pulse generators are at least twice the size of pacemaker generators (Fig. 26.1a).
- Subcutaneous ICD (S-ICD, Boston Scientific) is a device that is implanted in a pocket in the left lateral mid axillary chest wall with the lead tunneled subcutaneously into the anterior chest (Fig. 26.2c, d).

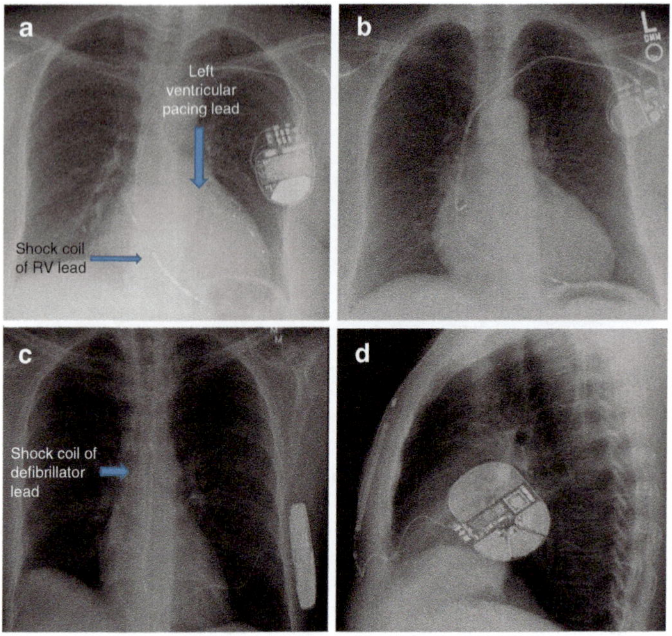

FIGURE 26.2 Various CIEDs on chest radiograph. (**a**) CRT-D device. (**b**) Dual-chamber pacemaker. (**c**) S-ICD in PA view. (**d**) S-ICD in lateral view [1]

Clinical Pearls

- All ICD devices have pacemaker capabilities in addition to delivery of therapies for tachycardia.
- S-ICDs are often considered in patients who are at high risk for bacteremia such as those on hemodialysis or have chronic endovascular indwelling catheters. Younger patients and those with challenging vascular access also benefit from S-ICD to avoid long-term complications of transvenous ICDs.
- There is no difference in efficacy of terminating VT or VF between S-ICDs and transvenous ICDs.

Indications

- Pacemakers are indicated for patients with symptomatic bradycardia. These symptoms include syncope, lightheadedness/dizziness, or fatigue/activity intolerance. Common conditions that can cause significant bradycardia include sinus node dysfunction and high-grade or complete AV block. Sinus node dysfunction can manifest as sinus pauses or inability to increase heart rate in relation to patient's activity (chronotropic incompetence) [2].
- ICDs are indicated both as secondary prevention of sudden cardiac death (SCD) in patients with prior ventricular fibrillation (VF) or sustained ventricular tachycardia (VT) and as primary prevention of SCD in high-risk patients such as those with systolic heart failure, certain channelopathies, and other familial conditions such as hypertrophic cardiomyopathy [3].
- CRTs are indicated to improve symptoms and survival in patients with evidence of severe systolic heart failure with LV ejection fraction (EF) of ≤35%, and left bundle branch block, especially when QRS duration is greater than 150 ms [4]. CRTs are also helpful in patients with AV block and LVEF less than 50%, irrespective of QRS duration if it is anticipated that they may require ventricular pacing >40% of the time [5].

Clinical Pearl

- Pacemakers are usually programmed to minimize ventricular pacing by promoting intrinsic AV conduction in patients without complete heart block. This is because chronic pacing of the right ventricle can lead to cardiomyopathy and worsening heart failure in up to 15–20% of patients. On the contrary, CRT devices are programmed to provide the maximum percentage of biventricular pacing in order to achieve the greatest benefit from the resynchronization therapy.

temporary pacemakers have automatic sensing threshold testing algorithms to adjust the sensitivity so that it is able to detect all intrinsic myocardial activity while filtering out noise or artifacts.

- CIEDs act on a sensed activity by either triggering or inhibiting pacing. The inability to sense appropriate intrinsic myocardial activity is termed *undersensing* (Fig. 26.3). This can occur when the sensitivity is programmed too low. If the sensitivity is programmed too high, the CIED may sense environmental noise or artifacts. This is termed *oversensing* (Fig. 26.4). Sensing abnormalities may also be an indication of lead malfunction.

Pacing and Capture

- Pacing occurs when the CIED delivers an electrical stimulus to the myocardium.

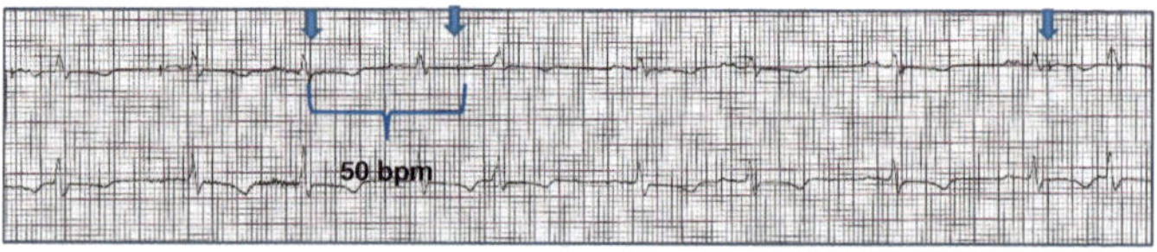

FIGURE 26.3 Atrial undersensing. Intrinsic P waves not sensed by the CIED as evidenced by atrial pacing (blue arrows) [1]

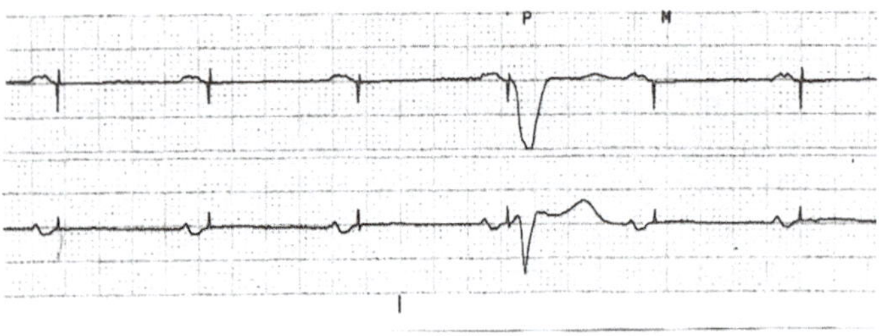

FIGURE 26.4 Ventricular oversensing. Ventricular pacing is inhibited by noise or artifact resulting in ventricular asystole [1]

- The successful depolarization and stimulation of the myocardium is termed *capture*, and the minimum electrical stimulus required to depolarize the myocardium is termed *capture threshold*.
- Contemporary pacemakers have automatic capture threshold testing algorithms and can adapt the programmed output according to improve battery longevity.
- The inability to depolarize myocardium despite delivery of pacing stimulus is termed *failure to capture* (Fig. 26.5). This problem may occur because the CIED pacing output is programmed below the capture threshold. It could also occur due to lead malfunction.

Event Markers

- Event markers are sensing and pacing indicators registered by the device and need to correlate with the surface ECG recording and intracardiac electrogram. An atrial or ventricular sensed marker coinciding with a native P wave or QRS, respectively, confirms proper sensing. Similarly, an atrial or ventricular paced marker indicates an electrical output is released by the device and if it is associated with an appropriate capture on the surface ECG confirms proper pacing.

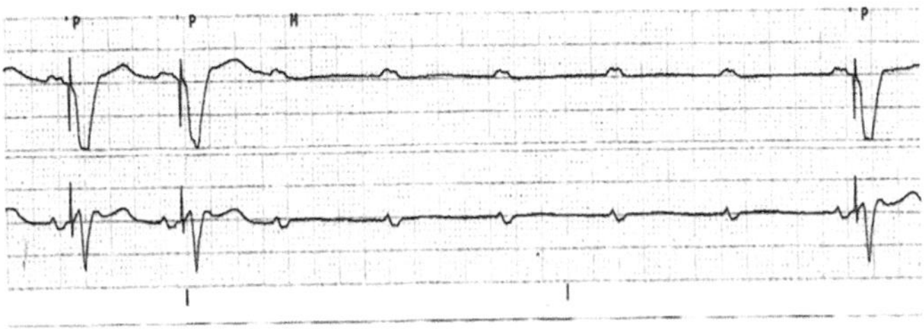

FIGURE 26.5 Loss of ventricular capture [1]

Clinical Pearl

- If the device registers a sensed-event marker that is not visible on the surface ECG, this could indicate inappropriate sensing, and further evaluation is required. The same is true if the device is undersensing and fails to respond by either triggering or inhibiting pacing.

Pacemaker Nomenclature

- The pacemaker nomenclature is often presented in a 4-digit code as described in Table 26.1.
- Rate responsiveness is the ability of the device to accelerate or decelerate its paced rate in relation to the patient's activity.
- Mode switching is the ability of the device to convert to a mode that no longer tracks the intrinsic atrial rate. This is useful in rapid atrial fibrillation to prevent rapid pacing of the ventricle.
- Pacemakers that are programmed DDD will pace and sense in both the atrium and ventricle and respond to a sensed event by either inhibiting or triggering pacing. DDD have four modes of pacing as presented below (Fig. 26.6).
- Pacemakers are programmed depending on the indication for pacing:
  - Patients with symptomatic sinus bradycardia who do not need frequent ventricular pacing are usually programmed DDD (or AAI with the ability to automatically switch to DDD when ventricular pacing is needed).
  - Patients with single-chamber ICD are typically programmed VVI with a backup rate of 40 beats per minute.

TABLE 26.1 Modified NASPE and BPEG (North American Society of Pacing and Electrophysiology/British Pacing and Electrophysiology Group) generic code for anti-bradycardia and multi-chamber pacing

I (chamber paced)	II (chamber sensed)	III (response to sensing)	IV (rate modulation)
A – Atria paced	A – Atria sensed	I – Inhibited	R – Rate responsive
V – Ventricle paced	V – Ventricle sensed	T – Triggered	
D – Dual (A + V)	D – Dual (A + V)	D – Dual (I + T)	
O – None	O – None	O – None	

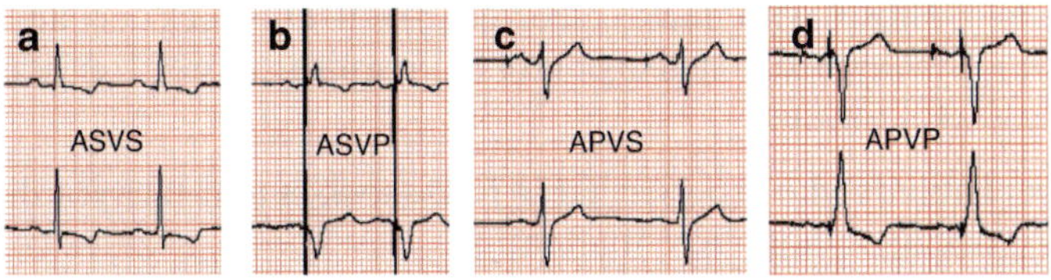

FIGURE 26.6 (**a**) Atrial-sensed, ventricular-sensed; (**b**) atrial-sensed, ventricular-paced; (**c**) atrial-paced, ventricular sensed; (**d**) atrial-paced, ventricular-paced [1]

Outpatient Device Management

- Pacemakers and defibrillators require regular routine interrogation through in-person office follow-up as well as remote device monitoring at home using a cellular network.
- Pacemaker/device interrogation includes evaluation of the following parameters:
  - Programmed pacing, therapies and parameters, and underlying native rhythm
  - Sensing and pacing/capture thresholds and lead impedance

- Events recorded including episodes of arrhythmias and all additional data collected
- Battery life and remaining longevity

- Patients who develop symptoms of shortness of breath, syncope/lightheadedness or dizziness, or palpitations that could potentially be secondary to an arrhythmia or device malfunction should be promptly referred for device interrogation.
- The frequency of follow-up interrogation depends on the type of device as well as the patient's clinical status:
  - Patients with a pacemaker or ICD who have not received any ICD therapies need to be followed up every 3–4 months with at least one in-person complete device interrogation annually.
  - Those who have received an ICD shock or anti-tachycardia pacing (ATP) require more frequent follow-ups.
- Patients who experienced an ICD shock or anti-tachycardia pacing require urgent attention.
  - If they had one shock and are otherwise asymptomatic and feel well, then they should be seen in clinic within 24–48 hours for complete evaluation. If this cannot be arranged, then the patient should be sent to the emergency department.
  - If they are symptomatic with syncope or dizziness or feel generally unwell, they need immediate medical attention and should be sent to the emergency department.
  - If they receive multiple ICD shocks in a span of minutes to hours, this is also considered a medical emergency, and they should be sent to the emergency department.
  - Clinicians should reassess and optimize medical management of these patients as ICD therapies are associated with higher mortality regardless if appropriate or inappropriate.

- Devices who have reached elective replacement indication (ERI) or end of life (EOL) need to be referred to the electrophysiologist for a pulse generator exchange.

References

1. Ayinde H, Sabayon MD, Lloyd MS. Pacemakers, defibrillators, and cardiac resynchronization therapy. In: Wells B, Quintero P, Southmayd G, editors. Handbook of inpatient cardiology. Cham: Springer; 2020. https://doi.org/10.1007/978-3-030-47868-1_7.
2. Kusumoto FM, Schoenfeld MH, Barrett C, Edgerton JR, Ellenbogen KA, Gold MR, Goldschlager NF, Hamilton RM, Joglar JA, Kim RJ, Lee R, Marine JE, McLeod CJ, Oken KR, Patton KK, Pellegrini CN, Selzman KA, Thompson A, Varosy PD. 2018 ACC/AHA/HRS Guideline on the Evaluation and Management of Patients With Bradycardia and Cardiac Conduction Delay: A Report of the American College of Cardiology/American Heart Association Task Force on Clinical Practice Guidelines and the Heart Rhythm Society. J Am Coll Cardiol. 2019;74(7):e51. Epub 2018 Nov 6.
3. Russo AM, Stainback RF, Bailey SR, Epstein AE, Heidenreich PA, Jessup M, Kapa S, Kremers MS, Lindsay BD, Stevenson LW. ACCF/HRS/AHA/ASE/HFSA/SCAI/SCCT/SCMR 2013 appropriate use criteria for implantable cardioverter-defibrillators and cardiac resynchronization therapy: a report of the American College of Cardiology Foundation appropriate use criteria task force, Heart Rhythm Society, American Heart Association, American Society of Echocardiography, Heart Failure Society of America, Society for Cardiovascular Angiography and Interventions, Society of Cardiovascular Computed Tomography, and Society for Cardiovascular Magnetic Resonance. J Am Coll Cardiol. 2013;61(12):1318–68. Epub 2013 Mar 1.
4. Epstein AE, JP DM, Ellenbogen KA, Estes NA 3rd, Freedman RA, Gettes LS, Gillinov AM, Gregoratos G, Hammill SC, Hayes DL, Hlatky MA, Newby LK, Page RL, Schoenfeld MH, Silka MJ, Stevenson LW, Sweeney MO, Tracy CM, Epstein AE, Darbar D, JP DM, Dunbar SB, Estes NA 3rd, Ferguson TB Jr, Hammill SC, Karasik PE, Link MS, Marine JE, Schoenfeld MH, Shanker AJ, Silka MJ, Stevenson LW, Stevenson WG, Varosy PD, American

College of Cardiology Foundation, American Heart Association Task Force on Practice Guidelines, Heart Rhythm Society. 2012 ACCF/AHA/HRS focused update incorporated into the ACCF/AHA/HRS 2008 guidelines for device-based therapy of cardiac rhythm abnormalities: a report of the American College of Cardiology Foundation/American Heart Association Task Force on Practice Guidelines and the Heart Rhythm Society. J Am Coll Cardiol. 2013;61(3):e6–75. Epub 2012 Dec 19.

5. Curtis AB, Worley SJ, Adamson PB, Chung ES, Niazi I, Sherfesee L, Shinn T, Sutton MS, Biventricular versus Right Ventricular Pacing in Heart Failure Patients with Atrioventricular Block (BLOCK HF) Trial Investigators. Biventricular pacing for atrioventricular block and systolic dysfunction. N Engl J Med. 2013;368(17):1585.

Part IX
Pericardial Disease

Chapter 27
Pericardial Diseases: Acute Pericarditis, Pericardial Effusion, and Cardiac Tamponade

Robert N. D'Angelo and Duane S. Pinto

Abbreviations

ACS	Acute coronary syndrome
CMR	Cardiac magnetic resonance imaging
CRP	C-reactive protein
CT	Computed tomography
ESR	Erythrocyte sedimentation rate
ILI	Influenza-like illness
IL-1	Interleukin-1
JVP	Jugular venous pressure
LGE	Late gadolinium enhancement
MI	Myocardial infarction
WBC	White blood cell

R. N. D'Angelo (✉) · D. S. Pinto
Department of Medicine, Division of Cardiology, Beth Israel Deaconess Medical Center, Harvard Medical School, Boston, MA, USA
e-mail: rdangelo@bidmc.harvard.edu; dpinto@bidmc.harvard.edu

A. A. Bhargava et al. (eds.), *Handbook of Outpatient Cardiology*, https://doi.org/10.1007/978-3-030-88953-1_27

Pericardial Disease

Anatomy and Physiology of the Pericardium

- The pericardium is a tough, two-layer sack that encases the heart.
  - Visceral pericardium is comprised of mesothelial cells and collagen/elastin fibers adherent to the epicardium (innermost layer).
  - Parietal pericardium is acellular and contains collagen/elastin fibers (outermost layer).
  - Pericardial space is contained between two layers and in normal circumstances contains up to 50 mL of serous fluid.
- The pericardium serves as an attachment point to the heart and a barrier to infection, although removal is generally without adverse effects [1].
- The pericardium is elastic at low stress, but then becomes stiff and non-compliant near the upper range of cardiac volume.
- When reserve volume of pericardial sac is exceeded, pressure is transmitted to the cardiac chambers, impairing cardiac function.
  - Fixed volume of the pericardium can lead to transmission of pressure from one chamber to the next, increasing diastolic interaction between chambers.
  - The pericardium can stretch and adapt if ventricular dilation or fluid accumulation is more gradual attenuating the effects of interdependence.

Acute Pericarditis

Definition

- Acute pericarditis is caused by inflammation of the pericardial layers and may be associated with pericardial effusion [2].

- Depending on the nature of symptoms and timing presentation, it can be further classified as acute, incessant, recurrent, or chronic (Table 27.1).

Etiology

- Infectious
  - Viral is most common, with many episodes preceded by influenza-like illness (ILI) or GI illness (e.g., adenovirus, coxsackievirus, Epstein-Barr virus, echovirus, HIV) [3–5].
  - Bacterial (e.g., *M. tuberculosis*, *Staphylococcus*, *Streptococcus*, Lyme disease, etc.).
  - Fungal (e.g., coccidioidomycosis, histoplasmosis).
  - Protozoal (e.g., toxoplasmosis).
- Inflammatory
  - Connective tissue disease (e.g., rheumatoid arthritis, systemic lupus erythematosus, Sjogren syndrome, scleroderma)

TABLE 27.1 Definition and diagnostic criteria for pericarditis

Classification	Definition
Acute	Inflammatory pericardial syndrome lasting <4–6 weeks with at least two of four criteria [3]: 1. Chest pain 2. Pericardial rub 3. Characteristic ECG changes (widespread ST elevation or PR depression) 4. Pericardial effusion (new or worsening) Additional supportive findings: Elevated inflammatory markers (CRP, ESR) Pericardial inflammation
Incessant	Pericarditis lasting >4–6 weeks, but <3 months without remission
Recurrent	Pericarditis after symptom-free interval >4–6 weeks
Chronic	Pericarditis lasting >3 months

  - Drug-induced (e.g., hydralazine, procainamide, cyclosporine)
  - Immunotherapy with checkpoint inhibitors (e.g., PD-1, CTLA-4 inhibitors) [6]
  - Genetic immune system disease (familial Mediterranean fever, tumor necrosis factor receptor-1-associated periodic syndrome (TRAPS))

- Post-cardiac injury

  - Post-pericardiotomy syndrome due to blunt or sharp trauma to the pericardium
  - Post-procedural including pacemaker insertion, radiofrequency ablation, and percutaneous coronary intervention

- Post-myocardial infarction

  - Early post-MI pericarditis can occur within 1–3 days immediately after MI, typically with large, transmural MIs due to absent or late reperfusion.
  - Late post-MI pericarditis (Dressler syndrome) occurs 1 week to 3 months after MI, usually with fever and chest pain. Often associated with pericardial effusion, although rarely pericardial tamponade [7].

- Other causes

  - Renal failure (uremia), malignancy (lymphoma, breast and lung carcinoma), radiation-induced

Clinical Pearl
In developed countries, 80–90% of acute pericarditis cases are idiopathic, presumed to be due to viral causes.

Clinical Presentation

- Criteria for diagnosis based on European Society of Cardiology (ESC) guidelines require at least two out of four of the following [8]:

    1. Chest pain (>85–90% cases): typically sharp and pleuritic and positional (better with leaning forward or sitting upright); can radiate to the neck, arms, and shoulders, mimicking ACS
    2. Pericardial rub (<33% cases): high pitched, best heard at the left lower sternal border
    3. Electrocardiogram (ECG) changes (up to 60% cases): diffused ST-segment elevation and PR-segment depression
    4. New or worsening pericardial effusion (up to 60% cases)

- May present with nonspecific symptoms accompanying chest pain including low-grade fever, tachycardia, cough, and occasionally hiccups.
- Past medical history, such as viral prodrome, history of malignancy or autoimmune disorder, or new medications can help to narrow differential diagnosis and guide diagnostic evaluation.
- Differential diagnosis is wide, although most important to exclude life-threatening causes including:

    - Acute coronary syndromes (ACS)
    - Pulmonary embolism
    - Aortic dissection
    - Pneumonia with pleurisy
    - Pneumothorax

Clinical Pearl
Chest pain is presenting symptom in more than 90% cases of acute pericarditis and is usually relieved with sitting up and leaving forward, commonly with pain that radiates to the trapezius ridge.

Diagnostics and Imaging

- Diagnosis is based primary on history of chest pain and friction rub and supported by laboratory, ECG, and imaging findings.
- ECG findings
  - Changes present in approximately 60% of isolated pericarditis, but in >90% cases with concomitant myocarditis [8]. Classically findings include diffuse ST-segment elevation and PR-segment depression, with evolution of ECG changes in the following stages (Fig. 27.1) [9]:
    1. PR depression and/or diffuse ST-segment elevation
    2. Normalization of ST segment (generally within 1 week)
    3. T-wave inversion with or without ST-segment depression
    4. Return to baseline (within weeks to months)
  - Low voltage (QRS amplitude <0.5 mV in limb leads) and electrical alternans suggest effusion.
- Laboratory findings

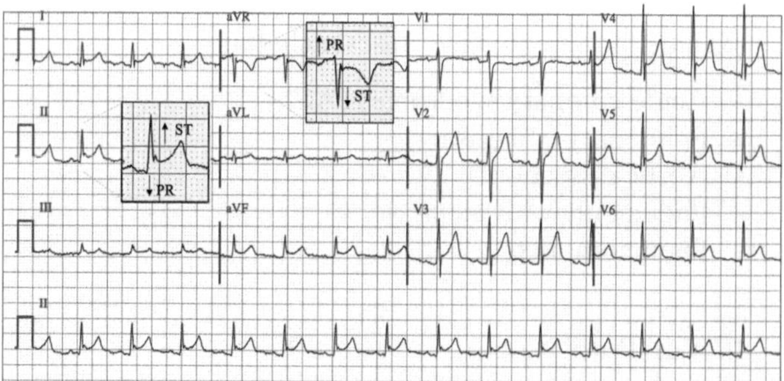

FIGURE 27.1 ECG findings in acute pericarditis, demonstrating diffuse ST-segment elevation and PR-segment depression, with PR-segment elevation and ST-segment depression in lead aVR

- Elevated inflammatory markers: leukocytosis, ↑ CRP, ↑ ESR.
- High-sensitivity C-reactive protein (hsCRP) is elevated in 3/4 of patients with acute pericarditis and normalizes typically within 1 week and in all cases by 4 weeks after diagnosis.
- Elevated cardiac biomarkers: elevated troponin and CK-MB seen in up to 30%, indicating myopericarditis.
- Additional labs not typically sent unless indicated by history and clinical suspicion: rheumatoid factor, ANA, thyroid function tests, anti-streptolysin O (ASO), viral panel.

• Imaging

- Chest X-ray (CXR)

  Typically normal, although helpful to evaluate other causes of pleuritic chest pain including pneumonia and pneumothorax

- Echocardiography

  Transthoracic echocardiogram (TTE) should be performed initially to evaluate for left ventricular dysfunction, pericardial effusion, tamponade physiology, and constrictive pericarditis [8, 10].

  Repeat TTE 1–2 weeks after treatment initiation is helpful to assess for developing or resolving effusion.

- Cardiac MRI (CMR)

  Useful to confirm diagnosis when echocardiogram images are ambiguous or if there is suggestion of myopericarditis. CMR demonstrates pericardial thickening and/or effusion.

  Late gadolinium enhancement (LGE) is up to 94% sensitive for the detection of pericardial inflammation, with increased signal in T2-weighted signal associated with acute inflammation [11].

- CT scan

  Useful for assessing pericardial thickening and often obtained otherwise to assess for pulmonary embolism

Clinical Pearl
A transthoracic echocardiogram should be performed at the time of initial diagnosis and 1–2 weeks after initiating treatment to assess for complications of acute pericarditis, including left ventricular dysfunction, pericardial effusion, pericardial tamponade, and constriction physiology. Cardiac MRI and CT can be useful as an adjunct to assess for pericardial inflammation.

Management

- Acute pericarditis is often self-limiting and generally resolves within 2–6 weeks, with anti-inflammatory drugs as the mainstay of treatment.
- Initial triage
  - Reliable patients with minimal or small effusion who respond well to initial treatment can usually be managed as outpatients.
  - Patients who respond poorly to therapy, are suspected to have causes other than idiopathic pericarditis, or present with factors predictive of poor prognosis (large pericardial effusion, high fever, cardiac tamponade, lack of response to treatment) should generally be hospitalized for evaluation and treatment.
- Activity restrictions
  - Athletic activity should be restricted until symptoms have resolved and CRP has normalized for those not involved in competitive sports.

- Competitive athletes should not return to sport until symptoms have resolved and other parameters have normalized (CRP, ECG, and echocardiogram). Expert consensus suggests limiting competitive sports for 3 months [12].

- Pharmacologic treatment
  - Nonsteroidal anti-inflammatory drugs (NSAIDs)

    Based on clinical experience as no clinical trial demonstrating benefit.
    Ibuprofen used most commonly, although naproxen and indomethacin are acceptable. If NPO, ketorolac can be used for up to 3 days initially.
    Aspirin recommended if patient has coronary artery disease or another indication for anti-platelet therapy.
    Patient should be treated for a minimum of 2 weeks with dose tapered over another 2–3 weeks (Table 27.2).
    Gastric protection with PPI while on high-dose NSAID.

  - Colchicine

    Colchicine plus aspirin led to statistically significant reduction in symptoms at 72 hours and recurrence rate in COPE (COlchicine for acute PEricarditis) trial, along with reduction in hospitalization rate in ICAP (Investigation on Colchicine for Acute Pericarditis) trial [13, 14].
    May be given with or without loading dose. When loading dose is used, typically 0.6–1.2 mg twice daily depending on patient's body weight.
    Daily maintenance dose is given for 3 months, with weight-based dosing (Table 27.2).
    Monitor for hepatotoxicity, myelosuppression, and myotoxicity: complete blood count (CBC), creatinine, transaminases, and creatinine kinase (CK).

TABLE 27.2 Anti-inflammatory treatment for acute and recurrent pericarditis

Drug	Dosage	Initial duration	Tapering schedule
Aspirin	750–1000 mg every 8 h	1–2 weeks	Decrease dose weekly for 2–3 weeks before discontinuation
Ibuprofen	600–800 mg every 8 h	1–2 weeks	Decrease dose every week for 2–3 weeks before discontinuation
Colchicine	0.6 mg once daily (<70 kg) or 0.6 mg twice daily (ε 70 kg)	3 months	Optional, 0.6 mg once daily or every other day over 2–3 weeks
Corticosteroids[a]	Starting dose 0.25–0.5 mg/kg/day	1–2 weeks	Over months, approximately 20% of the dose every 1–2 weeks
Anakinra[a]	100 mg once daily	Up to 6 months	None

[a]Generally used for recurrent pericarditis only

Gastrointestinal side effects (abdominal cramping, diarrhea, nausea, vomiting, or diarrhea) lead to discontinuation in 5–8% of patients [13, 14].

– Glucocorticoids

Should generally only be used for incomplete response to other anti-inflammatories or specific etiologies (e.g., immune checkpoint inhibitor-associated pericarditis, autoimmune disease) as use of corticosteroids has been associated with prolonged disease course and greater risk of recurrent pericarditis [13].

Low-dose corticosteroids recommended, generally 0.25–0.5 mg/kg/day to minimize complications (Table 27.2).

Taper slowly over months to reduce risk of recurrent pericarditis, using symptomatic response and CRP as guide [15].

- Interleukin-1 (IL-1) receptor antagonists

  IL-1 receptor antagonists (e.g., anakinra) beneficial for treatment recurrent pericarditis in AIRTRIP trial, with RCT (NCT03224585) ongoing to determine efficacy for treating acute pericarditis [16]

Recurrent Pericarditis

- Recurrence occurs in 15–30% of patients with idiopathic pericarditis [2, 8, 9].
- Diagnosis requires new symptoms and signs of disease after a 4- to 6-week symptom-free period (Table 27.1).
- Pharmacologic treatment with NSAIDs + colchicine as above and if disease is still refractory can add corticosteroids or anakinra (Table 27.2).
- Other immunosuppressives have been effective in refractory cases, including azathioprine, methotrexate, and mycophenolate.
- Pericardiectomy or pericardial window can be considered as a last resort for patients with refractory disease.

Clinical Pearl

Continue treatment for acute pericarditis until symptom resolution, and then taper slowly to avoid recurrence. IL-1 receptor antagonists (e.g., anakinra) have shown a benefit in the treatment of recurrent pericarditis.

Pericardial Effusion and Cardiac Tamponade

Definition

- Accumulation of fluid within the pericardial space beyond the 10–50 mL present, due to either inflammation (exudative effusion) or increased venous pressure (transudative effusion).
- Clinical presentation and implications depend on the speed and volume of fluid accumulated (Fig. 27.2).
  - Rapid accumulation of fluid can lead to hemodynamic compromise with small amounts of fluid (<250 mL) due to inability of the pericardium to accommodate.

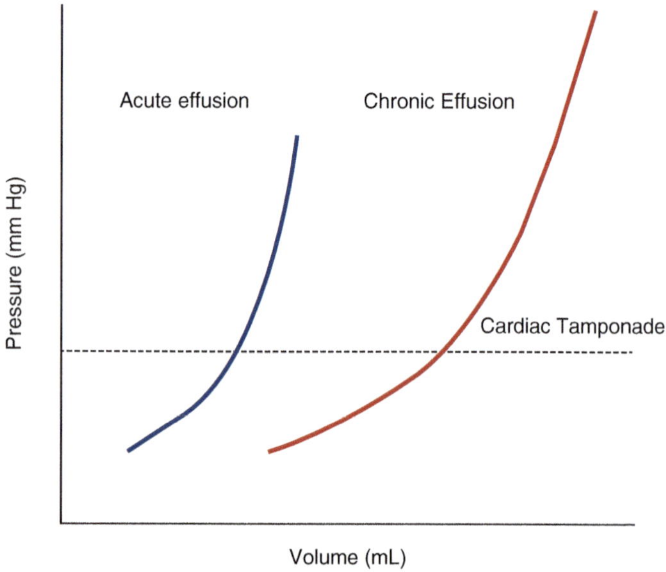

Figure 27.2 Relationship between pericardial volume and pericardial pressure in normal pericardium (left) and in stretched pericardium (right). The pericardium can accommodate more fluid before reaching tamponade if the fluid accumulation is gradual

  - Slow accumulation (days to weeks) can allow a large effusion to develop without symptoms.

- Cardiac tamponade is a life-threatening condition that occurs when a pericardial effusion inhibits cardiac filling, leading to hemodynamic instability.
  - Fluid, pus, blood, clots, or gas accumulates in the pericardial space, leading to pericardial pressures that exceed right ventricular filling pressures.
  - Right ventricular pressure overload leads to interventricular septum shifting to the left ventricle, decreasing diastolic filling, stroke volume, and cardiac output.

Etiology

- Effusions can be categorized as serous or hemorrhagic, although there is overlap between the groups.
- Serous pericardial effusion [17]
  - Idiopathic pericarditis
  - Malignancy
  - Acute pericarditis
  - Post-pericardiotomy
  - Autoimmune disorders
  - Hypothyroidism
  - Uremia
- Hemorrhagic pericardial effusion [18]
  - Post-pericardiotomy (e.g., coronary artery bypass surgery, valve replacement)
  - Complications of MI (free wall rupture and thrombolysis)
  - Aortic dissection
  - Idiopathic pericarditis
  - Malignancy
  - Tuberculosis
  - Uremia

Clinical Presentation

- Presentation depends on speed of fluid accumulation
  - Often minimally symptomatic initially
  - Dyspnea with exertion, progressing to orthopnea, chest pain, and chest fullness
  - Compression of local structures leading to nausea (diaphragm), dysphagia (esophagus), hoarseness (recurrent laryngeal nerve), and hiccups (phrenic nerve) [8]
  - Nonspecific symptoms including fever, particularly if related to underlying pericarditis, malignancy, or autoimmune process
- Cardiac tamponade characterized by the presence of:
  - Beck's triad

    Hypotension
    Muffled heart sounds
    Elevated jugular venous pressure (JVP)

  - Kussmaul's sign

    Distention of jugular veins with inspiration
    Usually seen with constrictive pericarditis, but also seen with tamponade and right ventricular failure

  - Pulsus paradoxus

    Defined as exaggerated drop in systolic pressure during inspiration, >10 mmHg
    Measurement as the following:

    - Use a sphygmomanometer, and then inflate cuff 20 mm Hg above systolic pressure.
    - Deflate cuff until the first Korotkoff sound is heard (only during expiration).
    - Deflate cuff until Korotkoff sounds heart equally with inspiration and expiration.
    - If difference >10 mm Hg, pulsus paradoxus is present.

- Differential diagnosis: cardiac tamponade, constrictive pericarditis, pulmonary embolism, severe asthma/COPD.

> **Clinical Pearl**
> Rapid accumulation of fluid in the pericardial space can lead to cardiac tamponade even at low volumes of fluid due to inability of the pericardium to adapt in the short term.

Diagnostics

- ECG (Fig. 27.3)
  - Low voltage (limb leads <5 mm and precordial leads <10 mm): Nonspecific, can also be caused by emphysema, infiltrative disease, or pneumothorax
  - Electrical alternans: Caused by anteroposterior swinging of the heart; specific but not sensitive
  - May see signs of pericarditis

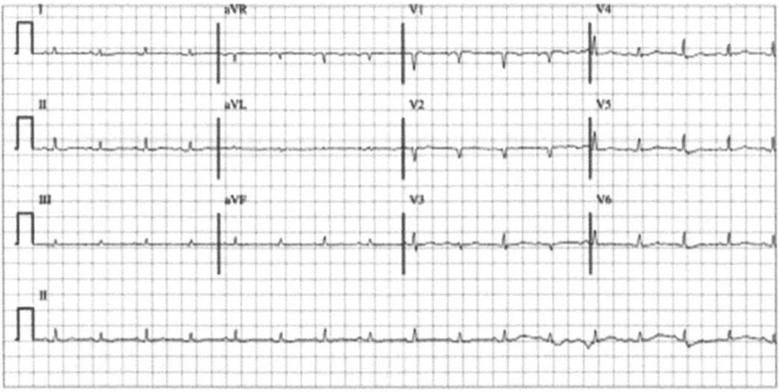

FIGURE 27.3 ECG from a patient with pericardial tamponade showing characteristic findings, including sinus tachycardia, electrical alternans (visible in lead II and lead V3), and low voltage

- CXR
  - Normal until effusions are moderate or larger
  - With larger effusions, can assume rounded appearance of the heart
- Echocardiography (TTE)
  - Perform urgent TTE if signs of pericardial effusion to assess for:

    Pericardial effusion

    - 2D echocardiography to assess size of effusion and location.
    - Circumferential effusion graded in diastole as small (<10 mm), medium (10–20 mm), or large (>20 mm) [9].
    - Assess quality of effusion and whether it is circumferential or loculated as this will guide options for drainage and/or pericardial window if indicated.

    Tamponade physiology

    - Late diastolic indentation or collapse of the right atrium
    - Early diastolic collapse of the right ventricle
    - Exaggerated respiratory variation in RV and LV size
    - Respiratory-phasic changes in tricuspid (>40%) and mitral (>25%) inflows
    - Dilated inferior vena cava (IVC) with <50% collapse with inspiration
- CT and MRI
  - Can be used to assess for pericardial thickening/effusion, calcifications, and co-occurring myopericarditis
  - Helpful to assess regional localization with loculated effusions

- Diagnostic procedures
  - Diagnostic pericardiocentesis should be considered in patients with large effusion or suspicion for malignancy, tuberculosis, or infection.
  - Pericardial biopsy should be considered in patients with recurrent effusions or malignant effusion.

Management

- Triage
  - Assess size, hemodynamic significance (particularly presence of tamponade), and associated conditions.
  - Admission is recommended for high-risk patients.
- Hemodynamically stable patients with pericardial effusion
  - Treatment should be targeted to the underlying cause.
  - If effusion is associated with pericarditis, treat the same as pericarditis (Table 27.1).
  - If symptomatic without evidence of inflammation or resolution in 1–2 weeks, consider pericardiocentesis.
  - If pericardial drain is placed, it is left in place until output <50 to 100 mL over 24 hours [2, 9, 14].
- Cardiac tamponade
  - Volume resuscitation emergently as patient is preload dependent.
  - Urgent drainage of pericardial effusion, preferentially with needle pericardiocentesis and drain placement under either echocardiographic or fluoroscopic guidance.
  - Surgical drainage may be necessary if the effusion is small, loculated, or unable to access through subxiphoid or apical approach (e.g., posterior effusion).
  - Can refer to surgery for pericardial window if recurrent effusions or risk of reaccumulation as with malignancy.

Key Learning Points

- Pericarditis is idiopathic in 80–90% of cases, usually in the setting of viral illness.
- Pericarditis can be managed safely as an outpatient unless high-risk features are present, including poor response to initial, conditions other than idiopathic etiologies, or signs of hemodynamic compromise.
- Treatment for acute pericarditis involves NSAIDs and colchicine and should be continued until there is symptom resolution with a slow taper to avoid risk of recurrent pericarditis.
- Pericardial effusion can present with minimal symptoms when it develops slowly due to the ability of the pericardium to stretch over time, although rapid accumulation can lead to cardiac tamponade even with minimal volumes.
- Pericardiocentesis should be considered, particularly when there are signs and/or symptoms of cardiac tamponade.

References

1. Gillaspie EA, Stulak JM, Daly RC, et al. A 20-year experience with isolated pericardiectomy: analysis of indications and outcomes. J Thorac Cardiovasc Surg. 2016;152(2):448–58. https://doi.org/10.1016/j.jtcvs.2016.03.098.
2. Chiabrando JG, Bonaventura A, Vecchié A, et al. Management of acute and recurrent pericarditis: JACC state-of-the-art review. J Am Coll Cardiol. 2020;75(1):76–92. https://doi.org/10.1016/j.jacc.2019.11.021.
3. Imazio M, Brucato A, Mayosi BM, et al. Medical therapy of pericardial diseases: Part I: idiopathic and infectious pericarditis. J Cardiovasc Med. 2010:712–22. https://doi.org/10.2459/JCM.0b013e3283340b97.
4. Imazio M. Evaluation and management of pericarditis. Expert Rev Cardiovasc Ther. 2011:1221–33. https://doi.org/10.1586/erc.11.111.

5. Maisch B, Rupp H, Ristic A, Pankuweit S. Pericardioscopy and epi- and pericardial biopsy – a new window to the heart improving etiological diagnoses and permitting targeted intrapericardial therapy. Heart Fail Rev. 2013;18(3):317–28. https://doi.org/10.1007/s10741-013-9382-y.
6. Altan M, Toki MI, Gettinger SN, et al. Immune checkpoint inhibitor–associated pericarditis. J Thorac Oncol. 2019;14(6):1102–8. https://doi.org/10.1016/j.jtho.2019.02.026.
7. Foris LA, Bhimji SS. Dressler syndrome. StatPearls Publishing; 2018.
8. Adler Y, Charron P, Imazio M, et al. ESC Guidelines for the diagnosis and management of pericardial diseases. Eur Heart J. 2015;2015:2921–64. https://doi.org/10.1093/eurheartj/ehv318.
9. Lewinter MM, Imazio M. 83 – pericardial diseases. Eleventh E: Elsevier Inc.; 2020.
10. Klein AL, Abbara S, Agler DA, et al. American society of echocardiography clinical recommendations for multimodality cardiovascular imaging of patients with pericardial disease: endorsed by the society for cardiovascular magnetic resonance and society of cardiovascular computed tomography. J Am Soc Echocardiogr. 2013;26(9):965–1012.e15. https://doi.org/10.1016/j.echo.2013.06.023.
11. Young PM, Glockner JF, Williamson EE, et al. MR imaging findings in 76 consecutive surgically proven cases of pericardial disease with CT and pathologic correlation. Int J Cardiovasc Imaging. 2012:1099–109. https://doi.org/10.1007/s10554-011-9916-0.
12. Pelliccia A, Solberg EE, Papadakis M, et al. Recommendations for participation in competitive and leisure time sport in athletes with cardiomyopathies, myocarditis, and pericarditis: Position statement of the Sport Cardiology Section of the European Association of Preventive Cardiology (EAPC). Eur Heart J. 2019;40(1):19–33. https://doi.org/10.1093/eurheartj/ehy730.
13. Imazio M, Bobbio M, Cecchi E, et al. Colchicine in addition to conventional therapy for acute pericarditis: results of the COlchicine for acute PEricarditis (COPE) trial. Circulation. 2005;112(13):2012–6. https://doi.org/10.1161/CIRCULATIONAHA.105.542738.
14. Imazio M, Brucato A, Cemin R, et al. A randomized trial of colchicine for acute pericarditis. N Engl J Med. 2013;369(16):1522–8. https://doi.org/10.1056/nejmoa1208536.

15. Imazio M, Brucato A, Cumetti D, et al. Corticosteroids for recurrent pericarditis: high versus low doses: a nonrandomized observation. Circulation. 2008;118(6):667–71. https://doi.org/10.1161/CIRCULATIONAHA.107.761064.
16. Brucato A, Imazio M, Gattorno M, et al. Effect of anakinra on recurrent pericarditis among patients with colchicine resistance and corticosteroid dependence: the AIRTRIP randomized clinical trial. JAMA – J Am Med Assoc. 2016;316(18):1906–12. https://doi.org/10.1001/jama.2016.15826.
17. Ben-Horin S, Bank I, Guetta V, Livneh A. Large symptomatic pericardial effusion as the presentation of unrecognized cancer: a study in 173 consecutive patients undergoing pericardiocentesis. Medicine (Baltimore). 2006;85(1):49–53. https://doi.org/10.1097/01.md.0000199556.69588.8e.
18. Atar S, Chiu J, Forrester JS, Siegel RJ. Bloody pericardial effusion in patients with cardiac tamponade. Is the cause cancerous, tuberculous, or iatrogenic in the 1990s? Chest. 1999;116(6):1564–9. https://doi.org/10.1378/chest.116.6.1564.

Part X
Miscellaneous Topics

Chapter 28
Simple Adult Congenital Heart Disease

Logan Eberly and Maan Jokhadar

Abbreviations

CHD	Congenital heart disease
ASD	Atrial septal defect
ECG	Electrocardiogram
TTE	Transthoracic echocardiogram
TEE	Transesophageal echocardiogram
Qp:Qs	Ratio of pulmonary to systemic flow
SVC	Superior vena cava
IVC	Inferior vena cava
PFO	Patent foramen ovale
VSD	Ventricular septal defect
PVR	Pulmonary vascular resistance
TOF	Tetralogy of Fallot

L. Eberly (✉) · M. Jokhadar
Department of Medicine, Division of Cardiology, Emory University School of Medicine, Atlanta, GA, USA
e-mail: LMEBERL@emory.edu; maan.jokhadar@emory.edu

A. A. Bhargava et al. (eds.), *Handbook of Outpatient Cardiology*, https://doi.org/10.1007/978-3-030-88953-1_28

Atrial Septal Defect (ASD)

A. Introduction

a. ASDs account for approximately 10% of CHD.
b. Typically result in a left-to-right shunt.
c. There are four different sub-types (Fig. 28.1).

B. Ostium Secundum ASD

a. Definition/Presentation

i. Ostium secundum ASDs are defects of the fossa ovalis and account for about 60% of all ASDs.
ii. Patients with an isolated ostium secundum ASD may not have symptoms for years and therefore often first present in adulthood, depending on the size.

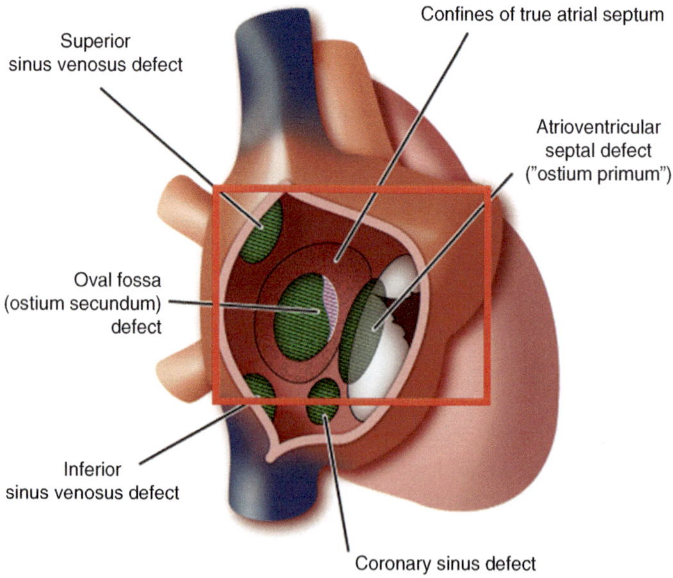

Figure 28.1 Schematic diagram outlines the different types of interatrial shunting that can be encountered. (With permissions from Zipes et al. [1])

iii. Patients may be asymptomatic at diagnosis (diagnosed by physical exam; see below); if symptomatic, they most commonly present with progressive exertional dyspnea and/or palpitations.

Clinical Pearl
Consider ASD in your differential diagnosis of an adult patient with otherwise unexplained exertional dyspnea and/or palpitations.

iv. Complications include:

1. Atrial fibrillation/flutter
2. Right heart failure
3. Pulmonary hypertension
4. Paradoxical embolism

v. Any condition that increases left atrial pressure (such as left ventricular dysfunction or mitral valve disease) increases the left-to-right shunt and worsens symptoms.

b. Physical Exam

i. Findings include:

1. Loud S1
2. Widely split and fixed S2
3. Pulmonary systolic ejection murmur loudest at the left upper sternal border
4. Tricuspid mid-diastolic murmur loudest at the left lower sternal border (due to increased flow across the tricuspid valve)

ii. If right-sided heart failure/pulmonary hypertension is present, exam may show signs of elevated jugular venous pressure and right ventricular heave.

c. Investigations

i. On electrocardiogram (ECG), one should look for sinus node dysfunction, prolonged PR interval, right axis deviation, rSr’ pattern in V1, and large P waves.

ii. On transthoracic echocardiogram (TTE), one should evaluate for color flow across the inter-atrial septum (as well as positive bubble study) and/or a dilated right ventricle. Doppler estimate of pulmonary artery pressure and an assessment for associated defects should be performed.
iii. Transesophageal echocardiogram (TEE) can often best characterize the ASD (precise size, margins, etc.) as well as identify the pulmonary veins (to assess for associated partial anomalous pulmonary venous return).
iv. Cardiac catheterization is performed to calculate pulmonary vascular resistance and determine the ratio of pulmonary to systemic flow (Qp:Qs). It is also often performed to evaluate for concomitant coronary artery disease prior to ASD repair.

d. ASD Closure

i. Indications for ASD closure include:

1. Evidence of right heart volume overload
2. Left-to-right shunt ratio greater than or equal to 1.5:1
3. Size greater than 10mm
4. Prevention of recurrent paradoxical embolism

ii. Contradictions to ASD closure include:

1. Significant pulmonary vascular disease
2. Severe left ventricular dysfunction
3. Significant mitral valve disease

iii. Ostium secundum ASDs can often be closed percutaneously or surgically.

C. Ostium Primum ASD

a. Ostium primum ASDs fall within the spectrum of endocardial cushion defects. They rarely occur in isolation and are typically seen as part of an atrioventricular septal defect (also referred to as an atrioventricular canal defect). Detailed discussion of atrioventricular septal defects is beyond the scope of this text.

D. Sinus Venosus ASD

a. Sinus venosus ASDs are caused by defects of the infolding of the atrial wall at the site of the superior vena cava (SVC) or inferior vena cava (IVC). Superior sinus venosus ASDs are more common than inferior sinus venosus ASDs.
b. With a superior sinus venosus ASD, the defect in the atrial wall leads to the SVC communicating with both atria; it is invariably associated with anomalous right-sided pulmonary venous return whereby the right-sided pulmonary veins drain into the SVC near its junction with the right atrium.
c. Sinus venosus ASDs account for approximately 2–3% of ASDs.
d. They can be associated with an ectopic atrial pacemaker (if the defect occurs in the area of the sinoatrial node); this can be seen on ECG as a leftward P wave axis and inverted P wave in lead III.
e. Presentation is similar to that of ostium secundum ASDs.
f. TEE should be performed both to evaluate the defect and to identify anomalous pulmonary venous drainage; MRI or CT may be required if the pulmonary venous return is not clearly seen on TEE.
g. The indications for closure are the same as for ostium secundum ASDs; however, sinus venosus ASDs are not suitable for percutaneous closure because of the lack of rim around the defect as well as the associated anomalous pulmonary venous return.

E. Coronary Sinus Defect

a. A coronary sinus defect is the rarest type of ASD. It is due to a defect that results in lack of separation between the coronary sinus and the left atrium.

b. The term unroofed coronary sinus is used to describe the variation of coronary sinus defect whereby the roof separating the coronary sinus and the left atrium is completely absent. This is usually associated with a persistent left SVC that drains into the coronary sinus, which results in right-to-left shunting and cyanosis.
c. TEE and cardiac catheterization are needed for further evaluation, and closure is done surgically.

Patent Foramen Ovale (PFO)

A. PFO is common and found in up to 25% of the population and is usually clinically silent.
B. PFO results from failure of fusion of the valve of the foramen ovale with the inter-atrial septum after birth when the left atrial pressure exceeds that of the right atrium; unlike ASDs, there is no defect in atrial septal tissue.
C. Most PFOs are found incidentally; however, paradoxical embolism can be a cause of cryptogenic stroke, particularly in young adults.
D. A PFO can be detected on contrast echocardiogram, whereby agitated saline is injected intravenously while an echocardiogram is obtained (can be done with TTE or TEE). A PFO is likely if, with Valsalva, bubbles appear within the left atrium within five heartbeats.
E. Patients with a diagnosed PFO who have had prior embolic stroke and have risk factors for venous thrombosis appear to benefit from PFO closure (which can be done percutaneously similar to ostium secundum ASD closure). However, a thorough evaluation of risk factors for alternative etiology of stroke should be performed prior to PFO closure.

Clinical Pearl
PFOs are commonly diagnosed on echocardiogram during the inpatient workup for stroke. However, one must complete a comprehensive evaluation to identify possible alternative etiologies for stroke before referral for PFO closure. If an alternative etiology is found, the patient is unlikely to benefit from PFO closure.

Ventricular Septal Defect (VSD)

A. Definition/Prevalence

a. The interventricular septum is composed of four parts: inlet septum, outlet septum, muscular (also known as trabecular) septum, and membranous septum. VSDs can arise from defects in any of these components (Fig. 28.2).
b. VSD is the most common congenital heart defect. Membranous VSDs are the most common type.
c. They can occur in isolation, in association with other lesions, or as part of a more complex condition (such as tetralogy of Fallot).

B. Presentation

a. The manner in which VSDs present clinically is dependent upon the size and hemodynamic effects of the defect.
b. Restrictive VSDs describe small defects with a high-pressure gradient between the left and right ventricles and a small shunt of no hemodynamic significance.
c. Larger defects are hemodynamically significant and cause left ventricular volume overload and progressive increase in pulmonary vascular resistance (PVR).

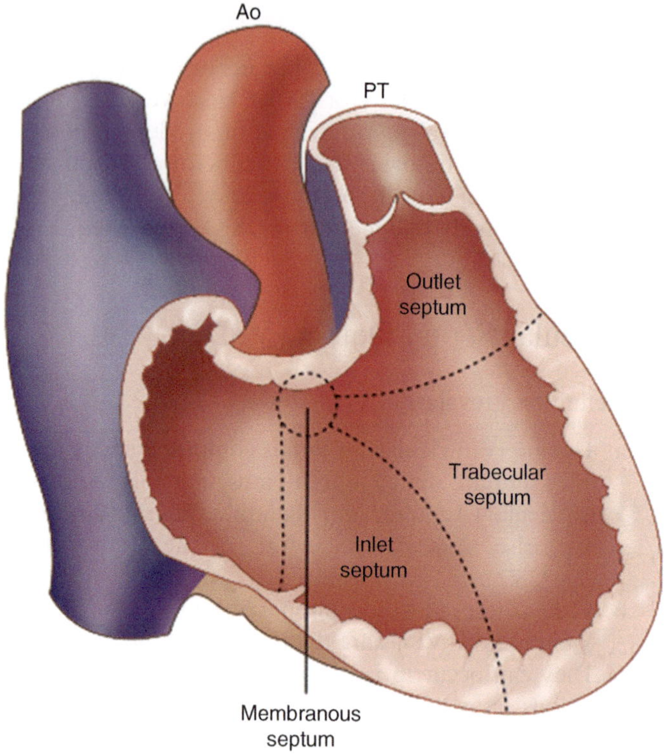

FIGURE 28.2 Four components of the ventricular septum are shown here from the right ventricular aspect. (*Ao* aorta, *PT* pulmonary trunk. With permissions from Zipes et al. [1])

d. In adults, un-operated restrictive VSDs are often asymptomatic, but a loud murmur is detected. Survivors of large un-operated VSDs are likely to have developed significant pulmonary hypertension and possibly Eisenmenger syndrome.

C. Physical Exam

a. Small restrictive VSDs cause a high-frequency pansystolic murmur loudest at the left sternal border.

b. Moderate-to-large nonrestrictive VSDs cause a displaced cardiac apex and a pan-systolic murmur, as well as an apical diastolic murmur and S3 (from increased flow through the mitral valve).

Clinical Pearl
The intensity of the systolic murmur due to a VSD is inversely proportional to the size of the VSD because of the increased turbulence and flow velocity produced by a smaller defect.

D. Investigations

a. With large defects, ECG may show right axis deviation and biventricular hypertrophy. The ECG is often unremarkable in small defects.
b. TTE is used to characterize the size, location, and hemodynamic consequences of the VSD, as well as to identify associated lesions. Moderate-sized VSDs cause left atrial and left ventricular volume overload, which leads to dilation of these chambers. Large VSDs that have already resulted in increased PVR cause right ventricular pressure overload, which leads to right ventricular hypertrophy.
c. Cardiac catheterization is performed to calculate the size of the shunt as well as PVR.

E. VSD Closure

a. Indications for closure include symptoms and Qp:Qs greater than 1.5:1, ventricular dysfunction with right ventricular pressure or left ventricular volume overload, or a previous episode of endocarditis.
b. Selected membranous and muscular VSDs are suitable for percutaneous closure; however, surgical repair is usually necessary when indicated.
c. It should be noted that damage to the conduction system is relatively common during VSD closure (either

percutaneous or surgical), especially for membranous VSDs. Right bundle branch block is common post-procedure, and complete heart block can occur, and if it is persistent, a pacemaker is required.

Tetralogy of Fallot (TOF)

A. Introduction

  a. The underlying abnormality in TOF is the antero-cephalad deviation of the outlet ventricular septum. This leads to the four features (Fig. 28.3).

    i. VSD
    ii. Sub-pulmonary stenosis
    iii. Aorta that overrides the interventricular septum
    iv. Secondary right ventricular hypertrophy

  b. TOF is the most common cyanotic congenital heart defect.

B. Natural History (Un-operated)

  a. If un-operated, survival past 40 years of age is rare.
  b. Survival into adulthood without repair is dependent upon mild right ventricular outflow tract obstruction in childhood. Patients with severe obstruction will have cyanosis early in life and will not survive to adulthood without repair.
  c. Complications from un-operated TOF include the following:

    i. Cyanosis
    ii. Arrhythmia (atrial or ventricular)
    iii. Ascending aortic dilation and aortic regurgitation

      1. Aortic regurgitation leads to volume overload of both ventricles and biventricular failure.

    iv. Endocarditis

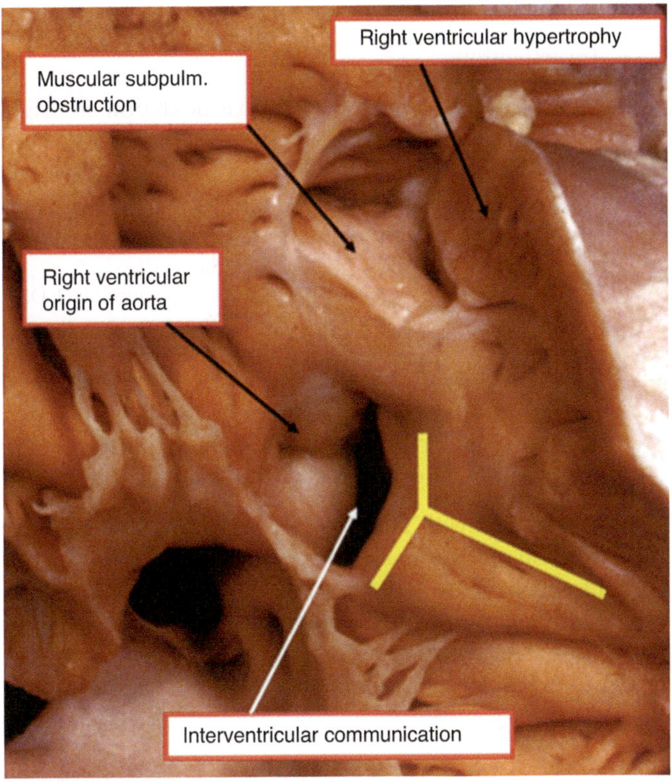

FIGURE 28.3 The photograph, taken from the apex of the right ventricle looking toward the base, shows the features of tetralogy of Fallot. The infundibulum is inserted to the antero-cephalad limb of the septomarginal trabeculation (*yellow* Y). (With permissions from Wernovsky et al. [2])

d. Physical exam findings of patients with un-operated TOF include the following:

   i. Cyanosis and clubbing
   ii. Right ventricular heave
   iii. Palpable thrill and loud systolic ejection murmur (from the right ventricular outflow tract obstruction)

iv. Soft P2

e. Investigations

i. ECG typically shows right axis deviation and right ventricular hypertrophy.
ii. Chest x-ray may show a boot-shaped heart and decreased pulmonary vascularity.
iii. Echocardiography makes the diagnosis.

C. TOF Repair

a. Surgical repair involves the following:

i. Patch closure of the VSD
ii. Resection of the infundibular stenosis
iii. Transannular patch to enlarge the pulmonary valve annulus in most patients

b. Most adults with TOF have undergone repair and have a good prognosis. However, lifetime follow-up is required due to increased risk of complications, particularly relating to the pulmonary valve and the need for pulmonary valve replacement.
c. Sequelae of repair can include the following:

i. Right bundle branch block

1. This occurs in almost all patients after repair because the right bundle runs in the floor of the VSD and is damaged during surgery.

ii. Pulmonary regurgitation (more on this below)
iii. Late complete heart block
iv. Residual right ventricular outflow tract obstruction
v. Aortic dilation and aortic regurgitation
vi. Endocarditis
vii. Arrhythmia and arrhythmogenic sudden death

D. Pulmonary Regurgitation After Repair

a. Most patients with TOF repair have severe pulmonary regurgitation that results from the relief of pulmonary stenosis and RVOT obstruction at the time of repair (transannular patch). Severe pulmonary regurgitation is usually well tolerated for several years or decades but most will eventually require pulmonary valve replacement. Pulmonary valve replacement is not a usual part of initial TOF repair.
b. Signs of severe pulmonary regurgitation include the following:
    i. Loss of sinus rhythm
    ii. Signs of right heart failure (elevated jugular venous pressure, hepatomegaly, peripheral edema, etc.)
    iii. Right ventricular heave
    iv. Soft or absent P2 (single S2)
    v. To and fro systolic and diastolic murmur of pulmonary regurgitation (the diastolic murmur is often missed when it is short with rapid decrescendo)
c. Investigations
    i. With few exceptions, ECG shows RBBB with QRS widening. Varying degrees of atrioventricular block can also be present. Longer QRS duration is associated with more severe RV dilation and arrhythmia risk.
    ii. In addition to demonstrating the severe pulmonary regurgitation, echocardiography is important to evaluate for other abnormalities, including:
        1. Ventricular dysfunction
        2. Paradoxical interventricular septal motion
        3. Residual VSD
        4. Aortic root dilation
        5. Aortic regurgitation
        6. Residual right ventricular outflow tract obstruction

iii. Cardiopulmonary exercise testing is often beneficial to objectively quantify exercise intolerance.

d. Indications for pulmonary valve replacement

i. Severe pulmonary regurgitation and any of the following:

1. Increasing symptoms
2. Impaired exercise tolerance on cardiopulmonary exercise testing
3. Arrhythmias
4. Progressive right ventricular dilation or dysfunction

Clinical Pearl
Severe pulmonary regurgitation after TOF repair can be asymptomatic for years. Indications for referral for pulmonary valve replacement include worsening symptoms, objective evidence of exercise intolerance, or right ventricular dilation or dysfunction.

Cyanotic Heart Disease: The Basics

A. Introduction

a. There are many specific defects that cause cyanosis other than TOF. Discussion of the details of each specific condition is beyond the scope of this text. Nevertheless, there are some general principles that apply to the care of the cyanotic patient with which adult providers should be familiar. These patients are typically followed at tertiary referral centers; however, they often live far away from these centers and may be co-managed with a local outpatient provider. This underlies the need for these providers to have a basic understanding of cyanotic heart disease.

b. Cyanosis is present when there is a right-to-left shunt. The shunt can occur at any level—intra-cardiac, between the great vessels, or intrapulmonary.
c. Cyanosis is typically clinically detectable when oxygen saturations are less than 85%.
d. It is important to remember that cyanosis is a multi-system disorder.

B. General Principles for Patients with Cyanotic Heart Disease

a. Supplemental oxygen should be used primarily for symptom relief and/or to maintain baseline oxygen saturations; oxygen is a pulmonary vasodilator, and depending on the patient's anatomy, excessive oxygen may cause pulmonary edema.
b. One should use 0.22 micron air filters on all intravenous lines and use infusion pumps with a bubble detector to prevent paradoxical bubble emboli.
c. Adequate hemoglobin concentration should be maintained to optimize oxygen-carrying capacity.
d. Phlebotomy should only be performed if there are signs and symptoms of hyperviscosity (headache, confusion, etc.) due to very high hemoglobin concentration. Phlebotomy can cause a relative iron deficiency anemia, which can increase thromboembolic risk.
e. Vasodilators should only be used with caution and under the supervision of an adult congenital cardiologist.

Clinical Pearl
One must be aware of the common pitfalls in caring for cyanotic patients—avoid the following: (1) excessive supplemental oxygen, (2) vasodilators, and (3) excessive phlebotomy.

C. Causes of Clinical Deterioration in Cyanotic Heart Disease

a. Tachyarrhythmias

    i. Atrial arrhythmias are often atypical.
    ii. Tachyarrhythmias are often not well tolerated, and prompt restoration of sinus rhythm may be required.
    iii. Electrical cardioversion is often safer and more effective than anti-arrhythmic therapy.

b. Hemoptysis

    i. Hemoptysis can be life-threatening and warrants inpatient admission. It is one of the leading causes of death in cyanotic patients, especially in those with pulmonary hypertension.
    ii. Chest CT should be obtained to identify the site of bleeding.
    iii. Possible sources of hemoptysis include:

        1. Pulmonary artery thrombus
        2. Bleeding from a pulmonary arteriovenous malformation
        3. Bleeding collateral vessels
        4. Chest infection

Key Learning Points

1. There are currently more adults than children living with CHD in the United States; therefore, adult outpatient providers need to be familiar with commonly encountered congenital heart defects.
2. ASDs comprise about 10% of CHD, and the diagnosis should be considered in patients with otherwise unexplained exertional dyspnea.
3. VSD is the most common congenital heart defect, and auscultation of the systolic murmur can lead to the diagnosis in asymptomatic patients.
4. Severe pulmonary regurgitation is common after TOF repair, and pulmonary valve replacement will eventually be needed in most patients, once indica-

tions arise, which include signs or symptoms of RV dilation and dysfunction.

5. For patients with cyanotic CHD, excessive oxygen supplementation, unnecessary phlebotomy, and vasodilators should be avoided, and 0.22 micron air filters should be used on all IVs. Arrhythmias should be treated aggressively, and hemoptysis can be life-threatening and warrants inpatient admission.

References

1. Zipes DP, Libby P, Bonow RO, Mann DL, Tomaselli GF, Braunwald E. Braunwalds heart disease a textbook of cardiovascular medicine. Philadelphia, PA: Elsevier; 2019.
2. Wernovsky G, Anderson RH, Kumar K, Mussatto K, Redington AN, Tweddell JS, et al. Anderson's pediatric cardiology. 4th ed. Elsevier; 2020.

Chapter 29
Pregnancy and Heart Disease

Mariana Garcia, An Young, and Gina Lundberg

Abbreviations

ACS	Acute coronary syndrome
ACOG	American College of Obstetricians and Gynecologists
CV	Cardiovascular
CHD	Coronary heart disease
HF	Heart failure
HCM	Hypertrophic cardiomyopathy
LV	Left ventricular
PPCM	Peripartum cardiomyopathy
VHD	Valvular heart disease
VT	Ventricular tachycardia

M. Garcia (✉) · A. Young · G. Lundberg
Department of Medicine, Division of Cardiology, Emory University School of Medicine, Atlanta, GA, USA
e-mail: mgarc40@emory.edu; an.young@emory.edu; gina.lundberg@emory.edu

A. A. Bhargava et al. (eds.), *Handbook of Outpatient Cardiology*, https://doi.org/10.1007/978-3-030-88953-1_29

Cardiac Disorders and Pregnancy

- Cardio-obstetrics is a growing field of expertise among cardiologists who care for high-risk pregnancies due to underlying heart disease or heart disease development as a complication or adverse pregnancy outcome.
- A team-based approach is used in caring for these women, based on proper training and experience as well as collaboration between obstetrics, primary care, cardiologists, and the cardio-obstetrics team [1, 2].
- Patients with known heart disease should request advice regarding future pregnancy. Patient education, preferably prior to conception, is key. Before referring to a cardiac preconception consultant, the following issues can be discussed with your patient:
- Maternal risk during pregnancy.
- Potential risks to the fetus, including adverse effects of cardiac medications.
- The risk of transmission of heart disease to the fetus.
- Important considerations for the management of antepartum and postpartum risks.
- Long-term risk to the mother and possible effect on maternal lifespan.
- Recommendations on safe birth control, interventions, or medications when appropriate to reduce maternal or fetal risk prior to pregnancy.

Normal Physiologic Changes During Pregnancy and the Puerperium

- Pregnancy involves marked physiologic changes that affect the cardiovascular (CV) system, with significant blood volume and hemodynamics changes.
- These changes can represent a "stress test" to the heart and cardiac function and reserve.
- More physicians, including primary care providers, are involved in the care of pregnant women with established heart disease today, due in part to pregnancy at an older

age and the increasing number of women with congenital heart disease who reach childbearing age.

A comprehensive understanding of the physiologic changes of pregnancy and their potential impact on maternal outcomes is critical. Table 29.1 summarizes hemodynamic changes with term pregnancy, labor and delivery, and the postpartum period.

TABLE 29.1 Cardiovascular changes associated with pregnancy

Physiologic parameter	Term pregnancy	Labor and delivery	Postpartum
Cardiac output	Increases 30–50%	Increases 50%	Increases 60–80% within 15–20 minutes, returns to pre-labor values within 1 hour of delivery
Blood volume	Increases 34–70% (50% average)	Additional 300–500 mL with each contraction	Decreases to baseline
Heart rate	Increases 15–20 bpm	Increase dependent on stress and pain relief	Decreases to baseline
Blood pressure	By mid-pregnancy, decreases 15–20 mm hg	Increase dependent on stress and pain relief	Decreases to baseline
Systemic vascular resistance	Decreases	Increases	Decreases to baseline
Oxygen consumption	Increases by 20%	Increases with stress of labor and delivery	Decreases to baseline
Red blood cell mass	Increases by 15–33%	---	---

Pregnant Women and Common Cardiac Symptoms

- The evaluation of heart disease in pregnancy may be problematic given the normal physiologic changes of the cardiovascular system.
- These changes can lead to signs and symptoms that can either simulate or obscure cardiac disease. A list of the various signs and symptoms of normal versus abnormal pregnancy, adapted from the American College of Obstetricians and Gynecologists (ACOG) 2019 Guideline, is included in Table 29.2.

Additional diagnostic tools are needed to obtain objective and reliable cardiac status information in many cases. The selection of such tools should be influenced by their diagnostic yield and the potential risk to the fetus. Table 29.3 summarizes clinical pearls as they relate to potential diagnostic tools in pregnancy [3].

TABLE 29.2 Signs and symptoms of normal vs abnormal pregnancy. Adapted from the 2019 American College of Obstetricians and Gynecologist Practice Bulletin

Normal	**Abnormal**
Dyspnea, fatigue, exercise intolerance, peripheral edema	S4 and diastolic murmurs
Right ventricle dilation	Sustained tachycardia with heart rate ≥120
Increased splitting of S2 due to increased volume on the right side of the heart	Ventricular tachycardias
Systolic ejection murmur, S3, or venous hum	Brady-arrhythmias
Mild left axis deviation on EKG	Elevated jugular venous pressure
Limited ectopy: Atrial or ventricular premature beats, supraventricular tachycardias	Gallop
	Marked edema
	Exertional or unprovoked syncope
	Systolic blood pressure ≥160

TABLE 29.3 Diagnostic tools for cardiovascular disease in pregnancy

Diagnostic tool	Clinical pearls	Findings during normal pregnancy
Chest x-ray	Radiation associated is minimal; however, due to the risks associated with fetal exposure to ionizing radiation should not be used casually	Straightening of the left upper cardiac border due to prominence of the pulmonary conus Horizontal position of the heart due to elevated diaphragm Increased lung marking seen with increased pulmonary venous pressure due to increased left atrial pressure Small pleural effusion in early postpartum period
EKG	Numerous studies have reported on changes in EKG in normal pregnant women as compared to nonpregnant women These changes may be due to change in position of the maternal heart in relation to the chest wall as a result of elevation of the diaphragm, changes in cardiac chambers size and wall thickness, and changes in the electrical properties of the myocardium due to sympathetic and hormonal effects	Left QRS axis deviation Q wave in leads II, III, and AVF T wave abnormalities (flattening or inversion in leads III, V1–V3) ST-segment and T wave changes (in tocolysis, cesarean section, anesthesia) Sinus tachycardia Atrial and ventricular premature beats Increased R/S ratio in leads V1 and V

(continued)

TABLE 29.3 (continued)

Diagnostic tool	Clinical pearls	Findings during normal pregnancy
Echocardiography	Transthoracic echocardiography is the favored diagnostic tool during pregnancy due to its availability and safety There is limited information on the safety of transesophageal echocardiograms in pregnancy, and there are no category A drugs used for sedation for patients undergoing one	Mildly increased left ventricular diastolic and systolic dimensions Unchanged left ventricular ejection fraction or fractional shortening Increased left ventricular radial and longitudinal strain Moderate increase in left atrium diameter and volume Moderate increase in right atrial and ventricular size Progressive dilatation of pulmonary, tricuspid, and mitral valve annuli Functional pulmonary, tricuspid, and mitral regurgitation Small pericardial effusion
Stress test	Useful in establishing ischemic heart disease in pregnancy or assessing functional capacity in known disease Submaximal exercise protocols such as the Naughton and the modified Bruce treadmill protocol are preferred over a regular Bruce protocol during pregnancy	

TABLE 29.3 (continued)

Diagnostic tool	Clinical pearls	Findings during normal pregnancy
Cardiac catheterization	May be indicated in cardiac decompensation during pregnancy when alternative noninvasive measures have failed Consider only when benefit outweighs risk, because it is associated with increased risk of iatrogenic coronary dissections	
Magnetic resonance imaging	Due to the absence of ionizing radiation, MRI is a favored imaging modality in pregnant women with congenital heart disease and for evaluation of the aorta in patients at risk for aortic dilatation and dissection	
Cardiovascular computed tomography	May be considered during pregnancy to rule out pulmonary embolism and aortic dissection when information cannot be obtained by other imaging modalities or invasive procedures are not desired	
BNP and proBNP	Levels are somewhat higher during early postpartum period but is usually within normal range during pregnancy and postpartum and may thus be a useful tool	

Hypertension Disorders of Pregnancy

- Hypertension is a relatively common finding during pregnancy, occurring in 6% to 8% of pregnancies and contributing significantly to stillbirths and neonatal morbidity and mortality. Hypertensive disorders are categorized into four major classes (summarized in Table 29.4) according to the ACOG:

  1. Chronic hypertension.
  2. Gestational hypertension.

Table 29.4 Hypertensive disorders of pregnancy

Hypertensive disorder class	Definition/clinical pearls	Percentage of pregnancies
Chronic hypertension	Occurs before 20 weeks of gestation or persists >12 weeks postpartum	5%
Gestational hypertension	Elevated BP after 20 weeks of gestation without proteinuria or other features of preeclampsia	7%
Preeclampsia/ eclampsia	HTN after 20 weeks of gestation and proteinuria or end-organ dysfunction +/– proteinuria -proteinuria diagnosed with 300 mg of protein per 24-h urine or a urinary protein-to-creatinine ratio of greater than 0.3 Eclampsia includes seizures	Preeclampsia: 2–5% Eclampsia: 0.003%
Chronic hypertension with superimposed preeclampsia	Those with chronic HTN who develop worsening HTN with proteinuria or other features of preeclampsia	1% (20–25% of chronic HTN patients)

3. Preeclampsia/eclampsia.
4. Chronic hypertension with superimposed preeclampsia [4].

There is growing consensus that preeclampsia is associated with an increased overall risk of cardiovascular disease, including future incident coronary heart disease, composite cardiovascular disease, heart failure, stroke, and CV death [5–8].

ACOG Recommendations for the Management of Hypertension Disorders of Pregnancy

- Methyldopa, labetalol, and nifedipine are recommended as first-line oral medications for the management of hypertension during pregnancy [4].
- Total body volume is reduced in preeclampsia, and further diuresis may worsen a hypovolemic state, leading to placental hypoperfusion; therefore, diuretics are a second-line recommendation [9].
- Due to association between first trimester in utero exposure and hypospadias, as well as association with thrombocytopenia and neonatal lupus-like syndrome in third trimester exposure, hydralazine is also considered a second-line medication.
- Angiotensin-converting enzyme inhibitors and angiotensin receptor blockers (ARBs) are contraindicated throughout pregnancy due to risks of oligohydramnios, intrauterine growth restriction, hypocalvaria, renal dysplasia, anuria, and fetal demise [10].
- During pregnancy, hypertensive emergencies defined as systolic blood pressure $\geq$ 180 mmHg and/or diastolic blood pressure $\geq$ 120 mmHg may be treated with the intravenous agents labetalol, hydralazine, and nifedipine, which are recommended as acceptable medications [4].

Congenital Heart Disease and Pregnancy

- A growing number of women with congenital heart disease (CHD) are reaching childbearing age and contemplating pregnancy. These women are usually aware of their congenital diagnosis before pregnancy; however, on occasion, the hemodynamic stress of pregnancy will unmask a previously unrecognized lesion.

- It is important for pregnant patients with CHD to be followed at a center that has expertise in both pregnancy and heart disease. A multidisciplinary team is always advisable to optimize outcomes.
- All caregivers should have access to the management plans for following the pregnancy, labor and delivery, and postpartum surveillance.
- Postpartum surveillance is particularly important because many cardiac complications occur during this period.
- Guidelines and scientific statements to assist in pregnancy care of women with CHD are available from the American Heart Association/American College of Cardiology [11, 12] and the European Society of Cardiology [13].

Clinical Pearl
Risk of Congenital Disorders

- In general, low-risk lesions include atrial septal defects (repaired or unrepaired), ventricular septal defects (repaired or unrepaired), and patent ductus arteriosus (repaired or unrepaired).
- Intermediate-risk lesions include repaired coarctation of the aorta, repaired tetralogy of Fallot, Ebstein anomaly (repaired or unrepaired), and arterial switch operation (Jatene operation).
- High-risk lesions include arterial switch operation (Mustard or Senning operation), Fontan operation, and Eisenmenger syndrome.

Native Valvular Heart Disease in Pregnancy

- Valvular heart disease (VHD) due to both congenital and acquired etiologies in pregnant patients continues to be a challenging aspect of patient care [14].

- The management for this group of patients should ideally begin before conception. A complete preconception evaluation includes:
  - Careful history and physical examination.
  - 12-lead EKG
  - Echocardiogram.
  - Exercise stress test for objective assessment of functional capacity.

Referral to a cardiologist with expertise in pregnancy management and a high-risk obstetrician is important for individualized discussion of the anticipated risk of pregnancy. Table 29.5 summarizes the optimal management of specific valvular disorders.

Peripartum Cardiomyopathy

- The European Society of Cardiology Working Group on Peripartum Cardiomyopathy (PPCM) has recently expanded the definition of PPCM to "an idiopathic cardiomyopathy presenting with heart failure (HF) secondary to left ventricular (LV) systolic dysfunction toward the end of pregnancy or in the months following delivery, where no other cause of heart failure is found" [15]. Predisposing factors include:
  - Multiparity.
  - Multifetal pregnancy.
  - Preeclampsia.
  - Advanced age.
  - African-American race.
  - Diabetes.
  - Malnutrition [16].
- PPCM is a diagnosis of exclusion and should be considered whenever a patient, without a prior history of congestive heart failure, presents with paroxysmal nocturnal dyspnea, new regurgitant murmurs, pulmonary edema,

TABLE 29.5 Management of specific valvular disorders. Adapted from Elkayam et al. Cardiac Problems in Pregnancy [44]

	Pregnancy not advised	Pregnancy management	Delivery
Mitral stenosis	Moderate to severe mitral stenosis (valve area <1.5 cm2) History of systemic embolism New-onset atrial fibrillation Increased pulmonary artery pressure (systolic pulmonary arterial pressure > 50 mmHg	*Laboratory* Close follow-up with frequent monitoring of symptoms, BNP or NT-ProBNP levels, echocardiographic pulmonary pressures *Physiology* Reduction of heart rate with β-blockers (β-1 selective preferred, like metoprolol or atenolol, high dose often required) *Rhythm* Cardioversion to sinus rhythm in new atrial fibrillation and rapid ventricular response *Anticoagulation* For paroxysmal or permanent atrial fibrillation or sinus rhythm with a history of thromboembolic events, left atrial thrombus *Invasive* Percutaneous mitral balloon commissurotomy (PMBC) in non-responding symptomatic patients Surgical mitral valve replacement in cases not amenable to PMBC	Vaginal delivery at term recommended C-section in case of fetal or maternal clinical deterioration

Mitral regurgitation	Symptomatic patients with severe mitral regurgitation Asymptomatic patients with LV dysfunction, pulmonary hypertension, or markedly reduced exercise tolerance Surgery should be considered before pregnancy in asymptomatic patients with preserved LVEF (>60%) and LVESD 40–44 mm with likelihood of durable repair	*Laboratory* Frequent monitoring of symptoms and BNP or NT-ProBNP levels *Volume* Diuretics for heart failure *Physiology* β-Blockers and oral vasodilators (hydralazine and isosorbide dinitrate) for patients with reduced LVEF	Vaginal delivery at term preferred C-section in case of fetal or maternal clinical deterioration
Aortic stenosis	Severe aortic stenosis Symptomatic Asymptomatic patients with markedly decreased exercise tolerance Impaired LV systolic function Aortic diameter >5 cm	*Laboratory* BNP or NT-ProBNP levels *Invasive* Percutaneous balloon valvuloplasty (PCBV) in severe uncontrolled symptoms TAVR Surgical valve replacement if PCBV not possible or not successful	Vaginal delivery at term preferred C-section in case of fetal or maternal clinical deterioration
Aortic regurgitation	Symptomatic aortic regurgitation LVEF <50% Asymptomatic severe AR with LVEDD >70 mm or LVESD >50 mm	*Laboratory* BNP or NT-ProBNP levels *Volume* Salt restriction, diuretics for heart failure *Physiology* Vasodilators and digoxin for LV systolic dysfunction	Vaginal delivery at term preferred C-section in case of fetal or maternal clinical deterioration

elevated jugular venous pressure, and hepatomegaly during the peripartum period.

- Available information in the United States demonstrates normalization of LV function in >50% of women with PPCM, mostly occurring within 2 to 6 months after diagnosis with later recovery occurring in some patients [17].
- In general, the treatment of HF in patients with PPCM should follow recent guideline recommendations.
- Certain drug therapies may need to be altered during pregnancy and lactation because of potential detrimental effects on the fetus or the lactating infant. The essential therapies for patients with acute PPCM have been summarized under the BOARD label: bromocriptine, oral heart failure therapies, anticoagulants, vasorelaxing agents, and diuretics [18].
- Subsequent pregnancies in women with history of PPCM are associated with a risk for recurrent and persistent cardiac dysfunction and even mortality. The risk is substantially higher in patients with persistent LV dysfunction before subsequent pregnancy [19].

Hypertrophic Cardiomyopathy and Pregnancy

- Hypertrophic cardiomyopathy (HCM), the most common inherited cardiovascular disorder, affects roughly 1 in 500 people worldwide [20].
- It is defined by the presence of increased LV wall thickness that is not solely explained by abnormal loading conditions [21, 22].
- Genetic linkage studies in familial HCM have demonstrated autosomal dominant disease loci in several chromosomal sites. Most of the genetic loci in familial HCM encode one of the myocardial contractile proteins of the cardiac sarcomere. Mutations in the cardiac myosin binding protein-C gene and cardiac beta-myosin heavy chain gene are the two most common mutations that account for 70% of identifiable mutations in HCM [23, 24].

- Echocardiography is safely used in pregnancy and is considered a definitive test for the diagnosis of HCM. The following echocardiographic criteria are used to establish the diagnosis:

  (i) Unexplained maximal wall thickness exceeding 15 mm in any myocardial segment.
  (ii) Septal/posterior wall thickness ratio >1.3 in normotensive patient.
  (iii) Septal/posterior wall thickness ratio >1.5 in hypertensive patient [25].

- It is of utmost importance to obtain a detailed evaluation prior to conception to establish the possible risks related to pregnancy and develop a treatment plan aimed at minimizing risks to both mother and fetus.
- Important discussions will be needed in advance regarding the possible effects of the disease on pregnancy safety for both mother and fetus, the potential fetal risks due to medications that may be required during pregnancy, and the possible need for premature delivery in case of clinical deterioration. Lastly, the likelihood of genetic inheritance of HCM to the fetus should be discussed, as well as the small risk of maternal sudden death during and after pregnancy.
- Detailed evaluation of HCM patients includes:

  - Comprehensive medical and family history.
  - Physical examination.
  - 12-lead EKG
  - Transthoracic echocardiogram.
  - B-type natriuretic peptide (BNP) or NT-proBNP levels.
  - Treadmill or bicycle exercise testing.

- Frequently, a cardiac consultation with expertise in pregnancy will be needed and can help to decide if additional evaluation, such as cardiopulmonary exercise test, 48-hour ambulatory EKG monitoring, and/or cardiovascular magnetic resonance imaging, is needed.

- According to available data, the majority of patients with HCM tolerate pregnancy with no issues and have a very low risk of mortality. Nonetheless, adverse outcomes, including heart failure, chest pain, palpitations, and atrial and ventricular arrhythmias, are not uncommon and can result in maternal and fetal morbidity [26–28].

Acute Myocardial Infarction in Pregnancy

- Acute coronary syndrome (ACS) complicating pregnancy is rare but accounts for a considerable proportion of cardiovascular-related mortality in pregnancy [29].

Clinical Pearl

- The etiology of coronary artery disease (CAD) in pregnancy frequently has a non-atherosclerotic mechanism, including spontaneous coronary artery dissection (43%), angiographically normal coronary arteries (18%), and coronary thrombosis (17%) [30].

Management of ACS During Pregnancy

- ACS management in pregnancy is similar to that in the general population. Percutaneous coronary intervention (PCI) can be performed safely in pregnancy due to low fetal radiation dose (<0.1 Gy) [31].
- In the event of maternal cardiac arrest, resuscitation and delivery should be performed per existing guidelines [32].
- Low-dose aspirin appears to be safe, and in general, clopidogrel is only used when strictly needed (after stenting). Glycoprotein IIb/IIIa inhibitors and statins should be avoided [30]. The benefits of short-term heparinization during PCI outweigh the risk of bleeding complications.
- Dual antiplatelet therapy with clopidogrel does not increase risk of fetal bleeding; however, it can cause bleeding if administered within 7 days of surgery. Some experts

recommend discontinuation 1 week before delivery [33]. The risk of stent thrombosis from early cessation of dual antiplatelet therapy should be weighed against the risk of bleeding at delivery.

- In pregnancy, coronary artery bypass grafting (CABG) is generally avoided due to elevated fetal mortality associated with cardiopulmonary bypass [34]. However, bypass grafting is sometimes necessary in cases of hemodynamic instability, obstructed coronary blood flow, or PCI failure. Bypass grafting without cardiopulmonary bypass or delivery before CABG can be considered during pregnancy [35].

Arrhythmias in Pregnancy

- Pregnancy is associated with a higher incidence of arrhythmias, partly explained by hemodynamic changes and increased sympathetic tone in pregnancy.
- Common arrhythmias in pregnancy include premature atrial and ventricular complexes, while ventricular tachycardia (VT) or fibrillation are extremely rare [36].

The initial step in the evaluation of pregnant patients with palpitations or syncope should include a 12-lead EKG and Holter monitoring [37]. Table 29.6 provides a summary of key management strategies based on ESC guidelines [38].

Management of Arrhythmias During Pregnancy

- If indicated, adenosine and direct cardioversion are considered safe during pregnancy [39].
- Pregnant women who require a cardioversion during the third trimester should be intubated prior to the procedure to decrease risk of aspiration [37].
- Pregnant women with atrial fibrillation and no structural heart disease with CHA2DS2VASC score ≥ 2 are candidates for systemic anticoagulation for thromboprophylaxis

TABLE 29.6 Management of arrhythmias in pregnancy

Arrhythmia	Initial management	Secondary management
Limited PAC or PVC without underlying cardiac disease	Reassurance	β-Blocker (if symptomatic)
SVT	Vagal stimulation if stable β-Blockers and digoxin if recurrent	Adenosine and cardioversion if unstable Flecainide, propafenone Rule out structural heart disease
SVT or atrial fibrillation with WPW	Cardioversion in acute situations	Flecainide, propafenone for long-term control
Atrial fibrillation Atrial flutter	β-1 selective blocker Anticoagulation	Cardioversion Rule out thyroid disease
Ventricular tachycardia Ventricular fibrillation	Cardioversion	EKG to rule out long QT Echocardiogram to rule out peripartum cardiomyopathy β-Blocker, anti-arrhythmic Implantable cardioverter-defibrillator
High-degree AV block	Temporary pacing in acute situation	Check for structural heart disease or myocarditis Pacemaker if persistent

Adapted from the European Society of Cardiology 2018 Guidelines for Management of Cardiovascular Disease in Pregnancy
Abbreviations: *PAC*, premature atrial tachycardia; *PVC*, premature ventricular tachycardia; *SVT*, supraventricular tachycardia; *WPW*, *Wolff-Parkinson-white*; *AV*, atrioventricular

and may be reasonable even in women without other risk factors due to the hypercoagulable state of pregnancy [40–42].

- Women with long QT syndrome are at increased risk of VT and require treatment with β-blockers throughout pregnancy and at least 40 weeks postpartum [43].

Clinical Pearl

- Amiodarone should be avoided due to risk of fetal thyroid suppression [42].

Key Learning Points

- For most women of reproductive age, pregnancy and the postpartum period provide an early "stress test" to identify underlying, often undiagnosed cardiovascular risk factors that identify future risk of CVD or unmasked established heart disease.
- Preventive medicine is a cornerstone of primary care. Medical care in the outpatient setting has a unique opportunity to improve outcomes in this patient population through earlier identification and management of these well-documented risk factors for CVD to preserve and improve long-term health.

Acknowledgments We would like to acknowledge the support of the Byron William Jr., MD Fellowship Fund.

References

1. Mehta LS, Warnes CA, Bradley E, Burton T, Economy K, Mehran R, et al. Cardiovascular considerations in caring for pregnant patients: A scientific statement from the American Heart Association. Circulation. 2020;141(23):e884–903.
2. Grodzinsky A, Florio K, Spertus JA, Daming T, Lee J, Rader V, et al. Importance of the cardio-obstetrics team. Curr Treat Options Cardiovasc Med. 2019;21(12):84.

3. Committee Opinion No. 723. Guidelines for diagnostic imaging during pregnancy and lactation. Obstet Gynecol. 2017;130(4):e210–e6.
4. Hypertension in pregnancy. Report of the American college of obstetricians and gynecologists' task force on hypertension in pregnancy. Obstet Gynecol. 2013;122(5):1122–31.
5. Bellamy L, Casas JP, Hingorani AD, Williams DJ. Pre-eclampsia and risk of cardiovascular disease and cancer in later life: systematic review and meta-analysis. BMJ. 2007;335(7627):974.
6. Ghossein-Doha C, van Neer J, Wissink B, Breetveld NM, de Windt LJ, van Dijk AP, et al. Pre-eclampsia: an important risk factor for asymptomatic heart failure. Ultrasound Obstet Gynecol. 2017;49(1):143–9.
7. Theilen LH, Meeks H, Fraser A, Esplin MS, Smith KR, Varner MW. Long-term mortality risk and life expectancy following recurrent hypertensive disease of pregnancy. Am J Obstet Gynecol. 2018;219(1):107.e1–e6.
8. Wu P, Haththotuwa R, Kwok CS, Babu A, Kotronias RA, Rushton C, et al. Preeclampsia and future cardiovascular health. Circ Cardiovasc Qual Outcomes. 2017;10(2):e003497.
9. Al-Balas M, Bozzo P, Einarson A. Use of diuretics during pregnancy. Can Fam Physician. 2009;55(1):44–5.
10. Cooper WO, Hernandez-Diaz S, Arbogast PG, Dudley JA, Dyer S, Gideon PS, et al. Major congenital malformations after first-trimester exposure to ACE inhibitors. N Engl J Med. 2006;354(23):2443–51.
11. Canobbio MM, Warnes CA, Aboulhosn J, Connolly HM, Khanna A, Koos BJ, et al. Management of Pregnancy in patients with complex congenital heart Disease: A scientific statement for healthcare professionals from the American Heart Association. Circulation. 2017;135(8):e50–87.
12. Warnes CA, Williams RG, Bashore TM, Child JS, Connolly HM, Dearani JA, et al. ACC/AHA 2008 guidelines for the Management of Adults with congenital heart Disease: a report of the American College of Cardiology/American Heart Association task force on practice guidelines (writing committee to develop guidelines on the management of adults with congenital heart disease). Circulation. 2008;118(23):e714–833.
13. Regitz-Zagrosek V, Blomstrom Lundqvist C, Borghi C, Cifkova R, Ferreira R, Foidart JM, et al. ESC guidelines on the management of cardiovascular diseases during pregnancy: the task force on the Management of Cardiovascular Diseases during preg-

nancy of the European Society of Cardiology (ESC). Eur Heart J. 2011;32(24):3147–97.
14. Elkayam U, Goland S, Pieper PG, Silverside CK. High-risk cardiac Disease in pregnancy: part I. J Am Coll Cardiol. 2016;68(4):396–410.
15. Sliwa K, Hilfiker-Kleiner D, Petrie MC, Mebazaa A, Pieske B, Buchmann E, et al. Current state of knowledge on aetiology, diagnosis, management, and therapy of peripartum cardiomyopathy: a position statement from the heart failure Association of the European Society of cardiology working group on peripartum cardiomyopathy. Eur J Heart Fail. 2010;12(8):767–78.
16. Elkayam U. Clinical characteristics of peripartum cardiomyopathy in the United States: diagnosis, prognosis, and management. J Am Coll Cardiol. 2011;58(7):659–70.
17. Elkayam U, Akhter MW, Singh H, Khan S, Bitar F, Hameed A, et al. Pregnancy-associated cardiomyopathy: clinical characteristics and a comparison between early and late presentation. Circulation. 2005;111(16):2050–5.
18. Arrigo M, Blet A, Mebazaa A. Bromocriptine for the treatment of peripartum cardiomyopathy: welcome on BOARD. Eur Heart J. 2017;38(35):2680–2.
19. Codsi E, Rose CH, Blauwet LA. Subsequent pregnancy outcomes in patients with Peripartum cardiomyopathy. Obstet Gynecol. 2018;131(2):322–7.
20. Sen-Chowdhry S, Jacoby D, Moon JC, McKenna WJ. Update on hypertrophic cardiomyopathy and a guide to the guidelines. Nat Rev Cardiol. 2016;13(11):651–75.
21. Gersh BJ, Maron BJ, Bonow RO, Dearani JA, Fifer MA, Link MS, et al. 2011 ACCF/AHA guideline for the diagnosis and treatment of hypertrophic cardiomyopathy: a report of the American College of Cardiology Foundation/American Heart Association task force on practice guidelines. J Thorac Cardiovasc Surg. 2011;142(6):e153–203.
22. Members ATF, Elliott PM, Anastasakis A, Borger MA, Borggrefe M, Cecchi F, et al. 2014 ESC guidelines on diagnosis and management of hypertrophic cardiomyopathy: the task force for the diagnosis and Management of Hypertrophic Cardiomyopathy of the European Society of Cardiology (ESC). Eur Heart J. 2014;35(39):2733–79.
23. Maron BJ, Maron MS. Hypertrophic cardiomyopathy. Lancet. 2013;381(9862):242–55.

24. Richard P, Charron P, Carrier L, Ledeuil C, Cheav T, Pichereau C, et al. Hypertrophic cardiomyopathy. Circulation. 2003;107(17):2227–32.
25. Maron MS, Rowin EJ, Maron BJ. How to image hypertrophic cardiomyopathy. Circ Cardiovasc Imaging. 2017;10(7):e005372.
26. Tanaka H, Kamiya C, Katsuragi S, Tanaka K, Miyoshi T, Tsuritani M, et al. Cardiovascular events in pregnancy with hypertrophic cardiomyopathy. Circ J. 2014;78(10):2501–6.
27. Goland S, van Hagen IM, Elbaz-Greener G, Elkayam U, Shotan A, Merz WM, et al. Pregnancy in women with hypertrophic cardiomyopathy: data from the European Society of Cardiology initiated registry of pregnancy and cardiac disease (ROPAC). Eur Heart J. 2017;38(35):2683–90.
28. Lima FV, Parikh PB, Zhu J, Yang J, Stergiopoulos K. Association of cardiomyopathy with adverse cardiac events in pregnant women at the time of delivery. JACC Heart Fail. 2015;3(3):257–66.
29. Gibson P, Narous M, Firoz T, Chou D, Barreix M, Say L, et al. Incidence of myocardial infarction in pregnancy: a systematic review and meta-analysis of population-based studies. Eur Heart J Qual Care Clin Outcomes. 2017;3(3):198–207.
30. Elkayam U, Jalnapurkar S, Barakkat MN, Khatri N, Kealey AJ, Mehra A, et al. Pregnancy-associated acute myocardial infarction: a review of contemporary experience in 150 cases between 2006 and 2011. Circulation. 2014;129(16):1695–702.
31. Colletti PM, Lee KH, Elkayam U. Cardiovascular imaging of the pregnant patient. AJR Am J Roentgenol. 2013;200(3):515–21.
32. Jeejeebhoy FM, Zelop CM, Lipman S, Carvalho B, Joglar J, Mhyre JM, et al. Cardiac arrest in pregnancy: A scientific statement from the American Heart Association. Circulation. 2015;132(18):1747–73.
33. Chernoguz A, Telem DA, Chu E, Ozao-Choy J, Tammaro Y, Divino CM. Cessation of clopidogrel before major abdominal procedures. Arch Surg. 2011;146(3):334–9.
34. Bernal JM, Miralles PJ. Cardiac surgery with cardiopulmonary bypass during pregnancy. Obstet Gynecol Surv. 1986;41(1):1–6.
35. Sundaram V, Chaudhry SP, Reddy YN, Longenecker CT, Fang JC. Emergent cesarean section in the catheterization laboratory for spontaneous coronary artery dissection. Am J Cardiol. 2015;115(12):1777–8.
36. Vaidya VR, Arora S, Patel N, Badheka AO, Patel N, Agnihotri K, et al. Burden of arrhythmia in pregnancy. Circulation. 2017;135(6):619–21.

37. Enriquez AD, Economy KE, Tedrow UB. Contemporary management of arrhythmias during pregnancy. Circ Arrhythm Electrophysiol. 2014;7(5):961–7.
38. Regitz-Zagrosek V, Roos-Hesselink JW, Bauersachs J, Blomström-Lundqvist C, Cífková R, De Bonis M, et al. 2018 ESC guidelines for the management of cardiovascular diseases during pregnancy. Eur Heart J. 2018;39(34):3165–241.
39. Wang YC, Chen CH, Su HY, Yu MH. The impact of maternal cardioversion on fetal haemodynamics. Eur J Obstet Gynecol Reprod Biol. 2006;126(2):268–9.
40. Agewall S, Camm J. New ESC/EACTS guidelines for the management of atrial fibrillation. Eur Heart J Cardiovasc Pharmacother. 2017;3(2):71–2.
41. Lau E, DeFaria Yeh D. Management of high risk cardiac conditions in pregnancy: anticoagulation, severe stenotic valvular disease and cardiomyopathy. Trends Cardiovasc Med. 2019;29(3):155–61.
42. Halpern DG, Weinberg CR, Pinnelas R, Mehta-Lee S, Economy KE, Valente AM. Use of medication for cardiovascular disease during pregnancy: JACC state-of-the-art review. J Am Coll Cardiol. 2019;73(4):457–76.
43. Rashba EJ, Zareba W, Moss AJ, Hall WJ, Robinson J, Locati EH, et al. Influence of pregnancy on the risk for cardiac events in patients with hereditary long QT syndrome. LQTS Investigat Circulat. 1998;97(5):451–6.
44. Elkayam U. Native valvular heart disease and pregnancy. In: Cardiac problems in pregnancy; 2019. p. 75–89.

Chapter 30
Perioperative Cardiovascular Risk Assessment

Susan McIlvaine and Eli V. Gelfand

Abbreviations

AF	Atrial fibrillation
CABG	Coronary artery bypass grafting
CAD	Coronary artery disease
DASI	Duke Activity Status Index
DES	Drug-eluting stent
MACE	Major adverse cardiac event
MACCE	Major adverse cardiovascular and cerebrovascular events
MET	Metabolic equivalents
MI	Myocardial infarction
NSQIP	National Surgical Quality Improvement Program
NSTEMI	Non-ST-Elevation Myocardial Infarction
PAUSE	Perioperative Anticoagulation Use for Surgery Evaluation
RCRI	Revised Cardiac Risk Index
STEMI	ST-Elevation Myocardial Infarction

S. McIlvaine · E. V. Gelfand (✉)
Department of Medicine, Division of Cardiology, Beth Israel Deaconess Medical Center, Harvard Medical School, Boston, MA, USA
e-mail: smcilvai@bidmc.harvard.edu; egelfand@bidmc.harvard.edu

A. A. Bhargava et al. (eds.), *Handbook of Outpatient Cardiology*, https://doi.org/10.1007/978-3-030-88953-1_30

Introduction

What is the purpose of performing a perioperative cardiovascular risk assessment prior to non-cardiac surgery?

- The purpose of a perioperative cardiovascular risk assessment is to help risk stratify a patient (from a cardiovascular perspective) prior to an operative procedure.
- In some cases, a perioperative risk assessment results in further testing and/or intervention (either before or after the procedure for which the assessment was performed) aimed at decreasing the patient's cardiovascular risk.
- In most cases, this risk assessment can be performed by a patient's primary care provider, with referral to a cardiologist if further workup is required or if the patient has a significant cardiac history with active disease.

Framework for Perioperative Risk Assessment:

1. Determine baseline risk factors of the patient and the planned procedure.
2. Determine the patient's functional status.
3. Estimate the patient's risk of a major adverse cardiac event (MACE).
4. Decide whether the patient needs any further testing/intervention to mitigate their risk, either prior to or after surgery (Fig. 30.1).

Determine Risk Factors

What are potential sources of perioperative cardiovascular risk?

- The risk of a procedure from a cardiovascular standpoint depends on the *procedure* itself and on the *comorbidities* and clinical status of the patient. Retrospective data helps determine the approximate level of risk based on these various factors.

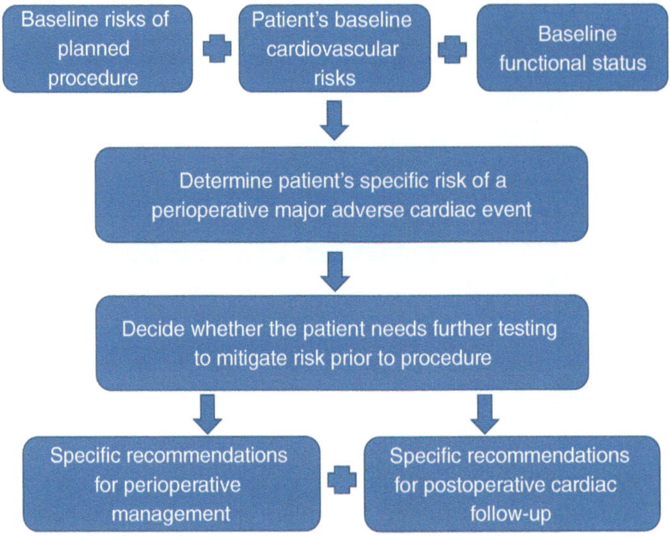

FIGURE 30.1 Framework for perioperative risk assessment

- Cardiovascular risk of non-cardiac surgery has decreased over time, driven mostly by a decline in frequency of perioperative death and acute MI [1].
- Not all perioperative morbidity/mortality is secondary to cardiovascular risk factors. The estimation of risk provided using the tools detailed below does not explicitly account for these other factors.

Procedure Risk Factors

- In a JAMA retrospective study of more than ten million patients undergoing non-cardiac surgery from 2004 to 2013, 3% of patients experienced a major adverse cardiovascular or cerebrovascular event (including perioperative death, myocardial infarction, and ischemic stroke). These major adverse events occurred most frequently in patients undergoing vascular, thoracic, and transplant surgery [1] (see Fig. 30.2).
- In the RCRI (see below), suprainguinal vascular, intraperitoneal, and intrathoracic surgeries are considered high risk [2].

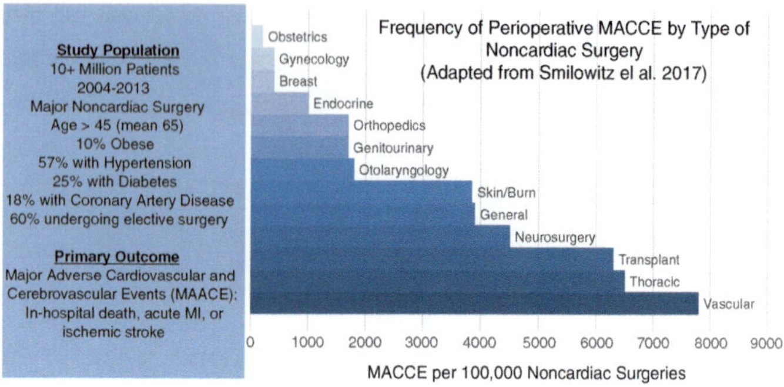

FIGURE 30.2 Frequency of perioperative MACE by type of noncardiac surgery

> **Clinical Pearl**
> Vascular, thoracic, and transplant surgeries have been shown to have higher rates of postoperative MACE. These are considered high-risk procedures.

Patient Risk Factors

- Cardiovascular conditions shown to be associated with MACE include:
  - Coronary artery disease.
  - Presence of a coronary stent.
  - Heart failure.
  - Arrhythmia.
  - Severe valvular heart disease.
  - Systemic arterial hypertension.
  - Pulmonary hypertension.
- History and physical should focus on elucidating whether any of these cardiac conditions are present at the time of evaluation or likely to be present at the time of the procedure.
- Patients with acute coronary syndrome (unstable angina or myocardial infarction), coronary stent placement within 6 months, acute decompensated heart failure, high-grade

arrhythmia (i.e., symptomatic tachy- or bradyarrhythmia), or symptomatic severe aortic stenosis should NOT undergo elective non-cardiac surgery until such issues are addressed.

Clinical Pearl
Contraindications to elective surgery include ACS, stent placement within 6 months, acute decompensated heart failure, high-grade arrhythmia, and symptomatic severe aortic stenosis.

Determine the Patient's Functional Status

- MET, or metabolic equivalent, refers to the amount of oxygen uptake required for certain activities. 1 MET is the resting oxygen uptake while sitting up. For perioperative risk assessment, a patient's functional status is most often defined with respect to how many METs the patient can achieve; this also serves as a reference standard used during exercise stress testing.
- If a patient can walk up a hill or climb two or more flights of stairs, they can perform at least 4 METs.
  - Patients who cannot perform 4 METs have double the risk for a perioperative MACE [3].
  - 4 to 10 METs suggest moderate functional capacity.
  - >10 METs suggest excellent functional capacity.
- Patients may overestimate their functional capacity. Subjective assessment is NOT predictive of postoperative morbidity or mortality [4].
- In addition to asking patients to subjectively assess their functional status, a validated tool like the Duke Activity Status Index (DASI) should preferably be used [5]. Wijeysundera et al. showed that DASI scores were associated with predicting death or MI within 30 days of surgery (see Table 30.1).

TABLE 30.1 The Duke Activity Status Index (DASI) is a validated way to assess a patient's functional status

Can you...	Weight
Take care of yourself (easting, dressing, bathing, using the toilet)?	2.75
Walk indoors, such as around your house?	1.75
Walk a block or 2 on level ground?	2.75
Climb a flight of stairs or walk up a hill?	5.50
Run a short distance?	8.00
Do light work around the house like dusting or washing dishes?	2.70
Do moderate work around the house like vacuuming, sweeping floors, or carrying in groceries?	3.50
Do heavy work around the house like scrubbing floors, or lifting or moving heavy furniture?	8.00
Do yardwork like raking leaves, weeding or pushing a power mower?	4.50
Have sexual relations?	5.25
Participate in moderate recreational activities like golf, bowling, dancing, doubles tennis, or throwing a baseball or football?	6.00
Participipiate in strenuous sports like swimming, singles tennis, football, basketball, or skiing?	7.50
Total DASI score:	______
[(DASI score x 0.43) + 9.6] / 3.5:	___ METs

Duke Activity Status Index (Adapted from Hlatky et al. [5])

Clinical Pearl

Patients may overestimate their functional status, which can lead to a misclassification of risk. Do not rely solely on a subjective assessment of functional status, but rather use a validated questionnaire like the DASI.

Estimate the Patient's Risk of a Major Adverse Cardiovascular Event

- There is no single "perfect" risk calculator. Several risk calculators have been derived using different retrospective data sets and predict various levels of risk. A clinician should understand the population used to derive and validate the specific risk calculator and ensure that her/his patient generally fits that population. The risk estimate must always be combined with an overall clinical impression.
- Common risk calculators include the Revised Cardiac Risk Index (RCRI), the American College of Surgeons NSQIP Surgical Risk Calculator (ACS-SRC), and the NSQIP perioperative MI and cardiac arrest calculator (MICA).
- The RCRI was published in 1999 [2] and has been validated and widely used in clinical practice. In 2017, Duceppe et al. combined data from five studies to calculate the pooled event rates for each RCRI score, which resulted in higher risk than was reported in the original study (likely due to validation studies using higher sensitivity troponin assays and including patients undergoing emergency surgery) (see Fig. 30.3).
- The RCRI has been shown to be less accurate at predicting risk in patients undergoing vascular surgery.
- The ACS-SRC may provide the best estimate of surgery-specific risk of MACE [6] but has not been validated in an external population. Given its inherent complexity, the authors have found the online version of the calculator to be particularly useful in daily practice. Visit http://www.riskcalculator.facs.org/RiskCalculator/ to use this calculator.

Clinical Pearl
There is no perfect risk calculator. The RCRI is validated and widely used and is a reasonable tool for risk assessment when combined with overall clinical judgment. An online version of the ACS-SRC can be helpful in daily clinical practice.

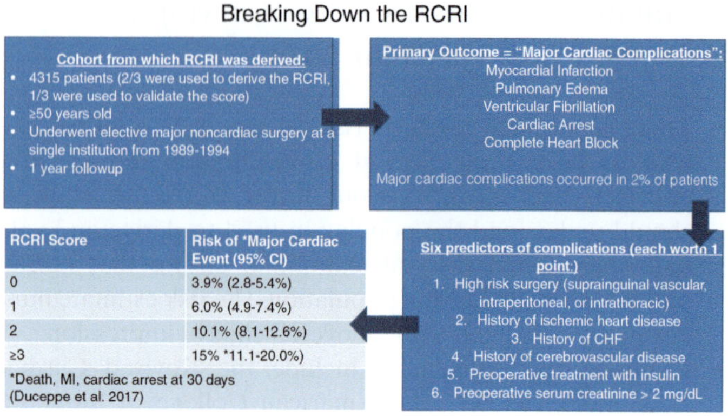

FIGURE 30.3 Breaking down the RCRI: knowledge of the study population and outcomes from which this score was derived can help providers decide whether this is the most appropriate tool to use for risk stratification

Further Testing/Intervention

ECG

- The purpose of a preoperative (within 1–3 months) ECG is to identify arrhythmia, prior MI, and to have a baseline ECG for comparison. However, there is no consensus as to the features of an abnormal ECG that portend prognostic significance in the perioperative setting [6].
- It is **not** necessary to obtain a preoperative ECG for patients undergoing low-risk surgeries (i.e., cataract or cosmetic surgery) regardless of their cardiac risk profile.
- 2014 ACC/AHA guidelines state that in patients undergoing anything other than low-risk surgery, it is reasonable to obtain a preoperative ECG if they have a history of CAD, arrhythmia, peripheral arterial disease, cerebrovascular disease, or other significant heart disease. ECG can be considered, but is not absolutely required, for asymptomatic patients with no known coronary disease undergoing moderate- or high-risk surgery [6].

Stress Testing

- Routine stress testing is NOT indicated for low-risk patients (i.e., those who can perform >4 METs).
- A stress test is only indicated if there is a separate reason *besides* the upcoming procedure to undergo cardiac risk stratification. An example is a patient with significant cardiac risk factors who is unable to perform 4 METs (or has an unknown functional status) [6].
- A stress test should only be performed if the results would change perioperative management (from either a medical or surgical perspective).

Coronary Angiography and Revascularization

- Indications for preoperative coronary angiography are similar to those when there is no plan for a patient to undergo surgery.
- Routine coronary revascularization in asymptomatic patients with unrevascularized coronary disease has not been shown to reduce perioperative risk [6].
- In patients who undergo coronary angiography and are subsequently recommended CABG, bypass surgery should be performed prior to any elective procedures.

Clinical Pearl
Patients undergoing low-risk procedures do not need a preoperative ECG. Routine preoperative stress testing in asymptomatic patients with good functional status is rarely warranted.

Special Cases

Patients with Coronary Stents

- Elective non-cardiac surgery should ideally be delayed until 1 year after DES placement, but can be considered 180 days after stent placement if the benefit of surgery outweighs the risk of stent thrombosis (see Table 30.2).

TABLE 30.2 Perioperative management of patients with drug-eluting coronary artery stents

Patients with Drug-Eluting Coronary Artery Stent(s) (Adapted from Fleisher et al. [6])				
Stent placed within 6 weeks	**Stent placed within 1 year (but not within 6 weeks)**		**Stent placed more than 1 year ago**	
Elective surgery: delay until 1 year after DES placement	*Risk of surgical delay > risk of DES thrombosis*: Proceed to surgery after 180 days	*Risk of surgical delay < risk of DES thrombosis*: Delay surgery until 1 year after DES placement	*Surgery does not require discontinuation of $P2Y_{12}$ inhibitors*: continue DAPT	*Surgery does require discontinuation of $P2Y_{12}$ inhibitors*: Continue ASA, restart P2Y12 ASAP

[a]*What is risk of stent thrombosis?* Risk is highest in the first 4-6 weeks after stent implantation. After 4-6 weeks, the risk is lower, but having surgery increases risk. Risk is of DES thrombosis with noncardiac surgery is likely stable 6 months after DES implantation

Patients on Anticoagulation and Bridging

- Patients undergoing most low-risk procedures can continue anticoagulation (e.g., cataract surgery, ICD placement, low-risk dental procedures).
- Per the PAUSE study [7], for patients with AF on a DOAC undergoing an elective procedure, a simple standardized perioperative management strategy that did not require the use of heparin bridging or preoperative coagulation function testing was associated with low rates of perioperative major bleeding and arterial thromboembolism. It should be noted that the average CHA2DS2-VASc scores were around 3.5 (see Table 30.3).

TABLE 30.3 DOAC guidelines for patients with AF undergoing elective surgery

PAUSE Study: Patients with AF undergoing elective surgery (Adapted from Douketis et al. [7])				
DOAC	**Surgical Bleeding Risk**	**Preoperative**	**Day of surgery**	**Postoperative**
Apixaban, Dabigatran, Rivaroxaban	Low	Hold DOAC for one day before surgical procedure	Hold DOAC	Resume DOAC on postoperative day 1
	High	Hold DOAC for two days before surgical procedure	Hold DOAC	Resume DOAC on postoperative day 2 or 3
Dabigatran in patients with creatinine clearance <50 mL/min	Low	Hold dabigatran for two days before surgical procedure	Hold DOAC	Resume DOAC on postoperative day 1
	High	Hold dabigatran for four days before surgical procedure	Hold DOAC	Resume DOAC on postoperative day 2 or 3

- For procedures where hemostasis is essential (i.e., major vascular surgery, spine surgery, epidural catheterization), discontinue anticoagulation for ≥48 hrs.
- In patients with AF who have a CHA2DS2-VASc score of 7 or 8 (i.e., high risk of thromboembolism), bridging with heparin or low molecular weight heparin is likely appropriate [8].
- Patients with mechanical **mitral** valve prosthesis should undergo bridging with unfractionated or low molecular weight heparin regardless of presence or absence of thrombosis/thromboembolic risk factors [6].
- Patients with mechanical **aortic** valve prosthesis should undergo bridging with heparin if at least one risk factor for thrombosis/thromboembolism is present (e.g., AF, prior VTE, hypercoagulable disorder, older mechanical valve) [6].
- Other scenarios where bridging anticoagulation may be appropriate include VTE or systemic embolic event within 3 months, coronary stenting within 12 weeks, or previous VTE during interruption of anticoagulation [9].

Clinical Pearl
Perioperative bridging should be considered in patients with AF at high risk for thromboembolism (CHA2DS2-VASc score of 7 or 8), patients with a mechanical mitral valve, and patients with a mechanical aortic valve that have an additional risk factor for thromboembolism.

Patients with Asymptomatic Severe Aortic Stenosis

- The hemodynamic stress of surgery can precipitate hypotension, heart failure, or frank cardiogenic shock in patients with severe aortic stenosis.
- However, the risk of surgery in patients with severe AS has declined over time due to advances in anesthesia and surgical approaches. In patients with asymptomatic severe AS, it is reasonable to perform elevated risk elective surgery if appropriate intraoprerative and postoperative hemodynamic monitoring is used [6].

Key Learning Points

1. The purpose of a perioperative cardiovascular risk assessment is to help risk stratify a patient (from a cardiovascular perspective) prior to an operative procedure.
2. The risk of a procedure from a cardiovascular standpoint depends on the procedure itself and on the comorbidities and clinical status of the patient. Retrospective data helps determine the approximate level of risk based on these various factors. Vascular, thoracic, and transplant surgeries are considered high-risk procedures.
3. Patients who cannot perform 4 METs have double the risk for a perioperative MACE.
4. There is no single "perfect" risk calculator. Several risk calculators have been derived using different retrospective data sets and predict various levels of risk. The RCRI has been validated and widely used in clinical practice and is a reasonable tool to use in combination with clinical judgment and an understanding of the limitations of this tool.
5. Routine stress testing is NOT indicated for low-risk patients (i.e., those who can perform >4 METs). A stress test is only indicated if there is a separate reason *besides* the upcoming procedure to undergo cardiac risk stratification.
6. Lower-risk patients with atrial fibrillation can likely stop their anticoagulation safely surrounding elective procedures without a heparin bridge. Perioperative bridging should be considered in patients with AF at high risk for thromboembolism (CHA2DS2-VASc score of 7 or 8), patients with a mechanical mitral valve, and patients with a mechanical aortic valve that have an additional risk factor for thromboembolism.

References

1. Smilowitz NR, Gupta N, Ramakrishna H, Guo Y, Berger JS, Bangalore S. Perioperative major adverse cardiovascular and cerebrovascular events associated with noncardiac surgery. JAMA Cardiol. 2017;2(2):181–7.
2. Lee TH, Marcantonio ER, Mangione CM, Thomas EJ, Polanczyk CA, Cook EF, Sugarbaker DJ, Donaldson MC, Poss R, Ho KK, Ludwig LE, Pedan A, Goldman L. Derivation and prospective validation of a simple index for prediction of cardiac risk of major noncardiac surgery. Circulation. 1999;100(10):1043–9.
3. Reilly DF, McNeely MJ, Doerner D, Greenberg DL, Staiger TO, Geist MJ, Vedovatti PA, Coffey JE, Mora MW, Johnson TR, Guray ED, Van Norman GA, Fihn SD. Self-reported exercise tolerance and the risk of serious perioperative complications. Arch Intern Med. 1999;159(18):2185–92.
4. Wijeysundera DN, Pearse RM, Shulman MA, Abbott TEF, Torres E, Ambosta A, Croal BL, Granton JT, Thorpe KE, Grocott MPW, Farrington C, Myles PS, Cuthbertson BH, METS Study Investigators. Assessment of functional capacity before major non-cardiac surgery: an international, prospective cohort study. Lancet. 2018;391(10140):2631–40.
5. Hlatky MA, Boineau RE, Higginbotham MB, Lee KL, Mark DB, Califf RM, Cobb FR, Pryor DB. A brief self-administered questionnaire to determine functional capacity (the Duke activity status index). Am J Cardiol. 1989;64(10):651–4.
6. Fleisher LA, Fleischmann KE, Auerbach AD, Barnason SA, Beckman JA, Bozkurt B, Davila-Roman VG, Gerhard-Herman MD, Holly TA, Kane GC, Marine JE, Nelson MT, Spencer CC, Thompson A, Ting HH, Uretsky BF, Wijeysundera DN, American College of Cardiology; American Heart Association. 2014 ACC/AHA guideline on perioperative cardiovascular evaluation and management of patients undergoing noncardiac surgery: a report of the American College of Cardiology/American Heart Association task force on practice guidelines. J Am Coll Cardiol. 2014;64(22):e77–137.
7. Douketis JD, Spyropoulos AC, Duncan J, Carrier M, Le Gal G, Tafur AJ, Vanassche T, Verhamme P, Shivakumar S, Gross PL, Lee AYY, Yeo E, Solymoss S, Kassis J, Le Templier G, Kowalski S, Blostein M, Shah V, MacKay E, Wu C, Clark NP, Bates SM, Spencer FA, Arnaoutoglou E, Coppens M, Arnold DM, Caprini

JA, Li N, Moffat KA, Syed S, Schulman S. Perioperative management of patients with atrial fibrillation receiving a direct oral anticoagulant. JAMA Intern Med. 2019;179(11):1469–78.
8. Douketis JD, Spyropoulos AC, Kaatz S, Becker RC, Caprini JA, Dunn AS, Garcia DA, Jacobson A, Jaffer AK, Kong DF, Schulman S, Turpie AG, Hasselblad V, Ortel TL, BRIDGE Investigators. Perioperative bridging anticoagulation in patients with atrial fibrillation. N Engl J Med. 2015;373(9):823–33.
9. Douketis JD. Perioperative management of patients who are receiving warfarin therapy: an evidence-based and practical approach. Blood. 2011;117(19):5044–9.

Chapter 31
Cardio-Oncology

Devinder S. Dhindsa and Anant Mandawat

Abbreviations

5-FU	5-Fluorouracil
ACE-i	Angiotensin-converting enzyme inhibitor
AF	Atrial fibrillation
AFL	Atrial flutter
ARB	Angiotensin receptor blocker
CT	Computed tomography
CV	Cardiovascular
CVD	Cardiovascular disease

D. S. Dhindsa (✉)
Department of Medicine, Division of Cardiology, Emory University School of Medicine, Atlanta, GA, USA
e-mail: devinder.singh.dhindsa@emory.edu

A. Mandawat
Department of Medicine, Division of Cardiology, Emory University School of Medicine, Atlanta, GA, USA

Winship Cancer Institute, Department of Hematology and Medical Oncology, Emory University School of Medicine, Atlanta, GA, USA
e-mail: Anant.mandawat@emory.edu

A. A. Bhargava et al. (eds.), *Handbook of Outpatient Cardiology*, https://doi.org/10.1007/978-3-030-88953-1_31

HER2	Human epidermal growth factor receptor 2
LVEF	Left ventricular ejection fraction
MRI	Magnetic resonance imaging
PAD	Peripheral arterial disease
VEGF	Vascular endothelial growth factor

Introduction

- As cancer survivorship continues to improve due to advancements in treatment and screening, a large number of cancer survivors are entering the population [1]. Many of these individuals are subject to cardiovascular (CV) complications, which are critical for practitioners to be aware of both at the time of and years after therapy [2].

Screening and Prevention

- Obtain a complete history and physical, including baseline clinical assessment based on established risk factors and anticipated cancer treatment [3].
- Optimize cardiac risk factors for all patients [4].
- Consider baseline assessment of left ventricular ejection fraction (LVEF) based on risk factors and anticipated cancer treatments [5].
- If there is baseline left ventricular dysfunction, engage cardiology and oncology providers regarding selection of chemotherapy options with lower risk of cardiotoxicity or additional cardioprotective drugs (e.g., beta-blocker or angiotensin-converting enzyme inhibitors [ACE-i]) [4, 6].

Cardiac Toxicities of Cancer Therapies

A. Heart Failure.

- Myocardial dysfunction can present early after exposure or several years after exposure due to myocardial injury that occurred at the time of oncological therapy [7–9].

- Cardiotoxicity is defined as a >10% decrease of LVEF to a value below the lower limit of normal (usually LVEF <50%) by echocardiography or nuclear cardiac imaging (MUGA).
- A >15% relative reduction from baseline of global longitudinal strain (GLS) can also suggest cardiotoxicity.

Clinical Pearl
Global longitudinal strain may help to detect more subtle myocardial dysfunction than monitoring for changes with LVEF.

- Chemotherapies associated with myocardial dysfunction and the incidence of LV dysfunction associated with each agent are presented in Table 31.1 [3]:
- Screening modalities for cardiotoxicity include:
  - Cardiac imaging: echocardiography, nuclear imaging, and cardiac magnetic resonance imaging.
  - Biomarkers: brain natriuretic peptide and troponin [7, 10–12].
  - Timing and frequency of monitoring depend on specific treatment, cumulative dose of chemotherapy, duration of therapy, and patient's baseline CV risk [3].
- Of note, LV dysfunction with immunotherapies, such as the anti-*HER2* monoclonal antibody trastuzumab, is usually reversible with interruption of chemotherapy and treatment with heart failure therapies; re-challenge is often well-tolerated. This is *in contrast* to the cardiotoxicity associated with anthracyclines, which often leads to an irreversible dilated cardiomyopathy.
- Immune checkpoint inhibitors (pembrolizumab, nivolumab, ipilimumab, tremelimumab, atezolizumab, avelumab, durvalumab) have an uncommon but severe association with myocarditis presenting within 3 months of starting therapy [13]. Patients presenting with this require cessation of the agent, high-dose steroids, and urgent cardiology/cardio-oncology consultation.

TABLE 31.1 Chemotherapies associated with myocardial dysfunction

Agents associated with myocardial dysfunction (incidence % of LV dysfunction)
Anthracyclines – Dose-dependent effect [e.g., doxorubicin (3–48%), idarubicin (5–18%), epirubicin (0.9–11.4%), mitoxantrone (2.6%)]
Alkylating agents [e.g., cyclophosphamide (7–28%), ifosfamide (0.5–17%)]
Antimetabolites [e.g., clofarabine (27%)]
Antimicrotubule agents [e.g., docetaxel (2.3–13%), paclitaxel (<1%)]
Monoclonal antibodies [e.g., *anti-HER2*: Trastuzumab (1.7–20.1%), pertuzumab (0.7–1.2%); *anti-VEGF:* Bevacizumab (1.6–4%)]
Small molecule tyrosine kinase inhibitors [e.g., sunitinib (2.7–19%), sorafenib (4–8%), dasatinib (2–4%), imatinib (0.2–2.7%)]
Proteosome inhibitors [e.g., carfilzomib (11–25%), bortezomib (2–5%)]
Immune checkpoint inhibitors – Associated with myocarditis in 1.1%

Clinical Pearl
Immune checkpoint inhibitor myocarditis is associated with a poor prognosis. Keep a high index of suspicion and treat early.

- If LV dysfunction or heart failure occurs during therapy, patients are likely to benefit from traditional heart failure management like ACE-i/ARB and beta-blocker therapy [6]. Recommend risk-benefit discussion with cardiology and oncology provider regarding interruption of cancer therapy or adjustment of chemotherapeutic strategy [5].

- In addition to managing overall cardiovascular risk, specific strategies to reduce chemotherapy-induced cardiotoxicity can vary by agent.
  - For anthracyclines and its analogs:
    Limit cumulative dose.
    Alter delivery system (e.g., liposomal doxorubicin).
    Use continuous infusions.
    Use dexrazoxane with anthracyclines to reduce anthracycline toxicity in appropriate patients.
    Use cardioprotective medications (ACE-i/ARBs, beta-blockers, statins).
    Encourage aerobic exercise to reduce the risk of cardiotoxicity.
  - For trastuzumab, cardioprotective medications (ACE-i/ARBs) are an important consideration [3].

B. Coronary Artery Disease/Therapy-Related Ischemia.

- Myocardial ischemia can occur through a number of mechanisms from cancer therapies, including vasospasm, endothelial injury, and acute arterial thrombosis, or through premature atherosclerosis [14–16].
- Therapies associated with myocardial ischemia are listed in Table 31.2 [14, 15, 17–20]:
- Baseline screening for pre-existing CVD is important as pre-existing CVD increases the risk of developing treatment-related CVD [16].

Clinical Pearl
When possible, avoid premature/unnecessary cessation as this may affect cancer curability. In addition to optimizing pre-existing cardiovascular disease/risk factors for patients receiving fluoropyrimidines, screening treadmill may not be sufficient, and coronary CT angiogram or left heart catheterization should be considered. Coronary spasm due to fluoropyrimidines is usually reversible but usually recurrent upon re-exposure if not treated with nitrates/calcium channel blockers.

TABLE 31.2 Therapies associated with myocardial ischemia

Therapy	Mechanism of ischemia
Pyrimidine analogs (e.g., 5-FU, capecitabine, gemcitabine)	Endothelial injury, vasospasm
Cisplatin	Procoagulant, direct endothelial toxicity
VEGF inhibitors (bevacizumab, sorafenib, sunitinib)	Endothelial injury, arterial thrombosis, vasospasm
Radiotherapy	Endothelial injury, plaque rupture, thrombosis

- For patients who develop signs or symptoms of ischemia on cancer therapy, in particular pyrimidine analogs (e.g., 5-FU, capecitabine), consider withholding treatment and referral to cardiology for evaluation and discussion with oncology regarding risk-benefit of continued use given high rates of symptom recurrence [3, 14, 21].
- Additionally, patients treated with radiation therapy can develop premature atherosclerotic disease. Consensus documents suggest regular screening beginning 5–10 years after receiving radiation therapy [22].
- Management with anti-platelets and anticoagulants is particularly challenging in this population given the prevalence of treatment-related thrombocytopenia [23]. An individualized risk-benefit discussion is recommended.

C. Valvular Disease.

- Radiation therapy can be associated with fibrosis and calcification of the aortic root or cardiac valves [16, 20, 24].
- Echocardiography is the imaging test of choice for the assessment of valvular disease, though cardiac MRI or computed tomography (CT) may also be used [25, 26].
- If valve repair is required, surgery is often challenging due to fibrosis and impaired wound healing. Transcatheter options may be a suitable alternative [27].

D. Arrhythmia.

- Patients treated with chemotherapy can experience a number of arrhythmias during their treatment course, including tachyarrhythmias or bradyarrhythmias and conduction disturbances [28].

- QT prolongation has been associated with arsenic trioxide and tyrosine kinase inhibitors, in particular vandetanib [29–31]. Management consists of correction of any electrolyte abnormalities (hypocalcemia, hypokalemia, hypomagnesemia) and avoidance or withdrawal of any QT-prolonging medication.
- Conduction disturbances, including complete heart block, have been noted with paclitaxel and thalidomide [32].
- Atrial fibrillation/flutter (AF/AFL) can occur due to comorbidities and malignancy, as well as with ibrutinib [33]. Management of this rhythm generally requires anticoagulation, though this can be challenging in this population due to thrombocytopenia.

E. Arterial Hypertension.

- Arterial hypertension can be associated with VEGF inhibitors [34]. Early and aggressive management is warranted with ACE-i/ARB, beta-blocker, or dihydropyridine calcium channel blocker to avoid CV complications, such as heart failure [35].
- If blood pressure remains uncontrolled, the VEGF inhibitor should be held or reduced until blood pressure is adequately controlled (<140/90 mmHg or lower in the case of overt proteinuria), at which point the VEGF inhibitor can be restarted [31, 35].

F. Thromboembolic Disease.

- Malignancy contributes to a prothrombotic state, placing cancer patients at risk for both arterial and venous thrombosis [36].
- Low molecular weight heparin had previously been preferred due to lower rates of recurrent venous thrombosis in those patients who are able to be anticoagulated (CLOT, 2003) [37].

- Newer evidence has shown noninferiority of apixaban to dalteparin in cancer-associated venous thrombosis without increased risk of major bleeding [38].
- If recurrence of thrombosis occurs despite therapy, the provider can consider adjusting anticoagulation strategy or consider placement of an inferior vena cava filter [39].

G. Peripheral Vascular Disease and Stroke.

- Severe atherosclerotic and non-atherosclerotic peripheral arterial disease can occur with nilotinib, ponatinib, or *BCR-ABL* tyrosine kinase inhibitors [40].
- Ischemic stroke has also been associated with head and neck radiotherapy [41, 42].
- Risk factor control is critical. In cases of severe PAD, the decision for revascularization should be individualized with multi-disciplinary input from cardio-oncology, vascular surgery, and hematology/oncology [43].
- Patients irradiated for head and neck cancer are at higher risk for developing cerebrovascular disease [44].

H. Pulmonary Hypertension.

- Pulmonary hypertension can occur following dasatinib therapy, stem cell bone marrow transplantation, or alkylating agent therapy (due to veno-occlusive disease) [45, 46].
- Baseline echocardiogram should be considered prior to dasatinib therapy [47].
- Signs of elevated pulmonary artery pressure may require cardiology or a pulmonary hypertension team assessment, as etiology of pulmonary hypertension may affect therapy.

Key Learning Points

- The CV effects of cancer and cancer-related therapies are a challenging reality of the treatment of these conditions.
- There should be a particular emphasis on screening and optimization of cardiac risk factors prior to receiving potentially cardiotoxic treatments.
- It is important to recognize that the CV effects can occur early or years after oncological treatment.

References

1. Shapiro CL. Cancer Survivorship. 2018;379(25):2438–50.
2. de Azambuja E, Ameye L, Diaz M, Vandenbossche S, Aftimos P, Bejarano Hernandez S, et al. Cardiac assessment of early breast cancer patients 18 years after treatment with cyclophosphamide-, methotrexate-, fluorouracil- or epirubicin-based chemotherapy. Eur J Cancer (Oxford, England: 1990). 2015;51(17):2517–24.
3. Zamorano JL, Lancellotti P, Rodriguez Muñoz D, Aboyans V, Asteggiano R, Galderisi M, et al. 2016 ESC position paper on cancer treatments and cardiovascular toxicity developed under the auspices of the ESC Committee for practice guidelines: the task force for cancer treatments and cardiovascular toxicity of the European Society of Cardiology (ESC). Eur Heart J. 2016;37(36):2768–801.
4. Barac A, Murtagh G, Carver JR, Chen MH, Freeman AM, Herrmann J, et al. Cardiovascular health of patients with cancer and cancer survivors: a roadmap to the next level. J Am Coll Cardiol. 2015;65(25):2739–46.
5. Cardinale D, Colombo A, Lamantia G, Colombo N, Civelli M, De Giacomi G, et al. Anthracycline-induced cardiomyopathy: clinical relevance and response to pharmacologic therapy. J Am Coll Cardiol. 2010;55(3):213–20.
6. Cardinale D, Colombo A, Bacchiani G, Tedeschi I, Meroni CA, Veglia F, et al. Early detection of anthracycline cardiotoxicity and improvement with heart failure therapy. Circulation. 2015;131(22):1981–8.

7. Armstrong GT, Plana JC, Zhang N, Srivastava D, Green DM, Ness KK, et al. Screening adult survivors of childhood cancer for cardiomyopathy: comparison of echocardiography and cardiac magnetic resonance imaging. J Clin Oncol. 2012;30(23):2876–84.
8. Hequet O, Le QH, Moullet I, Pauli E, Salles G, Espinouse D, et al. Subclinical late cardiomyopathy after doxorubicin therapy for lymphoma in adults. J Clin Oncol. 2004;22(10):1864–71.
9. Steinherz LJ, Steinherz PG, Tan CT, Heller G, Murphy ML. Cardiac toxicity 4 to 20 years after completing anthracycline therapy. JAMA. 1991;266(12):1672–7.
10. Cardinale D, Sandri MT. Role of biomarkers in chemotherapy-induced cardiotoxicity. Prog Cardiovasc Dis. 2010;53(2):121–9.
11. Ledwidge M, Gallagher J, Conlon C, Tallon E, O'Connell E, Dawkins I, et al. Natriuretic peptide-based screening and collaborative care for heart failure: the STOP-HF randomized trial. JAMA. 2013;310(1):66–74.
12. Mitani I, Jain D, Joska TM, Burtness B, Zaret BL. Doxorubicin cardiotoxicity: prevention of congestive heart failure with serial cardiac function monitoring with equilibrium radionuclide angiocardiography in the current era. J Nuclear Cardiol: Official Publication of the American Society of Nuclear Cardiology. 2003;10(2):132–9.
13. Mahmood SS, Fradley MG, Cohen JV, Nohria A, Reynolds KL, Heinzerling LM, et al. Myocarditis in patients treated with immune checkpoint inhibitors. J Am Coll Cardiol. 2018;71(16):1755–64.
14. Frickhofen N, Beck FJ, Jung B, Fuhr HG, Andrasch H, Sigmund M. Capecitabine can induce acute coronary syndrome similar to 5-fluorouracil. Annals of Oncology: Official Journal of the European Society for Medical Oncology. 2002;13(5):797–801.
15. Choueiri TK, Schutz FA, Je Y, Rosenberg JE, Bellmunt J. Risk of arterial thromboembolic events with sunitinib and sorafenib: a systematic review and meta-analysis of clinical trials. J Clin Oncol. 2010;28(13):2280–5.
16. Hull MC, Morris CG, Pepine CJ, Mendenhall NP. Valvular dysfunction and carotid, subclavian, and coronary artery disease in survivors of hodgkin lymphoma treated with radiation therapy. JAMA. 2003;290(21):2831–7.
17. Moore RA, Adel N, Riedel E, Bhutani M, Feldman DR, Tabbara NE, et al. High incidence of thromboembolic events in patients treated with cisplatin-based chemotherapy: a large retrospective analysis. J Clin Oncol. 2011;29(25):3466–73.

18. McEniery PT, Dorosti K, Schiavone WA, Pedrick TJ, Sheldon WC. Clinical and angiographic features of coronary artery disease after chest irradiation. Am J Cardiol. 1987;60(13):1020–4.
19. Virmani R, Farb A, Carter AJ, Jones RM. Comparative pathology: radiation-induced coronary artery disease in man and animals. Seminars in Intervent Cardiol: SIIC. 1998;3(3–4):163–72.
20. McGale P, Darby SC, Hall P, Adolfsson J, Bengtsson NO, Bennet AM, et al. Incidence of heart disease in 35,000 women treated with radiotherapy for breast cancer in Denmark and Sweden. Radiothera Oncol: J Eur Soc Therapeut Radiol Oncol. 2011;100(2):167–75.
21. Kosmas C, Kallistratos MS, Kopterides P, Syrios J, Skopelitis H, Mylonakis N, et al. Cardiotoxicity of fluoropyrimidines in different schedules of administration: a prospective study. J Cancer Res Clin Oncol. 2008;134(1):75–82.
22. Lancellotti P, Nkomo VT, Badano LP, Bergler J, Bogaert J, Davin L, et al. Expert consensus for multi-modality imaging evaluation of cardiovascular complications of radiotherapy in adults: a report from the European Association of Cardiovascular Imaging and the American Society of Echocardiography. J Am Soc Echocardiogr. 2013;26(9):1013–32.
23. Xu XR, Yousef GM, Ni H. Cancer and platelet crosstalk: opportunities and challenges for aspirin and other antiplatelet agents. 2018;131(16):1777–89.
24. Hering D, Faber L, Horstkotte D. Echocardiographic features of radiation-associated valvular disease. Am J Cardiol. 2003;92(2):226–30.
25. Plana JC, Galderisi M, Barac A, Ewer MS, Ky B, Scherrer-Crosbie M, et al. Expert consensus for multimodality imaging evaluation of adult patients during and after cancer therapy: a report from the American Society of Echocardiography and the European Association of Cardiovascular Imaging. Eur Heart J Cardiovasc Imaging. 2014;15(10):1063–93.
26. Groarke JD, Nguyen PL, Nohria A, Ferrari R, Cheng S, Moslehi J. Cardiovascular complications of radiation therapy for thoracic malignancies: the role for non-invasive imaging for detection of cardiovascular disease. Eur Heart J. 2014;35(10):612–23.
27. Nishimura RA, Otto CM, Bonow RO, Carabello BA, Erwin JP, Fleisher LA, et al. 2017 AHA/ACC focused update of the 2014 AHA/ACC guideline for the Management of Patients with Valvular Heart Disease. A Report of the American College of Cardiology/American Heart Association Task Force on Clinical Practice Guidelines. 2017;70(2):252–89.

28. Tamargo J, Caballero R, Delpon E. Cancer chemotherapy and cardiac arrhythmias: a review. Drug Saf. 2015;38(2):129–52.
29. Soignet SL, Frankel SR, Douer D, Tallman MS, Kantarjian H, Calleja E, et al. United States multicenter study of arsenic trioxide in relapsed acute promyelocytic leukemia. J Clin Oncol. 2001;19(18):3852–60.
30. Shah RR, Morganroth J, Shah DR. Cardiovascular safety of tyrosine kinase inhibitors: with a special focus on cardiac repolarisation (QT interval). Drug Saf. 2013;36(5):295–316.
31. Chandrasekhar S, Fradley MGJCTOIO. QT interval prolongation associated with cytotoxic and targeted cancer therapeutics. 2019;20(7):55.
32. Lenihan DJ, Kowey PR. Overview and management of cardiac adverse events associated with tyrosine kinase inhibitors. Oncologist. 2013;18(8):900–8.
33. Farmakis D, Parissis J, Filippatos G. Insights into onco-cardiology: atrial fibrillation in cancer. J Am Coll Cardiol. 2014;63(10):945–53.
34. Izzedine H, Ederhy S, Goldwasser F, Soria JC, Milano G, Cohen A, et al. Management of hypertension in angiogenesis inhibitor-treated patients. Annals of Oncology : Official Journal of the European Society for Medical Oncology. 2009;20(5):807–15.
35. Maitland ML, Bakris GL, Black HR, Chen HX, Durand JB, Elliott WJ, et al. Initial assessment, surveillance, and management of blood pressure in patients receiving vascular endothelial growth factor signaling pathway inhibitors. J Natl Cancer Inst. 2010;102(9):596–604.
36. Rickles FR. Mechanisms of cancer-induced thrombosis in cancer. Pathophysiol Haemost Thromb. 2006;35(1–2):103–10.
37. Lee AYY, Levine MN, Baker RI, Bowden C, Kakkar AK, Prins M, et al. Low-Molecular-Weight Heparin versus a Coumarin for the Prevention of Recurrent Venous Thromboembolism in Patients with Cancer. 2003;349(2):146–53.
38. Agnelli G, Becattini C, Meyer G, Muñoz A, Huisman MV, Connors JM, et al. Apixaban for the treatment of venous thromboembolism associated with cancer. N Engl J Med. 2020;382(17):1599–607.
39. Barginear MF, Gralla RJ, Bradley TP, Ali SS, Shapira I, Greben C, et al. Investigating the benefit of adding a vena cava filter to anticoagulation with fondaparinux sodium in patients with cancer and venous thromboembolism in a prospective randomized clinical trial. Supportive Care in Cancer : Official Journal

of the Multinational Association of Supportive Care in Cancer. 2012;20(11):2865–72.
40. Valent P, Hadzijusufovic E, Schernthaner GH, Wolf D, Rea D, le Coutre P. Vascular safety issues in CML patients treated with BCR/ABL1 kinase inhibitors. Blood. 2015;125(6):901–6.
41. De Bruin ML, Dorresteijn LD, van't Veer MB, Krol AD, van der Pal HJ, Kappelle AC, et al. Increased risk of stroke and transient ischemic attack in 5-year survivors of Hodgkin lymphoma. J Natl Cancer Inst. 2009;101(13):928–37.
42. Plummer C, Henderson RD, O'Sullivan JD, Read SJ. Ischemic stroke and transient ischemic attack after head and neck radiotherapy: a review. Stroke. 2011;42(9):2410–8.
43. Fokkema M, den Hartog AG, Bots ML, van der Tweel I, Moll FL, de Borst GJ. Stenting versus surgery in patients with carotid stenosis after previous cervical radiation therapy: systematic review and meta-analysis. Stroke. 2012;43(3):793–801.
44. Gujral DM, Shah BN, Chahal NS, Senior R, Harrington KJ, Nutting CM. Clinical features of radiation-induced carotid atherosclerosis. Clinical Oncol (Royal College of Radiologists (Great Britain)). 2014;26(2):94–102.
45. Limsuwan A, Pakakasama S, Rochanawutanon M, Hong-eng S. Pulmonary arterial hypertension after childhood cancer therapy and bone marrow transplantation. Cardiology. 2006;105(3):188–94.
46. Montani D, Bergot E, Gunther S, Savale L, Bergeron A, Bourdin A, et al. Pulmonary arterial hypertension in patients treated by dasatinib. Circulation. 2012;125(17):2128–37.
47. Montani D, Bergot E, Günther S, Savale L, Bergeron A, Bourdin A, et al. Pulmonary arterial hypertension in patients treated by Dasatinib. Circulation. 2012;125(17):2128–37.

Index

A. A. Bhargava et al. (eds.), *Handbook of Outpatient Cardiology*, https://doi.org/10.1007/978-3-030-88953-1

B

T

U

V

W

GPSR Compliance

The European Union's (EU) General Product Safety Regulation (GPSR) is a set of rules that requires consumer products to be safe and our obligations to ensure this.

If you have any concerns about our products, you can contact us on ProductSafety@springernature.com

In case Publisher is established outside the EU, the EU authorized representative is:

Springer Nature Customer Service Center GmbH
Europaplatz 3
69115 Heidelberg, Germany

Batch number: 10732632

Printed by Printforce, the Netherlands